Community Pharmacy

Symptoms, Diagnosis and Treatment

Paul Rutter FFRPS MRPharmS PhD

Professor of Pharmacy Practice, School of Pharmacy and Biomedical Sciences, University of Central Lancashire, Preston, UK

FOURTH EDITION

KT-377-879

ELSEVIER

Edinburgh   London   New York   Oxford   Philadelphia   St Louis   Sydney   Toronto   2017

ELSEVIER

© 2017 Elsevier Ltd. All rights reserved.

No part of this publication may be reproduced or transmitted in any form or by any means, electronic or mechanical, including photocopying, recording, or any information storage and retrieval system, without permission in writing from the publisher. Details on how to seek permission, further information about the Publisher's permissions policies and our arrangements with organizations such as the Copyright Clearance Center and the Copyright Licensing Agency, can be found at our website: www.elsevier.com/permissions.

This book and the individual contributions contained in it are protected under copyright by the publisher (other than as may be noted herein).

First edition 2004
Second edition 2009
Third edition 2013
Fourth edition 2017

ISBN 978-0-7020-6997-0

Notices

Knowledge and best practice in this field are constantly changing. As new research and experience broaden our understanding, changes in research methods, professional practices, or medical treatment may become necessary.

Practitioners and researchers must always rely on their own experience and knowledge in evaluating and using any information, methods, compounds, or experiments described herein. In using such information or methods they should be mindful of their own safety and the safety of others, including parties for whom they have a professional responsibility.

With respect to any drug or pharmaceutical products identified, readers are advised to check the most current information provided (i) on procedures featured or (ii) by the manufacturer of each product to be administered, to verify the recommended dose or formula, the method and duration of administration, and contraindications. It is the responsibility of practitioners, relying on their own experience and knowledge of their patients, to make diagnoses, to determine dosages and the best treatment for each individual patient, and to take all appropriate safety precautions.

To the fullest extent of the law, neither the publisher nor the authors, contributors, or editors, assume any liability for any injury and/or damage to persons or property as a matter of products liability, negligence or otherwise, or from any use or operation of any methods, products, instructions, or ideas contained in the material herein.

 your source for books, journals and multimedia in the health sciences

www.elsevierhealth.com

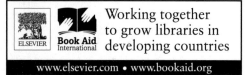

Working together to grow libraries in developing countries

www.elsevier.com • www.bookaid.org

For Elsevier:
Content Strategist: Pauline Graham
Content Development Specialist: Helen Leng
Project Manager: Andrew Riley
Designer: Christian Bilbow
Illustration Manager: Karen Giacomucci
Illustrator: PCA Creative

Printed in China
Last digit is the print number: 9 8 7 6 5 4 3 2 1

The Publisher's policy is to use **paper manufactured from sustainable forests**

Contents

Useful websites

Updated July 28th, 2015

Evidence-based Medicine

National Institute for Health and Care Excellence http://www.nice.org.uk/

Bandolier http://www.medicine.ox.ac.uk/bandolier/

Centre for Reviews and Dissemination http://www.york.ac.uk/crd/

Midlands Therapeutics Review and Advisory Committee http://www.centreformedicinesoptimisation.co.uk/mtrac/

Regional Drugs and Therapeutic Centre http://rdtc.nhs.uk/

Health Services Technology Assessment Texts (US site) http://www.ncbi.nlm.nih.gov/books/NBK16710/

King's Fund http://www.kingsfund.org.uk/

Medicines Information & Regulation

UK Medicines Information http://www.ukmi.nhs.uk/

Electronic Medicines Compendium http://www.medicines.org.uk/emc/

NICE Clinical Knowledge Summaries http://cks.nice.org.uk/#?char = A

Medicines & Healthcare products Regulatory Agency https://www.gov.uk/government/organisations/medicines-and-healthcare-products-regulatory-agency

European Medicines Agency http://www.ema.europa.eu/ema/

US Food and Drug Administration http://www.fda.gov/

Therapeutic Goods Administration (Australian) https://www.tga.gov.au/

Professional Bodies and Regulators

Royal Pharmaceutical Society http://www.rpharms.com/home/home.asp

General Pharmaceutical Council http://www.pharmacyregulation.org/

Pharmaceutical Society of Australia http://www.psa.org.au/

The British Medical Association https://www.bma.org.uk

The General Medical Council http://www.gmc-uk.org/

The Nursing and Midwifery Council http://www.nmc.org.uk/

Health and care Professions Council http://www.hpc-uk.org/

UK Pharmacy Organisations and Trade Bodies

National Pharmaceutical Association http://www.npa.co.uk/

Pharmaceutical Services Negotiating Committee http://psnc.org.uk/

Guild of Healthcare Pharmacists http://www.ghp.org.uk/

UK Clinical Pharmacists Association http://www.ukcpa.org/

Association of the British Pharmaceutical Industry http://www.abpi.org.uk/

The Proprietary Association of Great Britain http://www.pagb.co.uk/

British Pharmaceutical Students Association http://www.bpsa.com/

International Healthcare Organisations

International Pharmaceutical Federation (FIP) http://www.fip.org/

World Health Organisation http://www.who.ch/

Pharmacy Journals

Pharmaceutical Journal http://www.pharmj.com/

Chemist and Druggist http://www.chemistanddruggist.co.uk/

The Pharmacist http://www.thepharmacist.co.uk/

International Journal of Pharmacy Practice http://onlinelibrary.wiley.com/journal/10.1111/(ISSN)2042-7174

International Journal of Clinical Pharmacy http://www.springer.com/medicine/internal/journal/11096

Wider Healthcare Journals of Interest to Community Pharmacy

Journal of SelfCare http://www.selfcarejournal.com/

British Journal of General Practice http://www.bjgp.org/

British Medical Journal http://www.bmj.com/

Health Services Research http://www.hsr.org/

The Lancet http://www.thelancet.com/

Nursing Standard http://journals.rcni.com/journal/ns

General Health Sites for Healthcare Workers

Medscape http://emedicine.medscape.com/

Selfcare forum http://www.selfcareforum.org/

General Health Sites for Patients

http://www.patient.co.uk

http://www.healthfinder.gov/

http://www.mayoclinic.com/index.cfm?

http://www.evidence.nhs.uk

http://www.bbc.co.uk/health/

Preface

Demand on healthcare professionals to deliver high-quality patient care has never been greater. A multitude of factors impinge on healthcare delivery today, including an aging population, more sophisticated medicines, high patient expectation, health service infrastructure as well as adequate and appropriate staffing levels. In primary care the medical practitioner role is pivotal in providing this care and they remain the central member of the healthcare team, but demands on their time mean other models of service delivery are being adopted in the UK and in other developed countries that utilise other types of healthcare professionals.

This is leading to a breaking down of the traditional boundaries of care between doctors, nurses, and pharmacists. In particular, certain activities once seen as medical practitioner responsibility are now being performed by nurses and pharmacists as their scope of practice expands. The traditional role of supplying medicines safely and efficiently through community pharmacy still exists but greater patient-facing cognitive roles are now firmly established. Health prevention services are now routine, for example, smoking cessation, weight management and vaccination programmes. The pharmacy is now seen (by many governments) as a place where the general public can be managed for everyday healthcare needs without visiting a doctor. The most notable long-term global healthcare policy, which directly affects pharmacy, is the reclassification of Prescription-Only medicines to non-prescription status. In the UK between 1983 and 2015, over 90 Prescription-Only medicines have been reclassified as Pharmacy medicines. More recent switches have included products from new therapeutic classes, allowing community pharmacists to manage and treat a wider range of conditions.

Further deregulation of medicines to treat acute illness from different therapeutic areas seems likely, especially as healthcare professional opinion to acute medicine deregulation is broadly positive and the impact on general practice workload associated with dealing with minor ailments is high (and represents 100–150 million GP consultations per annum). Pharmacists, more than ever before need to demonstrate that they are competent practitioners and can be trusted with this additional responsibility. Therefore pharmacists require greater levels of knowledge and understanding about commonly occurring medical conditions. They will need to be able to recognise their signs and symptoms, and use an evidence-based approach to treatment.

This was, and still is, the catalyst for this book. Although other books targeted for pharmacists on diagnosis are published, this book aims to give a more in-depth view of minor conditions and how to differentiate them from more sinister pathology that may present in a similar way. The book is intended for all non-medical healthcare staff, but especially for pharmacists, from undergraduate students to experienced practitioners.

It is hoped that the information contained within the book is both informative and useful.

Introduction

Community pharmacists are the most accessible health-care professional. No appointment is needed to consult a pharmacist and patients can receive free, unbiased advice almost anywhere. A community pharmacist is often the first health professional the patient seeks advice from and, as such, provides a filtering mechanism whereby minor self-limiting conditions can be appropriately treated with the correct medication and patients with more sinister pathology referred on to the GP for further investigation. On a typical day a pharmacist practising in an 'average' community pharmacy can realistically expect to help between 5 and 15 patients a day who present with various symptoms for which they are seeking advice, reassurance, treatment or a combination of all three.

Probably of greatest impact to community pharmacy practice globally is the increased prominence of self-care. Self-care is not new; people have always taken an active role in their own health. What is different now is the attitude towards self-care by policy makers, healthcare organisations, not-for-profit agencies and front-line healthcare workers. Health improvements have been seen in people adopting health-enhancing behaviours rather than just through medical intervention. This has led to self-care being seen in a broader context than just the way in which people deal with everyday illness. In the UK the self-care forum (http://www.selfcareforum.org/), whose purpose is to promote self-care and embed it in everyday life, was established.

So what is self-care?

Fundamentally, the concept of self-care puts responsibility on individuals for their own health and well-being. The World Health Organisation defines self-care as '*the ability of individuals, families and communities to promote health, prevent disease, and maintain health and to cope with illness and disability with or without the support of a health-care provider*'.

Self-care has been described as a continuum (Fig. 1), starting with individual choices on health (e.g., taking exercise), moving through to managing their own ill health (e.g., self-medicating) either on their own or with help. As people progress along the continuum, more facilitation by others is required until a person needs fully managed care.

What is self-medication?

Self-medication is just one element of self-care and can be defined as the selection and use of medicines by individuals to treat self-recognised illness or symptoms. How these medicines are made available to the public vary from country to country but all have been approved by regulatory agencies as safe and effective for people to select and use without the need for medical supervision or intervention. In many countries (e.g., Australia, New Zealand, France, Sweden, Canada, UK) regulatory frameworks support reclassification of medicines away from prescription-only control by having a gradation in the level of medicine availability, whereby certain medicines can only be purchased at a pharmacy. These 'Pharmacy medicines' usually have to be sold either by the pharmacist or under his or her supervision. Over the last 30 years this approach to reclassification has seen a wide range of therapeutic agents made available to consumers, including proton pump inhibitors (US, EU-wide), orlistat (EU-wide), triptans (UK, Germany) and beta-2-agonists (Singapore, Australia).

'Facilitated self-medication'

The majority of purchases for non-prescription medicines are by the consumer alone, using product information from packaging to make an informed decision on whether to purchase. When consumers seek help at the point of purchase, this can be termed 'facilitated self-medication'. Where medicines are purchased through pharmacies, staff are in a strong position to facilitate self-care decision-making by consumers, as in most pharmacies the transaction takes place through a trained counter assistant or the pharmacist. Limited research has shown that consumer-purchasing decisions are affected by this

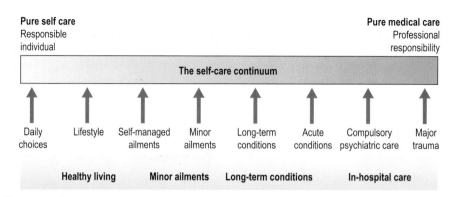

Fig. 1 The self-care continuum

'facilitation'. Nichol et al. and Sclar et al. both demonstrated that consumers (25% and 43%, respectively) altered their purchasing decision when proactively approached by pharmacy students. Furthermore, a small proportion of consumers did not purchase anything (13% and 8%) or were referred to their doctor (1% and 4%). These studies highlight how the pharmacy team are able to positively shape consumer decisions and help guide them to arguably better alternatives.

Community pharmacy and self-care

Increasing healthcare costs, changes in societal lifestyle, improved educational levels and increasing consumerism are all influencing factors on why people choose to exercise self-care. Of greatest importance are probably consumer-purchasing patterns and controlling costs.

Consumerism

Changes in society have led to people to have a different outlook on health and the way in which individuals perceive their own health/ill health. Today people have easy access to information; the creation of the Internet giving almost instantaneous access to limitless data on all aspects of health and care means that people across the globe have the means to query decisions and challenge medical opinion. This growing empowerment is also influenced by greater levels of education; having information is one thing but being able to understand it and utilise it is another. This has proved challenging to healthcare systems and workers, having to move from traditional structures and paternalistic doctrines (e.g., 'doctor knows best') to a patient-focused and centred type of care. This heightened public awareness about health, in the context of self-care, allows individuals to make informed choices and recognise that much can be done by themselves. The extent of

self-care is none better exemplified than by the level of consumer self-medication. The use of non-prescription medicines is the most prevalent form of medical care in the world. Sales are huge with the global market, estimated to be worth 73 billion Euros.

Despite the enormous sums of money spent on non-prescription medicines, approximately only 25% of people regularly purchase non-prescription medicines (25% tend to seek medical attention, and 50% do nothing). The extent to which this happens does vary from country to country, and in some markets, this is considerably higher, for example South Africa and the United States where 35% to 40% of people use OTC medications on a regular basis.

Many papers and commissioned reports show that access and convenience shape the purchasing patterns of consumers. These factors seem to be unaffected by country or time. Reports spanning thirty years have repeatedly concluded that these play an important part in consumer decision-making. The element of convenience does have a country context, for example, in Western countries this is primarily due to ease of access that negates the need for doctor seeking that often is associated with higher cost and increased time. In developing countries, 'convenience' is more associated with 'need' due to lower levels of health infrastructure and access to medical resources.

Costs

As populations across the globe live longer lives, whether through better hygiene, nutrition or advances in medicine, providing medical care is becoming more and more expensive. In an attempt to control costs many countries have gone through major healthcare reforms to maximise existing resources, both financial and staffing, to deliver effective and efficient healthcare. These reforms include integrating self-care into mainstream public health policy, including the management of long-term conditions.

Encouraging more people to exercise greater levels of self-care, either for acute or chronic problems, has the potential to shift costs away from professional care. Figures from the UK give some indication as to the magnitude of potential cost savings. Take primary care workload as an example. It is reported that approximately 20% to 40% of general practice (GP) workload constitutes patients seeking help for minor illness at a cost of £2 billion.

Contribution of community pharmacy to self-care

Community pharmacists are uniquely placed to provide support and advice to the general public compared with other healthcare professionals. The combination of location and accessibility mean that most consumers have ready access to a pharmacy where health professional advice is available on demand. A high level of public trust and confidence in pharmacists' ability to advise on non-prescription medicines is afforded to community pharmacists. Although there is a general global move to liberalise non-prescription markets, pharmacies in many countries still are the main supplier of non-prescription medicines. Pharmacists are therefore in a position to facilitate consumer self-care and self-medication, which needs to be built on and exploited.

References
Faculty for Self-care
http://www.collegeofmedicine.org.uk/faculties/
    faculty-self-care
Department of Health self-care week
http://socialcarebulletin.dh.gov.uk/tag/self-care-week/
Self-care connect
http://www.selfcareconnect.co.uk/
PSNC self-care and links
http://psnc.org.uk/services-commissioning/essential-services/
    support-for-self-care/

How to use the book

The book is divided into 11 chapters. The first chapter lays the foundations in how to go about making a diagnosis. This is followed by 9 systems-based chapters structured in the format shown in Fig. 2. The final chapter is product based and has a slightly different format. A list of abbreviations and a glossary are included at the end of the book.

Key features of each chapter

At the beginning of each chapter there is a short section addressing basic anatomy and history taking specific to that body system. A basic understanding of the anatomical location of major structures is useful when attempting to diagnose/exclude conditions from a patient's presenting complaint. It would be almost impossible to know whether to treat or refer a patient who presented with symptoms suggestive of renal colic if one does not know where the kidneys are. However, this is not intended to replace an anatomy text, and the reader is referred to further reading listed throughout the book for more detailed information on anatomical considerations.

Self-assessment questions

Twenty multiple choice questions and at least two case-study questions are presented at the end of each chapter. These are designed to test factual recall and applied knowledge. The type of multiple choice questions are constructed to mimic those set in the UK pre-registration examination set by the General Pharmaceutical Council. They start with simple traditional multiple choice questions in which the right answer has to be picked from a series of five possible answers, and work up to more complex questions which are interrelated.

The case studies challenge you with 'real-life' situations. All are drawn from practice and have been encountered by practising pharmacists, but have been modified for inclusion in the book.

Elements included under each condition

The same structure has been adopted for every condition. This is intended to help the reader approach differential diagnosis from the position of clinical decision-making (see Chapter 1). To help summarise the information, tables and algorithms are included for many of the conditions.

Arriving at a differential diagnosis

To contextualise how commonly conditions are seen by community pharmacists, a table listing the likelihood in which they are encountered is presented. This is designed to 'frame' the questions that should be asked from the point of working from the most likely cause of symptoms. To help a further table summarising the key questions that should be asked for each condition is included. The relevance (i.e., the rationale for asking the question) is given for each question. This will allow pharmacists to determine which questions should be asked to enable a differential diagnosis to be reached.

Primer for differential diagnosis

A 'primer for differential diagnosis' is available for a number of conditions covered. This algorithmic approach to differential diagnosis is geared towards nearly or recently qualified pharmacists. They are not intended to be solely relied upon in making a differential diagnosis but to act as an *aide memoire*. It is anticipated that the primers will be used in conjunction with the text, thus allowing a broader understanding of the differential diagnosis of the condition to be considered.

Trigger points indicative of referral

A summary box of trigger factors when it would be prudent to refer the patient to another healthcare practitioner is presented for each condition. In most instances a rationale for referral is presented. These trigger factors are not absolute and the pharmacist will have to use their professional judgement on a case-by-case basis. For example, a person with a cough of 3 days' duration might need referral if they are visibly poorly.

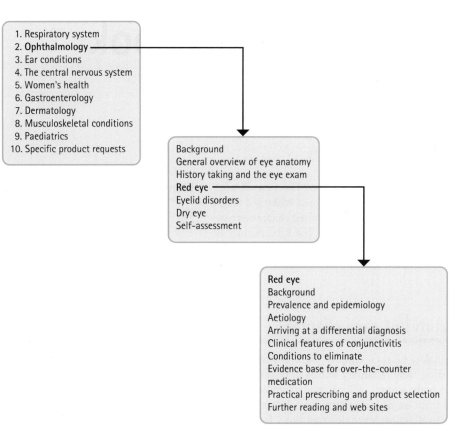

1. Respiratory system
2. Ophthalmology
3. Ear conditions
4. The central nervous system
5. Women's health
6. Gastroenterology
7. Dermatology
8. Musculoskeletal conditions
9. Paediatrics
10. Specific product requests

Background
General overview of eye anatomy
History taking and the eye exam
Red eye
Eyelid disorders
Dry eye
Self-assessment

Red eye
Background
Prevalence and epidemiology
Aetiology
Arriving at a differential diagnosis
Clinical features of conjunctivitis
Conditions to eliminate
Evidence base for over-the-counter
medication
Practical prescribing and product selection
Further reading and web sites

Evidence-based OTC medication and Practical prescribing and product selection

These two sections present the reader, first, with an evaluation of the current literature on whether over-the-counter medicine works, and second, with a quick reference to the dose of the medicine and when it cannot be prescribed. This does not replace standard textbooks such as *Martindale* or *Stockley's drug interactions,* but it does allow the user to find basic data in one text without having to reach for three or four other texts to answer simple questions.

The pregnancy and breast-feeding recommendations in this book are based largely on those from standard texts such as: Briggs' *Drugs in pregnancy and lactation* and, Schaefers' *Drugs in pregnancy and lactation.* Many manufacturers of over-the-counter medicines advise against their products being used in these groups, but where possible, in the summary tables reference is made to the recommendations made from these standard and trusted sources.

This hopefully will provide extra information for pharmacists when faced with queries from pregnant and lactating women and allow them to recommend products when faced with manufacturer information stipulating avoidance.

Hints and tips boxes

A summary box of useful information is provided near the end of each condition. This contains information that does not fall readily into any of the other sections but is nonetheless useful. For example, some of the hints and tips boxes give advice on how to administer eye drops, suppositories and other forms of medicines.

Further reading and websites

To supplement the text, at the end of each condition a list of selected references and reading is provided for those who wish to seek further information on the subject. Websites are also provided, and all sites have been checked and were active and relevant at the time of writing (Summer 2015).

Finally, all information presented in the book is accurate and factual as far as the author is aware. It is acknowledged that guidelines change, products become discontinued and new information becomes available over the lifetime of a book. Therefore if any information in the book is not current or valid, the author would be grateful of any feedback, positive or negative, to ensure that the next edition is as up to date as possible.

Electronic Resources

New to this edition is access to additional material hosted on Elsevier's electronic portal. The electronic resource holds additional material that includes:

- A chapter on evidence-based medicine
- Videos on physical examination
- Additional written case studies
- More multiple choice questions

Chapter 1

Making a diagnosis

Global healthcare policy now has a strong self-care focus and various strategies have been put in place to encourage consumers to have a more active role in exercising self-care.

Pharmacies unquestionably handle and manage large numbers of consumers who seek help and advice for minor illness, and advocates of pharmacy have argued that this will decrease doctor workload regarding minor illness, allowing them to concentrate more on 'complex' patient care.

The expansion of non-prescription medicines has undoubtedly contributed to the growth seen in the market and given consumers greater choice. It has also provided community pharmacy with an opportunity to demonstrate real and tangible benefits to consumers by facilitating patient self-care. For example, in the UK, Government-endorsed (and funded) schemes such as Minor Ailment Schemes have shown the positive impact community pharmacy can have on patient outcomes. However, research data on the impact community pharmacy makes to patient outcomes through facilitated self-medication is less convincing.

Community pharmacy performance when dealing with patients' signs and symptoms

Regardless what degree of control is placed on medicine availability in different countries, pharmacists can now manage and treat a wider number of conditions than ever

before. This raises the question as to whether pharmacists are capable to sell these medicines appropriately. Early research of pharmacist/consumer interactions in pharmacy practice did not address this but concentrated more on auditing questioning behaviour and analysing the advice people received. This body of work did illustrate the basic nature of performance; types of questions asked, frequency of advice provided and consumer perception to questioning. The findings were broadly critical of pharmacist performance. Over the same time period, covert investigation by the UK consumer organisation, 'Which', also concluded that pharmacists generally performed poorly. Further practice research (mainly from developed countries) has sought to determine the outcome of these interactions rather than the mechanics of the interaction. Findings from all papers raise questions over pharmacist ability to consistently perform at expected levels. Lamsam et al. (1998), found that in a third of interactions, the pharmacists made recommendations without assessing the patient's symptoms and in a further third of cases, recommendations were poor, which could have potentially caused harm. Horsley et al. (2004) found that the expected outcome was only reached in half of observed cases. Driesen et al. (2009) and Bilkhu et al. (2013) also report poor performance, and in each study (diarrhoea in a baby and allergic conjunctivitis in an adult) suggest that too few questions were asked. Tucker et al compared pharmacist performance to doctors and nurses across a spectrum of dermatological conditions. Pharmacists performed more poorly than doctors and only 40% of pharmacists were able to identify all lesions correctly. Data from developing countries is limited but a review by Brata et al. (2013) also highlighted inconsistent information gathering, leading to inappropriate recommendations.

Current pharmacy training in making a diagnosis

The use of protocols/guidelines and mnemonics seem to have been almost universally adopted by pharmacy. Many such mnemonics have been developed as highlighted in a 2014 review (Shealy, 2014). The use of these 'decision aids' seems to have had little impact on improving performance and recent research findings have shown that community pharmacists over rely on using this type of questioning strategy (Akhtar, 2014; Iqbal, 2013; Rutter, 2013).

Try not to use mnemonics

At best, these tools allow for standardising information gained from patients from and between pharmacists and the wider pharmacy team. The more fundamental and important question is not simply asking the questions but determining how that information is utilised. Having a set of data still requires interpretation and this inability to appropriately synthesise gathered information is where research has highlighted pharmacists' failings.

The use of mnemonics has been taught by many higher education institutions and adopted by commercial community pharmacy organisations. Mnemonics are rigid, inflexible and often inappropriate. Every patient is different and it is unlikely that a mnemonic can be fully applied, and more importantly, using mnemonics can mean that vital information is missed, which could shape decision-making. Some of the more commonly used mnemonics are discussed briefly in the next section.

WWHAM

This is the most common mnemonic in use and widely taught and used in the UK. It is the simplest to remember but also the worst to use. It gives the pharmacist very limited information from which to establish a differential diagnosis. If used, it should be used with caution and is probably only helpful to use as a basic information-gathering tool. WWHAM might be appropriate to allow for counter assistant staff to gain a general picture of the person's presenting complaint but should not be advocated as a tool to establish a diagnosis.

	Meaning of the letter	Attributes of the mnemonic
W	Who is the patient?	**Positive points**
W	What are the symptoms?	Establishes presenting complaint
H	How long have the symptoms been present?	**Negative points** Fails to consider general appearance of patient.
A	Action taken?	No social/lifestyle factors taken into account; no
M	Medication being taken?	family history sought; not specific or in-depth enough; no history of previous symptoms

Other examples of mnemonics that have been suggested as being helpful for pharmacists in differential diagnosis are ENCORE, ASMETHOD and SIT DOWN SIR. Although these are more comprehensive than WWHAM, they still are limited. None take into consideration all factors that might impinge on a differential diagnosis. All fail to establish a full history from the patient in respect to lifestyle and social factors or the relevance of a family history. They are very much designed to establish the nature and severity of the presenting complaint. This, in many instances, will be adequate but for intermittent conditions (e.g., irritable bowel syndrome, asthma, hay fever) or conditions where a positive family history is important (e.g., psoriasis, eczema), they might well miss important information that reduces the chances of gaining a correct diagnosis.

	Meaning of the letter	Attributes of the mnemonic
E	Explore	**Positive points**
N	No medication	'Observe' section suggests
C	Care	taking into account
O	Observe	the appearance of the
R	Refer	patient – does he or she
E	Explain	look poorly?
		Negative points
		Sections on 'No medication' and 'Refer' add little to the differential diagnosis process. No social/lifestyle factors taken into account; no family history sought

Meaning of the letter		Attributes of the acronym
A	Age/appearance?	**Positive points**
S	Self or someone else?	Establishes the nature of problem and if patient has suffered from previous similar episodes
M	Medication?	
E	Extra medicines?	
T	Time persisting?	**Negative points**
H	History?	Exact symptoms and severity of social/lifestyle factors not taken into account; no family history sought
O	Other symptoms?	
D	Danger symptoms?	

Meaning of the letter		Attributes of the acronym
S	Site or location?	**Positive points**
I	Intensity or severity?	Establishes the severity and nature of problem and if the patient has suffered from previous similar episodes
T	Type or nature?	
D	Duration?	
O	Onset?	
W	With (other symptoms)?	**Negative points**
N	Annoyed or aggravated?	Fails to consider general appearance of patient. No social/lifestyle factors taken into account; no family history sought
S	Spread or radiation?	
I	Incidence or frequency pattern?	
R	Relieved by? Have you tried anything already	

Clinical reasoning

Decision-making processes associated with clinical practice are an essential skill and are central to the practise of professional autonomy. It is a thinking process that allows the pharmacist to make wise decisions specific to individual patient context.

Whether we are conscious of it or not, most people will – at some level – use clinical reasoning to arrive at a differential diagnosis. Clinical reasoning relates to the decision-making processes associated with clinical practice. It is a thinking process directed towards enabling the pharmacist to take appropriate action in a specific context. It fundamentally differs from using mnemonics in that it is built around clinical knowledge and skills that are applied to the individual patient. It involves recognition of cues and analysis of data.

Steps to consider in clinical reasoning

1. Use epidemiology to shape your thoughts
   What is the presenting complaint? Some conditions are much more common than others. Therefore you can form an idea of what condition the patient is likely to be suffering from based on the laws of probability. For example, if a person presents with a cough then you should already know that by far the most common cause of cough is a viral infection. Other causes of cough are possible and need to be eliminated. Your line of questioning should therefore be shaped by thinking that this is the 'default' cause of the person's cough and ask questions based on this assumption (see 4. Hypothetico-deductive reasoning).

2. Take account of the person's age and sex
   Epidemiological studies show that age and sex will influence the likelihood of certain conditions. For example, it is very unlikely that a child who presents with cough will have chronic bronchitis, but the probability of an elderly person having chronic bronchitis is much higher. Likewise croup is a condition seen only in children. Sex can dramatically alter the probability of people suffering from certain conditions. For instance, migraines are five times more common in women than in men, yet cluster headache is nine times more common in men than in women. Use this to your advantage. It will allow you to internally change your thought processes as to which conditions are most likely for that person.

3. The general appearance of the patient
   Does the person look well or poorly? This will shape your thinking as to the severity of the problem. If a child is running around a pharmacy, they are likely to be healthier than a child who sat quietly on a chair not talking.

   Taking these three points into consideration, you should be able to form some initial thoughts as to the person's health status and ideas of what may be wrong with them. AT THIS POINT questions should be asked.

4. Hypothetico-deductive reasoning
   Based on this (limited) information, the pharmacist should arrive at a small number of hypotheses. The pharmacist should then set about testing these hypotheses by asking the patient a series of questions. Ask:

'The right question, at the right time, for the right reason'

   The answer to each question asked allows the pharmacist to narrow down the possible diagnosis by either eliminating particular conditions or confirming his or her suspicions of a particular condition. In effect the pharmacist asks questions with knowledge of what the answer is expected to be. For example, a confirmatory type of question asked to a patient suspected of having allergic conjunctivitis might be 'Do your eyes itch?' In this case the pharmacist is expecting the patient to say 'yes' and thus helps support your differential diagnosis. If a patient states 'no', then this is an unexpected answer that casts doubt on the differential diagnosis; therefore further questions will be asked and other diagnostic hypotheses explored. This cycle of testing and re-testing the hypotheses continues until you arrive at a differential diagnosis.

Good questioning following these principles will mean that you will end up at the right diagnosis about 80% of the time.

5. Pattern recognition
In addition, clinical experience (pattern recognition) also plays a part in the process. Certain conditions have very characteristic presentations and, once seen, it is a relatively straightforward task to diagnose the next case by recalling the appearance of the rash. Therefore much of daily practice will consist of seeing new cases that strongly resemble previous encounters and comparing new cases to old.

Pattern recognition is therefore much more commonly used by experienced or expert diagnosticians compared with novices. This is generally because there is a gap between the expert–novice knowledge and clinical experience store. Research has shown that experienced doctors tend to only use hypothetico-deductive strategies when presented with difficult cases.

6. Physical examinations
The ability to perform simple examinations (e.g., eye, ear, mouth and skin examinations) does increase the probability of arriving at the correct diagnosis. Where appropriate (provided pharmacists are suitably trained) examinations should be conducted. Seeing a rash or viewing an eardrum will provide much better data from which to base a decision than purely a patient description. Throughout this book, where examinations are possible, instruction is given in how to perform these examinations. Student Consult has some videos on how to perform these physical examinations.

7. Safety netting
Even if you are confident of your differential diagnosis, it is important to 'safety net'. You are not going to get it right all the time; making an incorrect diagnosis is inevitable. It has been reported that upward of 50% of patients do not receive a definitive diagnosis at the end of a consultation with a family doctor (Heneghan et al., 2009).

Many people will present to the pharmacist at an early stage in the evolution of their illness. This means that they may not present with classical textbook symptoms or have not yet developed any 'red flag'-type symptoms when seen by the pharmacist. For example, a child may have headache but no other symptoms yet later go on to develop a stiff neck and rash and be diagnosed with meningitis, or a person may have an acute cough that subsequently develops into pneumonia. Safety netting attempts to manage these situations.

This should take one of two forms:

- Conditional referrals
  This should be built into every consultation. It is more than a mere perfunctory 'If you don't get better come back to me or see the doctor'. It has to be tailored and specific to the individual and their symptoms. For example, if a person presents with a cough of 10 days' duration, after how many more days would you ask them to seek further medical help? Three days? Five days? Seven days? Longer?

  In this case knowledge on cough duration is important. If the differential diagnosis is a viral cough, then we know that this symptom typically lasts 10 to 14 days, but it is not unusual for the symptom to last 21 days. Longer than 21 days suggests that the cough is becoming chronic and requires further investigation. A conditional referral in this case would be anything between 5 and 10 days – in other words the person has had the cough for between 2 and 3 weeks, which is starting to become longer than one would expect for viral cough. Conversely, if the cough had been present for just 2 days, then a conditional referral after a further 2 more weeks would be appropriate.

- Advise patients on warning symptoms
  It is entirely reasonable to highlight to patients those signs and symptoms that they may develop subsequent to your consultation. For example, a child suffering with diarrhoea is managed by the pharmacist, but the pharmacist highlights the signs of dehydration to the child's parents. This would be good practice as the consequence of dehydration is clinically more significant than the diarrhoea itself.

Summary

In practice, family doctors tend to use a mixture of hypothetico-deductive reasoning and pattern recognition augmented with physical examination and, where needed, laboratory tests. It can seem to some patients that the doctor asks very few questions, spends very little time with them and closes the consultation even before they have 'warmed the seat'. In these circumstances the doctor is probably exhibiting very good clinical reasoning. Research has shown that, with greater experience, doctors tend to rely more on non-analytical decision-making (e.g., pattern recognition), whereas novice practitioners use analytical models (hypothetico-deductive reasoning) more frequently.

Most pharmacists will exhibit some degree of clinical reasoning but most likely at a sub-conscious level. The key to better performance is shifting this activity from the sub-conscious to conscious. Gaining clinical experience is fundamental to this process. Critical for pharmacists is the need to learn from uncertainty. When referrals are made, every attempt should be made to either follow-up with the doctor about the outcome of the referral or encourage the patient back to the pharmacy to see how they got on. Knowing what another person (usually a more experienced diagnostician) believed the diagnosis was allows you to build up experience and, when faced with similar presenting symptoms, have a better idea of what the cause is. Without this feedback, pharmacists reach a 'glass ceiling', where the outcome is always the same – referral – which might not be necessary.

Differential Diagnosis – an example

A 35-year-old female patient, Mrs JT, asks to speak to the pharmacist about getting some painkillers for her headache. She appears smartly dressed and in no obvious great discomfort but appears a little distracted.

1. STEP ONE: Use epidemiology to shape your thoughts
   In primary care, headache is a very common presenting symptom that can be caused by many conditions. Table 1.1 highlights the conditions associated with headache that can be seen by community pharmacists.

   From this background information you should already be thinking that the probability of Mrs JT's headaches

Table 1.1
Conditions associated with headache that can be seen by community pharmacists

Incidence	Cause
Most likely	Tension-type headache
Likely	Migraine, sinusitis, eye strain
Unlikely	Cluster headache, medication overuse headache, temporal arteritis, trigeminal neuralgia, depression
Very unlikely	Glaucoma, meningitis, sub-arachnoid haemorrhage, raised intracranial pressure

are going to be caused by the four conditions that are commonly seen by community pharmacists (tension-type headache, migraine, sinusitis and eye strain). This is not to say that it could not be caused by the other conditions, but the likelihood that they are the cause is much lower.

2. STEP TWO: Take account of the person's age and sex
   Does age or sex have any bearing on shaping your thoughts? The person is a woman – and we know migraines are more common in women compared with men. So although tension-type headache is the most common cause of headache, the chances of it being caused by migraine needs to be given more prominence in your thinking. Will age affect your thinking? In this case probably not as the common causes of headache do not really show any real variation with age.

   So at this point you should still be considering all four conditions as likely, but migraine as a cause should be now be thought of more seriously alongside the most common cause of headache, the tension type.

3. STEP 3: The general appearance of the patient
   Nothing obvious from her physical demeanour is constructive towards your thinking. Her 'distracted' state might be as a consequence of the pain from the headache and worth exploring.

4. STEP FOUR: Hypothetico-deductive reasoning
   Each question asked should have a purpose – again, it is about asking the **right question, at the right time and for the right reason**. In this case we are initially considering the conditions of tension-type headache, migraine, sinusitis and eye strain (listed in that sequence in terms of likelihood). It is important that your clinical knowledge is sufficiently sound to know how these different conditions present so that similarities and differences are known, allowing questions to be constructed to eliminate one type of headache from another. This will allow you to think of '**targeted questions**' to ask. Table 1.2 highlights associated signs and symptoms of these four conditions.

We can see that location and nature of pain for the four conditions vary as do the severity of pain experienced (although pain is subjective and difficult to measure reliably).

A reasonable first question then would be **LOCATION** of pain. If the patient says, 'It is bilateral and towards the back', this points towards the tension-type headache (other causes are frontal or unilateral).

Given this information if we asked about **NATURE** of pain next, and working on the hypothesis of tension-type headache, we would be expecting a response from the patient of an 'aching/non-throbbing headache', which might worsen as the day goes on. If patients describe symptoms similar to our expectation, this further points to tension-type headache as being the correct diagnosis.

Table 1.2
Associated signs and symptoms

	Duration	Timing and nature	Location	Severity (pain score from 0–10)	Precipitating factors	Who is affected?
Tension-type headache	Can last days	Symptoms worsen as day progresses. Non-throbbing pain	Bilateral; Most often at back of head	2–5	Stress due to changes in work or home environment	All age groups and both sexes equally affected
Migraine	Average attack lasts 24 h	Associated with menstrual cycle and weekends. Throbbing pain and nausea. Dislike of bright lights/loud noises	Usually unilateral	4–7	Food (in 10% of sufferers); Family history	3 times more common in women
Sinusitis	Days	Dull ache that begins as unilateral	Frontal	2–6	Valsalva movements	Adults
Eye strain	Days	Aching	Frontal	2–5	Close-vision work	All ages

To further confirm your thinking, you could ask about SEVERITY of pain. In tension-type headache we are expecting a response that does not suggest debilitating pain. Again if we found that the pain was bothersome but not severe, this would point to tension-type headache.

At this point we might want to ask other questions that RULE OUT other LIKELY CAUSES. We know migraine is associated with a positive family history. We would expect the patient to say there was no family history if our working differential diagnosis is tension-type headache. Likewise, asking about previous episodes of the same type of headache would help rule out migraine due to its episodic and recurrent nature. Similarly, eye strain is closely associated with close visual work. If the person has not been doing this activity more than normal, it tends to rule out eye strain. Finally, sinusitis is a consequence of upper respiratory tract infection so, if the person has not had a recent history of colds, this will rule out sinusitis.

So we are expecting certain responses to these questions if the symptoms are a consequence of suffering from a tension-type headache. If the patient answers in a contrary way, then this starts to cast doubt on your differential diagnosis. If this happens, you need to revisit your hypothesis and test another, – that is, think that the symptoms are caused by something else and 'recycle' your thought processes to test a hypothesis of a different cause of headache.

Consultation and communication skills

The ability of the community pharmacist to diagnose the patient's presenting signs and symptoms is a significant challenge given that, unlike most other healthcare professionals, community pharmacists do not normally have access to the patient's medical record and thus have no idea about what the person's problem is until a conversation is initiated.

For the most part, pharmacists will be totally dependent on their ability to question patients in order to arrive at a differential diagnosis. It is therefore vital that pharmacists possess excellent consultation and communication skills as a prerequisite to determining a differential diagnosis. This will be drawn from a combination of good questioning technique, listening actively to the patient and picking up on non-verbal cues.

Many models of medical consultation and communication have been developed. Probably the most familiar model and most widely used is the **Calgary-Cambridge model** of consultation. This model is widely taught in both pharmacy and medical education and provides an excellent platform in which to structure a consultation. The model is structured into:

- Initiating the session
  - Establishing initial rapport
  - Identifying the reason(s) for the consultation

- Gathering information
  - Exploration of problems
  - Understanding the patient's perspective
  - Providing structure to the consultation
- Building the relationship
  - Developing rapport
  - Involving the patient
- Explanation and planning
  - Providing the correct amount and type of information
  - Aiding accurate recall and understanding
  - Achieving a shared understanding: Incorporating the patient's perspective
  - Planning: Shared decision-making
- Closing the session

For more detailed information on this model, there are numerous Internet references available, and the authors of the model have written a book on communication skills (Silverman et al., 2013).

Conclusion

The way in which one goes about establishing what is wrong with the patient will vary from practitioner to practitioner. However, it is important that whatever method is adopted, it must be sufficiently robust enough to be of benefit to the patient. Using a clinical-reasoning approach to differential diagnosis allows you to build a fuller picture of the patient's presenting complaint. It is both flexible and specific to each individual, unlike the use of mnemonics.

References
Akhtar S, Rutter P. Pharmacists thought processes in making a differential diagnosis using a gastro-intestinal case vignette. Res Social Adm Pharm. http://dx.doi.org/10.1016/j.sapharm.2014.09.003.

Aradottir HAE, Kinnear M. Design of an algorithm to support community pharmacy dyspepsia management. Pharm World Sci 2008; 30:515-525.

Bertsche T, Nachbar M, Fiederling J, et al. Assessment of a computerised decision support system for allergic rhino-conjunctivitis counselling in German pharmacy. Int J Clin Pharm 2012; 34:17-22.

Bilkhu P, Wolffsohn JS, Taylor D, et al. The management of ocular allergy in community pharmacies in the United Kingdom. Int J Clin Pharm 2013; 35:190-194.

Brata C, Gudka S, Schneider CR, et al. A review of the information-gathering process for the provision of medicines for self-medication via community pharmacies in developing countries. Res Social Adm Pharm 2013; 9:370-383.

Cantrill JA, Weiss MC, Kishida M, et al. Pharmacists' perception and experiences of pharmacy protocols: A step in the right direction? Int J Pharm Pract 1997; 5:26-32.

Consumers' Association. Counter advice. Which Way to Health? 1999; 3:22-25.

Driesen A, Vandenplas Y. How do pharmacists manage acute diarrhoea in an 8-month-old baby? A simulated client study. Int J Pharm Pract 2009; 17:215-220.

Horsley E, Rutter P, Brown D. Evaluation of Community Pharmacists' Recommendations to Standardized Patient Scenarios. Ann Pharmacother 2004;38;1080-1085.

Iqbal N, Rutter P. Community Pharmacists Reasoning When Making a Diagnosis: A think-aloud study. Int J Pharm Pract 2013; 21: S2, 17-8.

Lamsam GD, Kropff MA. Community pharmacists' assessments and recommendations for treatment in four case scenarios. Ann Pharmacother 1998; 32:409-16.

Rutter P, Patel J. Decision making by community pharmacists when making an over-the-counter diagnosis in response to a dermatological presentation. SelfCare 2013;4:125-33.

Shealy KM. Mnemonics to assess patients for self-care: Is there a need? SelfCare. 2014;5:11-18.

Silverman J, Kurtz S, Draper J. Skills for Communicating with Patients, 3rd Edition. CRC Press; 2013.

Tucker R, Patel M, Layton AM, et al. An examination of the comparative ability of primary care health professionals in the recognition and treatment of a range of dermatological conditions. SelfCare 2013; 4:87-97.

Which? Can you trust your local pharmacy's advice? http://www.which.co.uk/news/2013/05/can-you-trust-your-local-pharmacys-advice-319886/ Accessed 17 March 2015.

Further Reading
Heneghan C, Glasziou P, Thompson M, et al. Diagnostic strategies used in primary care. Brit Med J 2009; 338: b946.

Rutter P. Role of community pharmacists in patients' self-care and self-medication. Journal of Integrated Pharmacy Research and Practice 2015; 4:57-65

Schneider C, Gudka S, Fleischer L, et al. The use of a written assessment checklist for the provision of emergency contraception via community pharmacies: A simulated patient study. Pharm Pract 2013; 11:127-131.

Schneider C, Emery L, Brostek R, et al. Evaluation of the supply of antifungal medication for the treatment of vaginal thrush in the community pharmacy setting: A randomized controlled trial. Pharm Pract 2013; 11:132-137.

Watson MC, Bond CM, Grimshaw JM, et al. Factors predicting the guideline compliant supply (or non-supply) of non-prescription medicines in the community pharmacy. Qual Saf Health Care. 2006; 15:53-57.

Lighter Reading
Helman C. Suburban Shaman - tales from medicine's frontline. Hammersmith Press Limited; Jan 2006. ISBN-10: 1905140088

Respiratory system

Background

Diseases of the respiratory tract are among the most common reasons for consulting a GP. The average GP sees approximately 700 to 1000 patients each year with respiratory disease. Although respiratory disease can cause significant morbidity and mortality, the vast majority of conditions are minor and self-limiting.

General overview of the anatomy of the respiratory tract

The basic requirement for all living cells to function and survive is a continuous supply of oxygen. However, a by-product of cell activity is carbon dioxide, which, if not removed, poisons and kills the cells of the body. The principal function of the respiratory system is therefore the exchange of carbon dioxide and oxygen between blood and atmospheric air. This exchange takes place in the lungs, where pulmonary capillaries are in direct contact with the linings of the lung's terminal air spaces: the alveoli. All other structures associated with the respiratory tract serve to facilitate this gaseous exchange.

The respiratory system is divided arbitrarily into the upper and lower respiratory tracts. In addition to these structures, the respiratory system also includes the oral cavity, rib cage and diaphragm.

Upper respiratory tract

The upper respiratory tract comprises those structures located outside the thorax: the nasal cavity, pharynx and larynx.

Nasal cavity

The internal portion of the nose is classed as the nasal cavity. The nasal cavity is connected to the pharynx through two openings called the internal nares. The cavity is divided into a larger respiratory region and a smaller olfactory region, which senses smells. The respiratory region is lined with cilia and plays an important part in respiration because it filters out large dust particles. The inhaled air circulates, allowing it to be warmed by close contact with blood from the capillaries. Mucous secreted from goblet cells also helps moisten the air.

Pharynx

The pharynx is divided into three sections:

- nasopharynx, which exchanges air with the nasal cavity and moves particulate matter towards the mouth
- oropharynx and laryngopharynx, which serve as a common passageway for air and food
- laryngopharynx, which connects with the oesophagus and the larynx and, like the oropharynx, serves as a common pathway for the respiratory and digestive systems.

Larynx (voice box)

The larynx is a short passageway that connects the pharynx with the trachea and lies in the midline of the neck. The glottis and epiglottis are located here and act like 'trap doors' to ensure that liquids and food are routed into the oesophagus and not the trachea.

Lower respiratory tract

The lower respiratory tract is located almost entirely within the thorax and comprises the trachea, bronchial tree and lungs.

Trachea (windpipe) and bronchi

The trachea lies in front of the oesophagus and extends from the larynx to the fifth thoracic vertebra where it divides into the right and left primary bronchi. The bronchi divide and subdivide into bronchioles, and these in turn divide to form terminal bronchioles, which give rise to alveoli where gaseous exchanges take place. The epithelial lining of the bronchial tree acts as a defence mechanism known as the mucociliary escalator. Cilia on the surface of cells beat upwards in organised waves of contraction, thus expelling foreign bodies.

Lungs

The lungs are paired, cone-shaped organs in the thoracic cavity, protected by the rib cage. Enclosing the lungs (and providing further protection) are the pleural membranes; the inner membrane covers the lungs and the outer membrane is attached to the thoracic cavity. Between the membranes is the pleural cavity, which contains fluid and prevents friction between the membranes during breathing.

History taking and physical examination

Cough, cold, sore throat and rhinitis often coexist, and an accurate history is therefore essential to differentially diagnose a patient who presents with symptoms of respiratory disease. A number of similar questions must be asked for each symptom, although symptom-specific questions are also needed (these are discussed under each heading that follow). Currently, examination of the respiratory tract is outside the remit of the community pharmacist, unless they have additional qualifications (e.g., independent prescriber status).

Cough

Background

Coughing is the body's defence mechanism in attempt to clear airways of foreign bodies and particulate matter. This is supplemented by the mucociliary escalator (the upward beating of the finger-like cilia in the bronchi that move mucous and entrapped foreign bodies to be expectorated or swallowed). Cough is the most common respiratory symptom and one of the few ways by which abnormalities of the respiratory tract manifest themselves. Cough can be very debilitating to the patient's well-being and can also be disruptive to family, friends and work colleagues.

Coughs can be described as either productive (chesty) or non-productive (dry, tight, tickly). However, many patients will say that they are not producing sputum, although they go on to say that they 'can feel it on their chest'. In these cases the cough is probably productive in nature and should be treated as such.

Coughs are either classified as *acute* or *chronic* in nature. The British Thoracic Society Guidelines (2006) recommend that:

- acute cough lasts less than 3 weeks
- chronic cough lasts more than 8 weeks

The guidelines acknowledge that a 'grey area' exists for those coughs lasting between 3 and 8 weeks as it is difficult to define their aetiological basis because all chronic coughs will have started as an acute cough. For community pharmacy practice this 'grey area' is rather academic, as any cough lasting longer than the accepted definition of acute should be referred to a medical practitioner for further investigation.

Prevalence and epidemiology

Statistics from UK general medical practice show that respiratory illness accounts for more patient visits than any other disease category. Acute cough is usually caused by a viral upper respiratory tract infection (URTI) and constitutes 20% of consultations. This translates to 12 million GP visits per year and represents the largest single cause of primary care consultation. These data are echoed elsewhere; for example, episodes of URTI are the most common acute condition seen in Australian general practice. In community pharmacy the figures are even higher, with at least 24 million visits per year (or 2000 visits per UK pharmacy each year).

Schoolchildren experience the greatest number of coughs, with an estimated 7–10 episodes per year (compared with adults with 2–5 episodes per year). Acute viral URTIs exhibit seasonality, with higher incidence seen in the winter months.

Aetiology

A five-part cough reflex is responsible for cough production. Receptors located mainly in the pharynx, larynx, trachea and bifurcations of the large bronchi are stimulated via mechanical, irritant or thermal mechanisms. Neural impulses are then carried along afferent pathways of the vagal and superior laryngeal nerves, which terminate at the cough centre in the medulla. Efferent fibres of the vagus and spinal nerves carry neural activity to the muscles of the diaphragm, chest wall and abdomen. These muscles contract and are followed by the sudden opening of the glottis, which causes coughing.

Arriving at a differential diagnosis

The most likely cause of acute cough in primary care for all ages is a viral infection. Recurrent viral bronchitis is most prevalent in preschool and young school-aged children, and is the most common cause of persistent cough in children of all ages. Table 2.1 highlights those conditions that can be encountered by community pharmacists and their relative incidence.

As viral infection is by far the most likely cause of cough in all age groups, it is logical to hypothesise that this will be the cause of the cough and questions should be directed to help confirm or refute this assumption (using hypothetico-deductive reasoning – see page 3) Asking symptom-specific questions will help the pharmacist establish a differential diagnosis (Table 2.2).

Table 2.1
Causes of cough and their relative incidence in community pharmacy

Incidence	Cause
Most likely	Viral infection
Likely	Upper airways cough syndrome (formerly known as postnasal drip and includes allergies), acute bronchitis
Unlikely	Croup, chronic bronchitis, asthma, pneumonia, ACE-inhibitor induced
Very unlikely	Heart failure, bronchiectasis, tuberculosis, cancer, pneumothorax, lung abscess, nocardiasis, GORD

Clinical features of acute viral cough

Viral coughs typically present with sudden onset and associated fever. Sputum production is minimal and symptoms are often worse in the evening. Associated cold symptoms are also often present; these usually last between 7 and 10 days. Duration of longer than 14 days might suggest 'postviral cough' or possibly indicate a bacterial secondary infection, but this is clinically difficult to establish without sputum samples being analysed. A common misconception is that cough with mucopurulent sputum is bacterial in cause and requires referral. This is almost never the case, and people should not be routinely referred to the GP for cough associated with mucopurulent sputum.

Conditions to eliminate

Likely causes

Upper airways cough syndrome (previously referred to as postnasal drip; also referred to as rhinosinusitis)
Postnasal drip has been broadened to include a number of rhinosinus conditions related to cough. The umbrella term of *upper airways cough syndrome* (UACS) is being adopted.

UACS is characterised by a sinus or nasal discharge that flows behind the nose and into the throat. Patients should be asked whether they are swallowing mucous or notice that they are clearing their throat more than usual, as these features are commonly seen in patients with UACS. Allergies are one cause of UACS. Coughs caused by allergies are often non-productive and worse at night. However, there are usually other associated symptoms, such as sneezing, nasal discharge/blockage, conjunctivitis and an itchy oral cavity. Cough of allergic origin might show seasonal variation, for example, hay fever. Other causes include vasomotor rhinitis (caused by odours and changes in temperature/humidity) and post-infectious UACS after a URTI. If UACS is present, it is better to direct treatment at the cause of the UACS (e.g., antihistamines or decongestants) rather than just treat the cough.

Acute bronchitis
Acute bronchitis affects over 4% of adults a year in the UK. Most cases are seen in autumn or winter, and symptoms are similar to viral URTI, but patients also tend to exhibit dyspnoea and wheeze. The cough usually lasts for 7 to 10 days but can persist for 3 weeks. The cause is normally viral, but sometimes bacterial. If bacterial in origin, symptoms usually resolve without antibiotic treatment.

<table>
<tr><td colspan="2">

?   Table 2.2
Specific questions to ask the patient: Cough
</td></tr>
</table>

Question	Relevance
Sputum colour	Mucoid (clear and white) is normally of little consequence and suggests that no infection is present Yellow, green or brown sputum normally indicates infection. **Mucopurulent sputum is generally caused by a viral infection and does not require automatic referral** Haemoptysis can either be rust coloured (pneumonia), pink tinged (left ventricular failure) or dark red (carcinoma). Occasionally, patients can produce sputum with bright red blood as one-off events. This is due to the force of coughing, causing a blood vessel to rupture. This is not serious and does not require automatic referral
Nature of sputum	Thin and frothy suggests left ventricular failure Thick, mucoid to yellow can suggest asthma Offensive foul-smelling sputum suggests either bronchiectasis or lung abscess
Onset of cough	A cough that is worse in the morning may suggest upper airways cough syndrome, bronchiectasis or chronic bronchitis

Duration of cough	Upper respiratory tract infection (URTI) cough can linger for more than 3 weeks and is termed 'postviral cough'. However, coughs lasting longer than 3 weeks should be viewed with caution, as the longer the cough is present, the more likely a serious pathology is responsible; for example, the most likely diagnoses of cough are as follows:
	    at 3 days' duration will be a URTI;
	    at 3 weeks' duration will be acute or chronic bronchitis;
	    and at 3 months' duration conditions such as chronic bronchitis, tuberculosis and carcinoma become more likely

Periodicity	Adult patients with recurrent cough might have chronic bronchitis, especially if they smoke Care should be exercised in children who present with recurrent cough and have a family history of eczema, asthma or hay fever. This might suggest asthma and referral would be required for further investigation
Age of the patient	Children will most likely be suffering from a URTI but asthma and croup should be considered With increasing age conditions such as bronchitis, pneumonia and carcinoma become more prevalent
Smoking history	Patients who smoke are more prone to chronic and recurrent cough. Over time this might develop in to chronic bronchitis and chronic obstructive pulmonary disease (COPD)

Unlikely causes

Laryngotracheobronchitis (croup)

Symptoms are triggered by a recent infection with parainfluenza virus and account for 75% of cases, although other viral pathogens include rhinovirus and respiratory syncytial virus. It affects infants aged between 3 months and 6 years and affects 2–6% of children. The incidence is highest between 1 and 2 years of age and occurs more in boys than in girls; it is more common in autumn and winter months. Symptoms occur in the late evening and night. The cough can be severe and violent, and is described as having a barking (seal-like) quality. In between coughing episodes the child may be breathless and struggle to breathe properly. Typically, symptoms improve during the day and often recur again the following night, with the majority of children seeing symptoms resolve in 48 hours. Warm moist air as a treatment for croup has been used since the 19th century. This is either done by moving the child to a bathroom and running a hot bath or shower, or by boiling a kettle in the room. However, current guidelines do not advocate humidification, as there is no evidence to support its use.

Croup management is based on an assessment of severity. Parents should be advised that if the child's symptoms persist beyond 48 hours or they exhibit any symptoms of stridor/distress, then medical intervention is required. Standard treatment for those children with stridor would be oral or intra-muscular dexamethasone or nebulised budesonide (Russell et al., 2011).

Chronic obstructive pulmonary disease (COPD)

Chronic bronchitis (CB), along with emphysema, is characterised by the destruction of lung tissue and collectively they are known as chronic obstructive pulmonary disease (COPD). The prevalence of COPD in the UK is uncertain. However, figures from the Health and Safety Executive (2014) estimate that over a million individuals currently have a diagnosis of COPD, which accounts for 25 000 deaths each year.

Patients with CB often present with a long-standing history of recurrent acute bronchitis in which episodes become increasingly severe and persist for increasing duration until the cough becomes continual. CB has been defined as coughing up sputum on most days for three or more consecutive months over the previous 2 years. CB is caused by chronic irritation of the airways by inhaled substances, especially tobacco smoke. A history of smoking is the single most important factor in the aetiology of CB. In non-smokers the likely cause of CB is UACS, asthma or gastro-oesophageal reflux. One study has shown that 99% of non-smokers with CB and a normal chest x-ray suffered from one of these three conditions.

CB starts with a non-productive cough that later becomes a mucopurulent productive cough. The patient should be questioned about smoking habit. If the patient is a smoker, the cough will usually be worse in the morning. Secondary infections contribute to acute exacerbations seen in CB. It typically occurs in patients over the age of 40 and is more common in men. Pharmacists have an important role to play in identifying smokers with CB, as this provides an excellent opportunity for health promotion advice and assessing the patient's willingness to stop smoking.

Asthma

The exact prevalence of asthma is unknown due to differing terminologies and definitions plus difficulties in correct diagnosis, especially in children, and co-morbidity with COPD in the elderly. Best estimates of adult asthma prevalence are approximately 4%, but it may be up to 10%. In children the figures are higher (10–15%) because a proportion of children will 'grow out' of it and be symptom free by adulthood.

Asthma is a chronic inflammatory condition of the airways characterised by coughing, wheezing, chest tightness and shortness of breath. Classically these symptoms tend to be variable, intermittent, worse at night and provoked by triggers. In addition, possible associated features are family or personal history of atopy and worsening symptoms after taking non-steroidal anti-inflammatory drugs (NSAIDs) – upward of 20% of people affected – or beta-blockers (although a 2002 Cochrane review by Salpeter concluded that cardioselective beta-blocker use in patients with reversible airway disease demonstrated no increase in adverse respiratory effects).

In the context of presentations to a community pharmacist, asthma can present as a non-productive cough, especially in young children where the cough is often worst at night. In these cases pay particular attention to other possible symptoms such as chest tightness, wheeze and difficulty in breathing, which may be frequent and recurrent, and occur even when the child does not have a cold.

Pneumonia (community acquired)

Every year between 0.5% and 1% of adults in the UK will have community-acquired pneumonia. Bacterial infection is usually responsible for pneumonia and most commonly caused by *Streptococcus pneumoniae* (80% of cases), although other pathogens are also responsible, e.g., *Chlamydia* and *Mycoplasma*. Initially, the cough is non-productive and painful (first 24–48 hours), but it rapidly becomes productive, with sputum being stained red. The intensity of the redness varies depending on the causative organism. The cough tends to be worst at night. The patient will be unwell, with a high fever, malaise, headache and breathlessness, and experience pleuritic pain (inflammation of pleural membranes, manifested as pain to the sides) that worsens on inspiration. Urgent referral to the doctor is required to conduct tests such as C-reactive protein to establish the need for antibiotics.

Medicine-induced cough or wheeze

A number of medicines may cause bronchoconstriction, which presents as cough or wheeze. Angiotensin-converting enzyme (ACE) inhibitors are most commonly associated with cough. Incidence might be as high as 16%; it is not dose related and time to onset is variable, ranging from a few hours to more than 1 year after the start of treatment. Cough invariably ceases after withdrawal of the ACE inhibitor but takes 3 to 4 weeks to resolve. Other medicines that are associated with cough or wheeze are NSAIDs and beta-blockers. If an adverse drug reaction (ADR) is suspected, then the pharmacist should discuss alternative medication with the prescriber, for example, the incidence of cough with angiotensin II receptor blockers is half that of ACE inhibitors.

Very unlikely causes

Cough is a symptom of many other conditions, although the majority will be rarely encountered in community pharmacy. However, it is important to be aware of these rare causes of cough to ensure that appropriate referrals are made.

Heart failure

Heart failure is a condition of the elderly. The prevalence of heart failure rises with increasing age; it is rare under 65, but thereafter increases rapidly with increasing age. Heart failure is characterised by insidious progression and diagnosing early mild heart failure is extremely difficult because symptoms are not pronounced. Often, the first symptoms patients experience are fatigue, shortness of breath, orthopnoea and dyspnoea at night. As the condition progresses from mild/moderate to severe heart failure, patients will show ankle swelling and might complain of a productive, frothy cough, which may have pink-tinged sputum.

Bronchiectasis

Bronchiectasis is caused by irreversible dilation of the bronchi. It might be under-diagnosed as people are often thought to have COPD. Characteristically, the patient has a chronic cough of very long duration. Over three quarters of patients will cough daily with sputum production. Breathlessness is a very common accompanying symptom. Approximately a third of patients will also suffer from wheeze and chest pain.

Tuberculosis

Tuberculosis (TB) is a bacterial infection caused by *Mycobacterium tuberculosis* and is transmitted primarily by inhalation. In 2013 UK figures showed that nearly 8000 cases were notified. TB remains concentrated in the most deprived populations, with almost half of cases associated with people not in employment. As in previous years, London accounted for the highest proportion of cases (38%), followed by the West Midlands area (12%). Three quarters of TB cases occurred among people born outside the UK.

TB is characterised by its slow onset and initial mild symptoms. The cough is chronic in nature and sputum production can vary from mild to severe with associated haemoptysis. Other symptoms of the condition are malaise, fever, night sweats and weight loss. However, not all patients will experience all symptoms. A patient with a productive cough for more than 3 weeks and exhibiting one or more of the associated symptoms should be referred for further investigation, especially if they are non-UK born (most UK cases originate from India, Pakistan and Somalia). Chest x-rays and sputum smear tests can be performed to confirm the diagnosis.

Carcinoma of the lung

A number of studies have shown that between 20% and 90% of patients will develop a cough at some point during the progression of carcinoma of the lung. The possibility of carcinoma increases in long-term cigarette smokers who have had a cough for a number of months or who develop a marked change in the character of their cough. The cough produces small amounts of sputum that might be blood streaked. If a person over the age of 40 has two or more of the following symptoms – cough, fatigue, shortness of breath, chest pain, weight loss or appetite loss – he or she needs to be referred to the GP for a chest x-ray.

Lung abscess

A typical presentation is of a non-productive cough with pleuritic pain and dyspnoea. It is more common in the elderly. Signs of infection such as malaise and fever can also be present. Later, the cough produces large amounts of purulent and often foul-smelling sputum.

Spontaneous pneumothorax (collapsed lung)

Rupture of the bullae (the small air or fluid-filled sacs in the lung) can cause spontaneous pneumothorax, but normally there is no underlying cause. It affects approximately 1 in 10 000 people, usually tall, thin men between 20 and 40 years old. Cigarette smoking and a family history of pneumothorax are contributing risk factors. This can be a life-threatening disorder, causing a non-productive cough and severe respiratory distress. The patient experiences sudden sharp unilateral chest pain that worsens on inspiration. The symptoms often begin quickly, and can occur during rest or sleep.

Gastro-oesophageal reflux disease

Gastro-oesophageal reflux disease (GORD) does not usually present with cough, but patients with this condition might cough when recumbent (lying down). The patient might show symptoms of reflux or heartburn. Patients with GORD have increased cough reflex sensitivity and respond well to proton pump inhibitors. GORD should always be considered in all cases of unexplained cough.

Nocardiasis

Nocardiasis is an extremely rare bacterial infection caused by *Nocardia asteroides;* it is transmitted primarily by inhalation. It is very unlikely a pharmacist will ever encounter this condition and it is included in this text for the sake of completeness. It has a higher incidence in the elderly population, especially in men. The sputum is purulent, thick and possibly blood tinged. Fever is prominent, and night sweats, pleurisy, weight loss and fatigue might also be present.

Fig. 2.1 will aid the differentiation between serious and non-serious conditions of cough in adults.

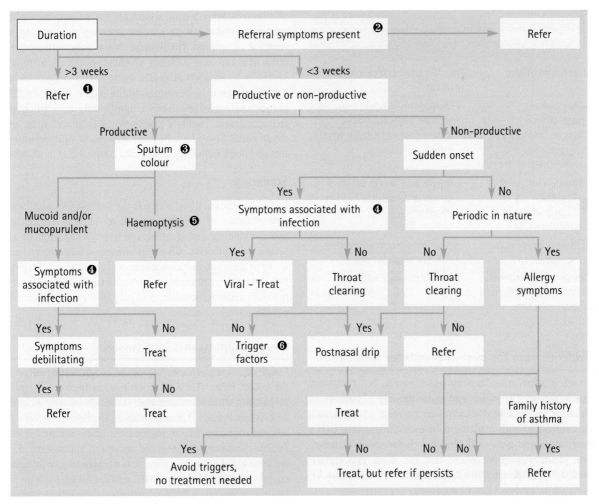

Fig. 2.1 Primer for differential diagnosis of cough in adults.

❶ Duration of cough
Coughs lasting longer than 3 weeks are considered chronic in nature. Most acute, self-limiting coughs usually resolve within 3 weeks; conditions with sinister pathology are more likely the longer the cough has been present. However, not all coughs that have lasted 3 weeks have to be referred automatically. Postnasal drip and seasonal allergies (e.g., hay fever) can persist for weeks and be managed by community pharmacists.

❷ Referral symptoms
Certain symptoms warrant direct referral to the GP or even casualty. For example, shortness of breath, breathlessness (possible asthma), chest pain (possible cardiovascular cause) or pain on inspiration (pleurisy or pneumothorax).

❸ Sputum colour
Sputum colour can be helpful in deciding when to refer. However, there is a common misconception that patients who present with green-yellow or brown sputum have a

bacterial infection; this is not the case – almost all will be viral in origin. If the cough has persisted for more than 7 to 10 days, it is possible that an initial viral infection has become secondarily infected with a bacterial infection. This could indicate referral, especially if the symptoms are debilitating or if the patient is elderly.

❹ Symptoms associated with infection
The patient might have associated symptoms of fever, rhinorrhoea and sore throat.

❺ Haemoptysis
Blood in the sputum requires further investigation, especially if the person has had the symptoms for a period of time.

❻ Trigger factors
Certain atmospheric factors can trigger cough. These factors include air-temperature changes, pollution (e.g., cigarette smoke) and dry atmospheres (e.g., air conditioning).

! TRIGGER POINTS indicative of referral: Cough

Symptoms/signs	Possible danger/reason for referral
Chest pain Haemoptysis Pain on inspiration Wheeze and/or shortness of breath	All symptoms suggest possible sinister pathology or severe cases of simple viral infection
Duration longer than 3 weeks Cough that recurs on a regular basis	Suggests non-acute cause of cough and requires further investigation
Debilitating symptoms in the elderly	This patient group at greater risk of complications
Persistent nocturnal cough in children	Suggests possible asthma

Evidence base for over-the-counter medication

Cough is often trivialised by practitioners, but coughing can impair quality of life and cause anxiety to parents of children with cough. Patients who exercise self-care will be confronted with a plethora of over-the-counter (OTC) medication and many will find the choice overwhelming. The pharmacist must ensure that the most appropriate medication is selected for the patient, but this must be done on an evidence-based approach.

All the active ingredients to treat cough were brought to the market many years ago when clinical trials suffered from flaws in study design compared with today's standards, thus clinical efficacy is therefore difficult to establish.

Expectorants

A number of active ingredients have been formulated to help expectoration, including guaifenesin, ammonium salts, ipecacuanha, creosote and squill. The majority of products marketed in the UK for productive cough contain guaifenesin, although products containing squill (e.g., Buttercup Syrup) and ipecacuanha (e.g., Covonia Herbal mucous Cough Syrup) are available. The clinical evidence available for any active ingredient is limited. Older ingredients, such as ammonium salts, ipecacuanha and squill, were traditionally used to induce vomiting as it was believed that at subemetic doses they would cause gastric irritation, triggering reflex expectoration; however, this has never been proven and belongs in the annals of folklore. Guaifenesin is thought to stimulate secretion of respiratory tract fluid, increasing sputum volume and decreasing viscosity so assisting in removal of sputum. Guaifenesin is the only active ingredient that has any evidence of effectiveness. Two studies identified by Smith et al. (2012) found conflicting results for guaifenesin as an expectorant. In the largest study ($n = 239$) participants stated guaifenesin significantly reduced cough frequency and intensity compared with placebo. In the smaller trial ($n = 65$) guaifenesin was found to have no effect on cough frequency or severity compared with placebo.

Summary

Based on studies, guaifenesin is the only expectorant with any evidence of effectiveness. However, trial results are not convincing and guaifenesin is probably little or no better than placebo. Given its proven safety record, absence of drug interactions, placebo properties and the public's desire to treat productive coughs with a home remedy, it would seem reasonable to supply OTC cough medicines containing guaifenesin.

Cough suppressants (antitussives)

Cough suppressants act directly on the cough centre to depress the cough reflex. Their effectiveness has been investigated in patients with acute and chronic cough as well as citric acid-induced cough. Although trials on healthy volunteers – in whom coughing was induced by citric acid – allowed reproducible conditions to assess the activity of antitussives, they are of little value because they do not represent physiological cough. Of greatest interest to OTC medication are trials investigating acute cough, because patients suffering from chronic cough should be referred to the doctor.

Codeine

Codeine is generally accepted as a standard or benchmark antitussive against which all others are judged. A review by Eddy et al. (1970) showed codeine to be an effective antitussive in animal models, and cough-induced studies in humans have also shown codeine to be effective. However, these findings appear to be less reproducible in acute and pathological chronic cough. More recent studies have failed to demonstrate a significant clinical effect of codeine compared with placebo in patients suffering with acute cough. Greater voluntary control of the cough reflex by patients has been suggested for the apparent lack of effect codeine has on acute cough.

Pholcodine

Pholcodine, like codeine, has been subject to limited clinical trials, with the majority being either animal models or citric acid-induced cough studies in man. These studies have shown pholcodine to have antitussive activity. A review by Findlay (1988) concluded that, on balance, pholcodine appears to possess antitussive activity but advocates the need for better, well-controlled studies.

Dextromethorphan

Trial data for dextromethorphan, like that for codeine and pholcodine, are limited. The Cochrane review of cough mixtures (Smith et al., 2014) identified three studies comparing dextromethorphan with placebo. Two studies found an improvement in cough counts and cough effort, which, in one study, equated to a difference of up to 8 to 10 coughing bouts every 30 minutes. The third study found no difference between dextromethorphan and placebo in terms of cough frequency and subjective cough scores. It appears to have limited abuse potential and fewer side effects than codeine.

Antihistamines

Antihistamines have been included in cough remedies for decades. Their mechanism of action is thought to be through the anticholinergic-like drying action on the mucous membranes and not via histamine. There are numerous clinical trials involving antihistamines for the relief of cough and cold symptoms, most notably with diphenhydramine.

Citric acid-induced cough studies have demonstrated significant antitussive activity compared with placebo and results from chronic cough trials support an antitussive activity for diphenhydramine. However, trials that showed a significant reduction in cough frequency suffered from having small patient numbers, thus limiting their usefulness. Additionally, poor trial design investigating the antitussive activity of diphenhydramine in acute cough makes assessment of its effectiveness difficult. A recent review concluded 'Presumptions about efficacy of diphenhydramine against cough in humans are not unequivocally substantiated in literature' (Bjornsdottir et al., 2007). Less sedating antihistamines have also not been shown to have any benefit in treating coughs compared with placebo (Smith et al., 2014).

Demulcents

Demulcents, such as simple linctus and honey, are pharmacologically inert and are used on the theoretical basis that they reduce irritation by coating the pharynx and so prevent coughing. A Cochrane review (Oduwole et al., 2014) involving three trials with honey stated that honey might be better than no treatment or placebo, although these trials were small and subject to bias.

Combination cough mixtures

Many OTC cough preparations are combinations of agents. Some of these include ingredients, such as decongestants, that target other aspects of the common cold. It should be noted that some combination products contain subtherapeutic doses of the active ingredients, while a few contain illogical combinations such as cough suppressants with an expectorant, or an antihistamine with an expectorant. If possible, these should be avoided.

Summary

Antitussives have been traditionally evaluated for efficacy in animal studies or cough-induced models on healthy volunteers. This presents serious problems in assessing their effectiveness because support for their antitussive activity does not come from patients with acute cough associated with URTI. Furthermore, there appear to be no comparative studies of sound study design to allow for judgements to be made on their comparable efficacy. Compounding these problems is the self-limiting nature of acute cough, which further hinders differentiation between clinical efficacy and normal symptom resolution.

Antitussives therefore have a limited role in the treatment of acute non-productive cough. Patients should be encouraged to drink more fluid and told that their symptoms will resolve in time on their own. If recommended, then side effect profile and abuse tendency rather than clinical efficacy will drive choice. On this basis, pholcodine and dextromethorphan would be first-line therapy and codeine, because of its greater side effect profile and tendency to be abused, should be reserved for second-line treatment. Antihistamines should not be used routinely, unless night-time sedation is perceived as beneficial to aid sleep.

Cough medication for children

Very few well-designed studies have been conducted in children. A review published in the Drug and Therapeutics Bulletin (Anonymous, 1999) identified just five trials of sound methodological design. However, of these five trials, one study used illogical drug combinations (expectorant combined with suppressant) and a further three studies used combination products not available on the UK market. In addition, there has been growing evidence of the potential harm that these agents can pose to young children, either due to adverse effects or from accidental inappropriate dosing (Isbister et al., 2010; Vassilev et al.,

2010). In 2014 a Cochrane review examining the treatment of acute cough in both adults and children concluded there was no good evidence to support the effectiveness of cough medicines in acute cough (Smith et al., 2014). Based on the lack of efficacy and potential harm, the MHRA advised (April, 2015) healthcare professionals that when prescribing or dispensing codeine-containing medicines for cough or cold, codeine is contraindicated in children under 12. In addition, codeine-containing medicines are not recommended for adolescents (aged 12–18) who have problems with breathing.

Practical prescribing and product selection

Prescribing information relating to the cough medicines reviewed in the section 'Evidence base for over-the-counter medication' is discussed and summarised in Table 2.3; useful tips relating to patients presenting with cough are given in 'Hints and Tips' in Box 2.1. Due to recent MHRA announcements on cough products, many manufacturers have taken the opportunity to revise their prescribing information and no longer recommend cough products in children under the age of 12.

Table 2.3
Practical prescribing: Summary of cough medicines

Name of medicine	Use in children	Likely side effects	Drug interactions of note	Patients in which care is exercised	Pregnancy & breastfeeding
Cough expectorants					
Guaifenesin	>6 years	None	None	None	OK
Cough suppressants					
Codeine	>18 years	Sedation, constipation	Increased sedation with alcohol, opioid analgesics, anxiolytics, hypnotics and antidepressants	Asthmatics	Pregnancy – best avoided in 3rd trimester
Pholcodine	>6 years	Possible sedation			Short periods OK in breastfeeding. Reports of dextromethorphan causing drowsiness and poor feeding in the baby
Dextromethorphan	>12 years				
Antihistamines					
Diphenhydramine	>6 years*	Dry mouth, sedation and constipation	Increased sedation with alcohol, opioid analgesics, anxiolytics, hypnotics and antidepressants	Glaucoma, prostate enlargement	Pregnancy – Standard references state OK, although some manufacturers advise avoidance Breastfeeding – OK, as amount secreted into breast milk is small. It may, however, reduce milk supply. Reports of poor feeding in the baby
Demulcents					
Simple linctus	>1 month	None	None	None	OK

*Included in some cough preparations (e.g., Benylin Children's Night Cough).

HINTS AND TIPS BOX 2.1: COUGH

Treatment for children under 6	Parents should be advised to make the child drink more fluid and potentially try a non-pharmacological cough mixture, such as a demulcent.
Insulin-dependent diabetics	People with insulin-dependent diabetes should be asked to monitor their blood glucose more frequently because insulin requirements increase during acute infections.
Avoid theophylline	Theophylline is available as a pharmacy only medicine, but it is best avoided because patients requiring medication to help with shortness of breath or wheeze need further assessment.
Avoid illogical combinations	Few cough remedies now have illogical medicine combinations. However, there are still a few on the market and these are best avoided. For example, combinations of expectorants and suppressants (e.g., Pulmo Bailey).

Cough expectorants

Guaifenesin

Almost all manufacturers include guaifenesin in their cough product ranges, including Benylin and Robitussin. Adults and children 12 years and over should take 200 mg four times a day, and the dose for children over the age of 6 is 100 mg four times a day, although most manufacturers do not recommend its use in those children under 12 years of age. Guaifenesin-based products have no cautions in their use and no side effects; they are also free from clinically significant drug interactions so can be given safely with prescribed medication. Sugar-free versions (e.g., Robitussin range) are available.

Cough suppressants (codeine, pholcodine, dextromethorphan)

Codeine, pholcodine and dextromethorphan are all opiate derivatives, and therefore – broadly – have the same interactions, cautions in use and side effect profile. They do interact with prescription-only medications (POMs) and also with OTC medications, especially those that cross the blood–brain barrier. Their combined effect is to potentiate sedation and it is important to warn the patient of this, although short-term use of cough suppressants with the interacting medication is unlikely to warrant dosage modification. Care should be exercised when giving cough suppressants to asthmatics because, in theory, cough suppressants can cause respiratory depression. However, in practice this is very rarely observed and does not preclude the use of cough suppressants in asthmatic patients. However, other side effects can occur (e.g., constipation), especially with codeine. If a cough suppressant is unsuitable, for example, in late pregnancy and children, then a demulcent can be offered.

Codeine

The dose for adults and children over 18 years of age is 5 mL three or four times a day.

Pholcodine

The adult dose is 5 to 10 mL (5–10 mg) three or four times a day. Most marketed products now state avoidance in children but British National Formulary (BNF) (70) still states that it can be given to children aged 6 years and over. Sugar-free versions (e.g., Pavacol-D) are available.

Dextromethorphan

For adults and children aged over 12, there are a number of products available (e.g., Benylin dry coughs non-drowsy; Covonia original Bronchial Balsam and Robitussin Dry medicine). The dosing for these listed products is standard – 10 mL four times a day.

Antihistamines

Routine use of antihistamines is unjustified in treating non-productive cough. However, the sedative side effects from antihistamines can, on occasion, be useful to allow the patient an uninterrupted night's sleep. Diphenhydramine is commonly included in products, especially in the Benylin range.

All antihistamines included in cough remedies are first-generation antihistamines and associated with sedation. They interact with other sedating medication, resulting in potentiation of the sedative properties of the interacting medicines. They also possess antimuscarinic side effects, which commonly result in dry mouth and possibly constipation. It is these antimuscarinic properties that mean patients with glaucoma and prostate enlargement should ideally avoid their use, because it could lead to increased intraocular pressure and precipitation of urinary retention.

Demulcents

Demulcents, for example, simple linctus and glycerin, provide a safe alternative for at-risk patient groups such as the elderly, pregnant women, young children and those taking multiple medication. They are increasingly used, as manufacturers have reformulated their cough products in light of restrictions placed on antitussives. They can act as useful placebos when the patient insists on a cough mixture. If recommended they should be given three or four times a day.

References

Anonymous. Cough medications in children. Drug and Therapeutics Bulletin 1999; 37:19–21

Bjornsdottir I, Einarson TR, Guomundsson LS, et al. Efficacy of diphenhydramine against cough in humans: a review. Pharm World Sci 2007;29(6):577–83.

Eddy NB, Friebel H, Hahn KJ, et al. Codeine and its alternatives for pain and cough relief. Geneva: World Health Organ 1970;1–253.

Findlay JWA. Review articles: pholcodine. J Clin Pharm Ther 1988;13:5–17.

Isbister GK, Prior F, Kilham HA. Restricting cough and cold medicines in children. Journal of Paediatrics and Child Health 2012;48:91–8.

Oduwole O, Meremikwu MM, O yo-Ita A, et al. Honey for acute cough in children. Cochrane Database of Systematic Reviews 2014, Issue 12. Art. No.: CD007094. http://dx.doi.org/10.1002/14651858.CD007094.pub4.

Russell KF, Liang Y, O'Gorman K, et al. Glucocorticoids for croup. Cochrane Database of Systematic Reviews 2011, Issue 1. Art. No.: CD001955. http://dx.doi.org/10.1002/14651858.CD001955.pub3.

Salpeter SR, Ormiston TM, Salpeter EE. Cardioselective beta-blockers for reversible airway disease. Cochrane Database of Systematic Reviews 2002, Issue 4. Art. No.: CD002992. http://dx.doi.org/10.1002/14651858.CD002992.

Smith SM, Schroeder K, Fahey T. Over-the-counter (OTC) medications for acute cough in children and adults in ambulatory settings. Cochrane Database of Systematic Reviews 2014, Issue 11. Art. No.: CD001831. http://dx.doi.org/10.1002/14651858.CD001831.pub5.

Vassilev ZP, Kabadi S, Villa R. Safety and efficacy of over-the-counter cough and cold medicines for use in children. Expert Opinion Drug Safety 2010;9(2):233–42.

Further reading

Dicpinigaitis PV, Colice GL, Goolsby MJ, et al. Acute cough: a diagnostic and therapeutic challenge. Cough 2009;5:11.

Knutson D, Aring A. Viral croup. Am Fam Physician 2004;69:535–40, 541–2.

Morice AH, McGarvey L, Pavord I. Recommendations for the management of cough in adults. Thorax 2006;61:S1–24.

NICE Guidance on TB. 2011, Available at: https://www.nice.org.uk/Guidance/CG117 (accessed 1 July 2015).

NICE Guidance- Suspected cancers recognition and referral. 2015, Available at: http://www.nice.org.uk/guidance/NG12/chapter/1-recommendations#lung-and-pleural-cancers (accessed 1 July 2015).

NICE Guidance on Pneumonia. 2014, Available at: http://www.nice.org.uk/guidance/cg191 (accessed 1 July 2015).

Pratter MR. Overview of common causes of chronic cough: ACCP evidence-based clinical practice guidelines. Chest 2006;129(1 Suppl):59S–62S.

Sahn S, Heffner J. Spontaneous pneumothorax. N Engl J Med 2000;342:868–74.

Websites

Action on Smoking and Health (ASH): http://www.ash.org.uk/
Asthma UK: http://www.asthma.org.uk/
British Lung Foundation: https://www.blf.org.uk/Home
The British Thoracic Society: www.brit-thoracic.org.uk/

The common cold

Background

Colds, along with coughs, represent the largest case load for primary healthcare workers. Because the condition has no specific cure and is self-limiting with two thirds of sufferers recovering within a week, it would be easy to dismiss the condition as unimportant. However, because of the very high number of cases seen, it is essential that pharmacists have a thorough understanding of the condition so that severe symptoms or symptoms suggestive of influenza are identified.

Prevalence and epidemiology

The common cold is extremely prevalent and, like cough, is caused by viral URTI. Children contract colds more frequently than adults, with on average five to six colds per year compared with two to four colds in adults, although in children this can be as high as 12 colds per year. Children aged between 4 and 8 years are most likely to contract a cold and it can appear to a child's parents that one cold follows another with no respite. By the age of

10, the number of colds contracted is half that observed in pre-school children. In the UK, colds peak in December and January, possibly due to increased crowding indoors during cold weather, especially among schoolchildren who promote transmission.

Aetiology

More than 200 different virus types can produce symptoms of the common cold, including rhinoviruses (accounting for 30–50% of all cases), coronaviruses, parainfluenza virus, respiratory syncytial virus and adenovirus. Transmission is primarily by the virus coming into contact with the hands, which then touch the nose, mouth and eyes (direct contact transmission). Droplets shed from the nose coat surfaces such as door handles and telephones. Cold viruses can remain viable on these surfaces for several hours and, when an uninfected person touches the contaminated surface, transmission occurs. Transmission by coughing and sneezing does occur, although it is a secondary mechanism. This is why good hygiene (washing hands frequently and using disposable tissues) remains the cornerstone of reducing the spread of a cold.

Once the virus is exposed to the mucosa, it invades the nasal and bronchial epithelia, attaching to specific receptors and causing damage to the ciliated cells. This results in the release of inflammatory mediators, which, in turn, leads to inflammation of the tissues lining the nose. Permeability of capillary cell walls increases, resulting in oedema, which is experienced by the patient as nasal congestion and sneezing. Fluid might drip down the back of the throat, spreading the virus to the throat and upper chest, causing cough and sore throat. Colds are most contagious during the first 1 to 2 days of symptoms.

Arriving at a differential diagnosis

It is extremely likely that someone presenting with cold symptoms will have a viral infection. Table 2.4 highlights those conditions that can be encountered by community pharmacists and their relative incidence.

Most people will accurately self-diagnose a common cold and it is the pharmacist's role to confirm this self-diagnosis and assess the severity of the symptoms as some patients, for example, the elderly, infirm and those with existing medical conditions, might need greater support and care. In the first instance, the pharmacist should make an overall assessment of the person's general state of health. Anyone with debilitating symptoms that effectively prevents him or her from doing normal day-to-day routines should be managed more carefully. Although it is likely that a patient will have a common cold, severe colds

Table 2.4
Causes of cold and their relative incidence in community pharmacy

Incidence	Cause
Most likely	Viral infection
Likely	Rhinitis, rhinosinusitis, otitis media
Unlikely	Influenza

Table 2.5
Specific questions to ask the patient: The common cold

Question	Relevance
Onset of symptoms	Peak incidence of flu is in the winter months; the common cold occurs any time throughout the year. Flu symptoms tend to have a more abrupt onset than the common cold – a matter of hours rather than 1 or 2 days. Summer colds are common, but they must be differentiated from seasonal allergic rhinitis (hay fever).
Nature of symptoms	Marked myalgia, chills and malaise are more prominent in flu than the common cold. Loss of appetite is also common with flu.
Aggravating factors	Headache/pain that is worsened by sneezing, coughing and bending over suggests sinus complications. If ear pain is present, especially in children, middle ear involvement is likely.

can mimic symptoms of flu, which is the only condition of any real significance that has to be eliminated before treatment can be given, although secondary complications associated with the common cold can occur. Asking symptom-specific questions will help the pharmacist establish a differential diagnosis (Table 2.5).

Clinical features of the common cold

Symptoms of the common cold are well known. However, the nature and severity of symptoms will be influenced by factors such as the causative agent, patient age and underlying medical conditions. Following an incubation period of between 1 and 3 days (although this can be as short as 10 to 12 hours), the patient develops a sore throat and sneezing, followed by profuse nasal discharge and congestion. Cough and UACS commonly follow. In addition, headache, mild to moderate fever (<38.9° C; 102° F) and general malaise may be present. Most colds resolve in 1 week, but up to a quarter of people will have symptoms lasting 14 days or more.

Conditions to eliminate

Likely causes

Rhinitis

A blocked or stuffy nose, whether acute or chronic in nature, is a common complaint. Rhinitis is covered in more detail on page 33 and the reader is referred to this section for differential diagnosis of rhinitis from the common cold.

Acute rhinosinusitis

Rhinosinusitis (formerly sinusitis) is inflammation of one or more of the paranasal sinuses. Up to 2% of patients will develop acute rhinosinusitis as a complication of the common cold. Anatomically the sinuses are described in four pairs: frontal sinuses, ethmoid sinuses, maxillary sinuses and sphenoid sinuses (Fig. 2.2). All are air-filled spaces that drain into the nasal cavity. Following a cold, sinus air spaces can become filled with nasal secretions, which stagnate because of a reduction in ciliary function of the cells lining the sinuses. Bacteria – commonly *Streptococcus* and *Haemophilus* – can then secondarily infect these stagnant secretions. It is clinically defined by at least two of these symptoms:

- blockage or congestion
- discharge or UACS
- facial pain or pressure
- reduction or loss of smell

The pain in the early stages tends to be relatively mild and localised, usually unilateral and dull, but becomes bilateral and more severe the longer the condition persists. Bending forward often exacerbates the pain (moving the eyes from side to side and coughing or sneezing can also increase the pain), and sinuses will be tender when gently palpated. If the ethmoid sinuses are involved, retro-orbital pain (behind the eye) is often experienced. Analgesics for pain relief and oral or nasal sympathomimetics can be tried to remove the nasal secretions. Antibiotics are not routinely recommended (UK guidelines, 2015) unless the person is systemically unwell or at risk of complications due to underlying medical conditions. If antibiotics are to be prescribed, then amoxicillin is first line (or doxycycline if the patient has a penicillin allergy).

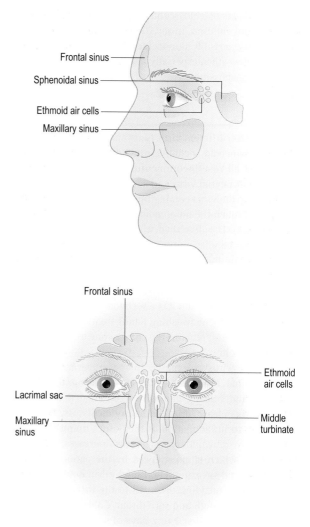

Fig. 2.2 Location of the sinuses

Acute otitis media

Acute otitis media is commonly seen in children following a common cold and results from the virus spreading to the middle ear via the Eustachian tube, where an accumulation of pus within the middle ear or inflammation of the tympanic membrane (eardrum) result. The overriding symptom is ear pain, but the child may rub or tug at the ear and become more irritable. Referral to the GP would be appropriate for auroscopical examination, unless the pharmacist is competent to perform this procedure. Examination reveals a bulging tympanic membrane, loss of normal landmarks and a change in colour (red or yellow). See Student Consult (https://studentconsult.inkling.com) for eardrum images. Rupture of the eardrum causes purulent discharge and relieves the pain. For management of acute otitis media, see page 84.

Unlikely causes

Influenza

There are two main types of influenza virus: type A and type B, of which there many different strains as they constantly alter their antigenic structure, necessitating yearly recommendations to which strains of influenza should be included in vaccines. Its spread is the same as the common cold – via droplet inhalation or having direct contact with an infected person's nasal secretions.

Patients often use the word 'flu' when describing a common cold. However, subtle differences in symptoms between the two conditions should allow for differentiation. It is helpful to remember that the 'flu' season tends to be between December and March, whereas the common cold, although more common in winter months, can occur at any time. The onset of influenza is sudden and the typical symptoms are shivering, chills, malaise, marked aching of limbs, insomnia, a non-productive cough (cough in the common cold is usually productive) and loss of appetite. Influenza is therefore normally debilitating, and a person with flu is much more likely to send a third party into a pharmacy for medication than present in person. Symptoms improve after approximately 5 days with resolution after a week or more. Flu vaccination programmes are the most important preventative measure to reduce flu cases and the associated complications of flu in at-risk populations.

> **!**
>
> **TRIGGER POINTS indicative of referral:**
> **The common cold**

Symptoms/signs	Possible danger/reason for referral
Acute sinus involvement that fails to respond to OTC decongestant therapy	Possible need for antibiotics
Middle ear pain that fails to respond to analgesia	
Patients with symptoms indicative of flu	Need an assessment of symptom severity by doctor
Vulnerable patient groups, such as the very elderly	

Evidence base for over-the-counter medication

Many of the active ingredients found in cold remedies are also constituents of cough products. Often they are combined and marketed as cough and cold or flu remedies. For information relating to cough ingredients, the reader is referred to the sections on OTC medication for coughs (page 16).

Antihistamines

A Cochrane review (De Sutter et al., 2009 – but subsequently withdrawn) found that antihistamines, when used as monotherapy, did not have significant benefit clinically in nasal congestion, rhinorrhoea or sneezing in older children and adults. Additionally, they appeared not to influence subjective improvement. Only two trials were evaluated in young children, the results of which were conflicting. However, the larger study, which was more robustly conducted, showed no benefit of antihistamines on the common cold.

Trials that used antihistamines in combination with other products such as decongestants and antitussives do show some beneficial global effects in adults and older children. Unfortunately, in most trials it was not possible to assess the clinical significance of these benefits because of insufficient data.

Sympathomimetics

Trial data specifically looking at the effects of decongestants in the common cold are limited. A Cochrane review (Taverner & Latte, 2009) identified seven trials that met their inclusion criteria, which involved topical oxymetazoline and oral pseudoephedrine and phenylpropanolamine (no longer used in the UK). The authors found a small (6%) but significant improvement in symptoms of nasal congestion in adults. However, data were lacking in children under 12 years. No difference in efficacy was found between topical or systemic products.

A systematic review of single-dose phenylephrine studies found a statistically significant improvement in nasal airway resistance at 60 minutes compared with placebo (Kollar et al., 2007). However, the studies did not measure clinical outcomes (e.g., subjective improvement in symptoms) and the difference was small (16% at 60 minutes). In addition, four of the eight studies showed no benefit for phenylephrine compared with placebo. Importantly the manufacturers of phenylephrine conducted this review and the studies included were from an FDA submission and have not been subject to peer review. A systematic review (Hatton et al., 2007) concluded that there was insufficient evidence for the efficacy of phenylephrine as a nasal decongestant.

Multi-ingredient preparations

There is no shortage of cold and flu remedies marketed. Many combine three or more ingredients. In the majority of cases either the patient will not require all the active ingredients to treat symptoms or the 'drug cocktail' administered will not contain active ingredients that have proven efficacy. A more sensible approach to medicine management would be to match symptoms with active ingredients with known evidence of efficacy. In many cases this can be achieved by providing the patient with monotherapy or a product containing two active ingredients. Preparations with multiple ingredients therefore have a very limited role to play in the management of coughs and colds. However, patients might perceive an 'all in one' medicine as better value for money and, potentially, compliance with such preparations might be improved. The only review conducted on combination therapies for the cold was by De Sutter et al. (2012). They investigated oral antihistamine–decongestant–analgesic combinations for the common cold. The review involved 27 trials and over 5000 patients, and concluded that, for adults, an antihistamine–decongestant combination was most effective.

Alternative therapies

Many products are advocated to help treat cold symptoms. Three products in particular have received much attention and are widely used.

Zinc lozenges

The argument for zinc as a plausible treatment in ameliorating symptoms of the common cold can be traced back to 1984. Since that time a number of studies have looked at zinc's effect on treating the common cold. A recent Cochrane review (Singh & Das, 2013) identified 15 randomised and controlled trials that compared zinc versus placebo. Findings demonstrated that zinc (lozenges or syrup) is beneficial in reducing the duration of the common cold by approximately 1 day, when taken within 24 hours of onset of symptoms. They also reported that people taking zinc lozenges (not syrup or tablet form) were more likely to experience adverse events, including bad taste and nausea. In conclusion, the authors were reluctant to make a general recommendation for the use of zinc in the treatment of the common cold because of variability in the dose, formulation and duration of use seen in the trials

reviewed. In April 2015 this review was withdrawn due to concerns regarding the analysis of data. It therefore seems prudent that until such time that data is re-analysed, zinc should not be recommended to treat the common cold.

Vitamin C

Vitamin C has been widely recommended as a 'cure' for the common cold by many sources, both medical and non-medical. However, controversy still remains whether it is an effective weapon in combating the common cold. A large number of clinical trials have investigated the effect of vitamin C on the prevention and treatment of the common cold.

A Cochrane review examining the role of vitamin C at doses higher than 200 mg per day in preventing and treating the common cold identified 29 studies involving 11 306 subjects (Hemilä et al., 2013). The review found that vitamin C prophylaxis had no effect on the incidence of the common cold in the general community, and a small effect on the duration of a cold. However, they found a halving of the incidence of the common cold in people undergoing high physical stress (marathon runners, skiers and soldiers on subarctic exercises) with the prophylactic use of vitamin C. The review found that the use of vitamin C, once a cold had started, had no consistent effect on the duration or the severity of the cold. The authors concluded that routine prophylaxis with vitamin C in the general community is unjustified, but could be beneficial to those exposed to brief periods of severe physical exercise.

Echinacea

The herbal remedy echinacea is marketed as a treatment for URTIs, including the common cold. Several reviews have reported echinacea's effect as inconsistent. This is in part due to the limited number of trials that are comparable, as different echinacea species are used as well as differing plant parts and extraction methods. A Cochrane review has attempted to take these factors into consideration (Karsch-Völk et al., 2014). The authors reviewed 24 trails involving 4631 participants in an attempt to determine echinacea's effectiveness in preventing and treating the common cold. Overall they concluded that evidence was weak for echinacea in preventing and treating colds, although stronger evidence exists as a preventative treatment.

Vapour inhalation

Steam inhalation has long been advocated to aid relief of symptoms of the common cold, usually with the addition of menthol crystals. Trial data (review of six trials [$n = 387$], all involving adults) shows conflicting evidence in symptom relief of the common cold (Singh & Singh, 2013). However, it is cheap and does not carry any significant risks apart from minor discomfort and irritation of the nose. It appears that steam is the key to symptom resolution, and not any additional ingredient that is added to the water.

Saline sprays

Saline sprays have been shown to work in observational studies. A Cochrane review exploring the use of saline irrigation on acute upper respiratory tract infections identified five randomised controlled trials involving 205 adults and 544 children (King et al., 2015). The studies generally found no difference between saline treatment and control, although one study involving children did demonstrate statistically significant reductions in nasal secretion scores. Whether this translates into clinical improvement is uncertain. The authors noted that there were no serious side effects, but saline irrigation could cause minor irritation and discomfort, with up to 40% of babies not tolerating saline nasal drops. In conclusion, it remains unclear if saline irrigation is beneficial.

Garlic

A Cochrane review (Lissiman et al., 2014) identified one trial that randomly assigned 146 participants to either a garlic supplement (with 180 mg of allicin content) or a placebo once daily for 12 weeks. The trial relied on self-reported episodes of the common cold and reported 24 occurrences of the common cold in the garlic intervention group compared with 65 in the placebo group (P value <0.001). This single trial does suggest that garlic may prevent occurrences of the common cold, but more studies are needed to substantiate these findings.

General summary

Evidence of efficacy for Western and alternative medicines in preventing and treating the common cold are weak. Decongestants used on a when-needed basis probably have the strongest evidence base in treating symptoms.

Practical prescribing and product selection

Prescribing information relating to cold medicines reviewed in the section 'Evidence base for over-the-counter medication' is discussed and summarised in Table 2.6, and useful tips relating to patients presenting with a cold are given in 'Hints and Tips' in Box 2.2.

Antihistamines

First-generation antihistamines are now included in relatively few cough and cold remedies. Further information on antihistamines can be found on page 17.

Sympathomimetics

Sympathomimetics serve to constrict dilated blood vessels and swollen nasal mucosa, easing congestion and helping breathing. Sympathomimetics interact with monoamine oxidase inhibitors (MAOIs) (e.g., phenelzine, isocarboxazid, tranylcypromine and moclobemide), which can result in a fatal hypertensive crisis. The danger of the interaction persists for up to 2 weeks after treatment with MAOIs is discontinued. In addition, systemic sympathomimetics can also increase blood pressure, which might, although unlikely with short courses of treatment, alter control of blood pressure in hypertensive patients and disturb blood glucose control in diabetics. However, coadministration of medicines, such as beta-blockers, is probably clinically unimportant and does not preclude patients on beta-blockers from taking a sympathomimetic. A topical sympathomimetic could be given to such patients to negate this potential interaction. The most likely side effects of sympathomimetics are insomnia, restlessness and tachycardia. Patients should be advised not to take a dose just before bedtime because their mild stimulant action can disturb sleep.

As with cough remedies, the MHRA/CHM has stated that sympathomimetics (oral or nasally administered) should not be given to children under 6 years of age, and for those aged between 6 and 12 duration of treatment should be limited to a maximum of 5 days. Additionally, maximum pack sizes are limited to 720 mg (the equivalent of 12 tablets or capsules of 60 mg or 24 tablets or capsules of 30 mg), and sales are restricted to one pack per person owing to concerns over illicit manufacture of methylamphetamine (crystal meth) from OTC sympathomimetics.

Systemic sympathomimetics
Phenylephrine
Phenylephrine is available in a number of proprietary cold remedies, for example, the Lemsip, Sudafed and Beecham ranges, in doses ranging between 5 and 12 mg three or four times a day for adults and children over the age of 12. It is often combined with paracetamol and other ingredients, and marketed as a cold and flu remedy.

Pseudoephedrine
Pseudoephedrine is widely available as either a single ingredient (e.g., Sudafed Decongestant Tablets) or in multiingredient products in cold and cough remedies (e.g., Benylin

Table 2.6
Practical prescribing: Summary of cold medicines

Name of medicine	Use in children	Likely side effects	Drug interactions of note	Patients in which care is exercised	Pregnancy & breastfeeding
Antihistamines					
Diphenhydramine	>6 years	Dry mouth, sedation and constipation	Increased sedation with alcohol, opioid analgesics, anxiolytics, hypnotics and antidepressants	Glaucoma, prostate enlargement.	Pregnancy – Standard references state OK, although some manufacturers advise avoidance. Breastfeeding – OK, as amount secreted into breast milk is small. It may, however, reduce milk supply
Systemic sympathomimetics					
Phenylephrine	>12 years	At OTC doses insomnia most likely. Possibly may cause tachycardia	Avoid concomitant use with MAOIs and moclobemide due to risk of hypertensive crisis. Avoid in patients taking beta-blockers and TCAs	Control of hypertension and diabetes may be affected, but a short treatment course is unlikely to be clinically important	Best avoided in pregnancy as mild foetal malformations have been reported. Breastfeeding – OK, as amount secreted into breast milk is small. It may, however, reduce milk supply
Pseudoephedrine	>6 years				
Topical sympathomimetics					
Oxymetazoline	>12 years	Possible local irritation in ~5% of patients	Avoid concomitant use with MAOIs and moclobemide due to risk of hypertensive crisis	None	Pregnancy – Not adequately studied, avoid. Breastfeeding – OK
Xylometazoline	>6 years (Otrivine Child Nasal Drops)				

MAOI, monoamine oxidase inhibitor; OTC, over-the-counter; TCA, tricyclic antidepressant.

HINTS AND TIPS BOX 2.2: THE COMMON COLD

Limiting viral spread	Use disposable tissues rather than handkerchiefs Wash hands frequently, especially after nose blowing Do not share hand towels Try to avoid touching your nose
Stuffy noses in babies	Saline nose drops can be used from birth to help with congestion. This would be a more suitable and safer alternative than a topical sympathomimetic
General Sales List cold remedies	Products such as the Lemsip and Beechams ranges contain paracetamol. It is important to ensure patients are not taking excessive doses of analgesia unknowingly. Also, many products contain subtherapeutic doses of sympathomimetics. If a sympathomimetic is needed, then these products are generally best avoided.
Administration of nasal drops	The best way to administer nose drops is to have the head in the downward position facing the floor. Tilting the head backward and towards the ceiling is incorrect, as this facilitates the swallowing of the drops. However, most patients will find the latter way of putting drops into the nose much easier than the former.

Four Flu Tablets). The standard adult dose is 60 mg three or four times a day, and half the adult dose (30 mg) is suitable for children between 6 and 12 years of age. Some products only recommend use in adults and children over 12.

Nasal sympathomimetics

Nasal administration of sympathomimetics represents the safest route of administration. They can be given to most patient groups, including pregnant women after the first trimester and patients with pre-existing heart disease, diabetes, hypertension and hyperthyroidism. However, a degree of systemic absorption is possible, especially when using drops, as a small quantity might be swallowed, and therefore they should be avoided in patients taking MAOIs. All topical decongestants should not be used for longer than 5 to 7 days (August 2015, BNF 70 states maximum of 5 days in children over 6 years of age), otherwise rhinitis medicamentosa (rebound congestion) can occur.

Ephedrine

Adults and children over 12 years should put 1 to 2 drops into each nostril up to four times daily when required.

Oxymetazoline and xylometazoline

These agents are longer acting than ephedrine and require less frequent dosing, typically two or three times a day. They are made by a number of manufacturers (e.g., Otrivine range, Sudafed Blocked Nose Spray and Vicks range) who all recommend use from 12 years upwards, except Otrivine Child Nasal Drops, which can be given to children over the age of 6 (1 or 2 drops into each nostril once or twice daily).

References

De Sutter AIM, Lemiengre M, Campbell H. Antihistamines for the common cold. Cochrane Database of Systematic Reviews 2009, Issue 4. Art. No.: CD001267. http://dx.doi.org/10.1002/14651858.CD001267.pub2.

De Sutter AIM, van Driel ML, Kumar AA, et al. Oral antihistamine-decongestant-analgesic combinations for the common cold. Cochrane Database of Systematic Reviews 2012, Issue 2. Art. No.: CD004976. http://dx.doi.org/10.1002/14651858.CD004976.pub3

Hatton RC, Winterstein AG, McKelvey RP et al. Efficacy and safety of oral phenylephrine: systematic review and meta-analysis. Ann. Pharmacother 2007;41(3):381–90.

Hemilä H, Chalker E. Vitamin C for preventing and treating the common cold. Cochrane Database of Systematic Reviews 2013, Issue 1. Art. No.: CD000980. http://dx.doi.org/10.1002/14651858.CD000980.pub4.

Karsch-Völk M, Barrett B, Kiefer D, et al. Echinacea for preventing and treating the common cold. Cochrane

Database of Systematic Reviews 2014, Issue 2. Art. No.: CD000530. http://dx.doi.org/10.1002/14651858.CD000530.pub3.

King D, Mitchell B, Williams CP, et al. Saline nasal irrigation for acute upper respiratory tract infections. Cochrane Database of Systematic Reviews 2015, Issue 4. Art. No.: CD006821. http://dx.doi.org/10.1002/14651858.CD006821.pub3

Kollar C, Schneider H, Waksman J, et al. Meta-analysis of the efficacy of a single dose of phenylephrine 10 mg compared with placebo in adults with acute nasal congestion due to the common cold. Clin Ther 2007; 29(6):1057–70.

Lissiman E, Bhasale AL, Cohen M. Garlic for the common cold. Cochrane Database of Systematic Reviews 2014, Issue 11. Art. No.: CD006206. http://dx.doi.org/10.1002/14651858.CD006206.pub4.

Singh M, Singh M. Heated, humidified air for the common cold. Cochrane Database of Systematic Reviews 2013, Issue 6. Art. No.: CD001728. http://dx.doi.org/10.1002/14651858.CD001728.pub5.

Taverner D, Latte GJ. Nasal decongestants for the common cold. Cochrane Database of Systematic Reviews 2009, Issue 2. Art. No.: CD001953. http://dx.doi.org/10.1002/14651858.CD001953.pub4.

Further reading

Aljazaf K, Hale TW, Ilett KF, et al. Pseudoephedrine: effects on milk production in women and estimation of infant exposure via breastmilk. Br J Clin Pharmacol 2003;56:18–24.

Chadha NK, Chadha R. 10-minute consultation: sinusitis. BMJ 2007;334:1165. http://dx.doi.org/10.1136/bmj.39161.557211.47.

Sanders S, Glasziou PP, Del Mar CB, et al. Antibiotics for acute otitis media in children. Cochrane Database of Systematic Reviews 2004, Issue 1. Art. No.: CD000219. http://dx.doi.org/10.1002/14651858.CD000219.pub2.

Scadding GK, Durham SR, Mirakian R, et al. BSACI guidelines for the management of rhinosinusitis and nasal polyposis. Clin. Exp. Allergy 2007;38(2):260–75.

Sore throats

Background

Any part of the respiratory mucosa of the throat can give rise to symptoms of throat pain. This includes the pharynx (pharyngitis) and tonsils (tonsillitis), yet clinical distinction between pharyngitis and tonsillitis is unclear and the term 'sore throat' is commonly used. Pain can range from irritation to severe pain. Sore throats are often associated with the common cold. However, in this section, people who present with sore throat as the principal symptom are considered.

Prevalence and epidemiology

Sore throats are extremely common. UK figures show that a GP with a list size of 2000 patients will see about 120 people each year with a throat infection. However, four to six times as many people will visit the pharmacy and self-treat. Figures from other countries such as New Zealand and Australia broadly support UK findings. On average an adult will experience two to three sore throats each year.

Aetiology

Viral infection accounts for between 70% and 90% of all sore throat cases. Remaining cases are nearly all bacterial; the most common cause being Group A beta-haemolytic *Streptococcus* (also known as *Streptococcus pyogenes*). A fuller account of the aetiology of viral and bacterial pathogens that affect the upper respiratory tract appears on page 20.

Arriving at a differential diagnosis

The overwhelming majority of cases will be acute and self-limiting URTI, whether viral or bacterial in origin. Clinically, differentiation between viral and bacterial infection is extremely difficult, although specific symptom clusters are suggestive for sore throat of bacterial origin (see conditions to eliminate), but these are by no means foolproof. Other causes of sore throat also need to be considered, and Table 2.7 highlights those conditions that can be encountered by community pharmacists and their relative incidence. Asking symptom-specific questions will help the pharmacist establish a differential diagnosis (Table 2.8).

Table 2.7
Causes of sore throat and their relative incidence in community pharmacy

Incidence	Cause
Most likely	Viral infection
Likely	Streptococcal infection
Unlikely	Glandular fever, trauma
Very unlikely	Carcinoma, medicines

Table 2.8
Specific questions to ask the patient: Sore throat

Question	Relevance
Age of the patient	Although viruses are the most common cause of sore throat, there are epidemiological variances with age: Under 3 years old, *Streptococcus* is uncommon. *Streptococcal* infections are more prevalent in people under the age of 30, particularly those of school age (5–10 years) and young adults (15–25 years old). Viral causes are the most common cause of sore throat in adults. Glandular fever is most prevalent in adolescents
Tender cervical glands	On examination patients suffering from glandular fever and streptococcal sore throat often have markedly swollen glands. This is less so in viral sore throat
Tonsillar exudate present	Marked tonsillar exudate is more suggestive of a bacterial cause than a viral cause
Ulceration	Herpetiform and herpes simplex ulcers can also cause soreness in the mouth, especially in the posterior part of the mouth

Physical examination

After questioning, the pharmacist should inspect the mouth and cervical glands (located just below the angle of the jaw) to aid the differential diagnosis (Fig. 2.3).

The examination requires a good light source (e.g., pen torch). These steps should be followed:

1. Get the person seated so that the examiner can be at eye level

2. Ask the patient to say 'ah'; this should allow you to see the posterior throat. Pay particular attention to the size of the tonsils. Are they red and swollen? Is there any exudate present? Is there any sign of ulceration?

3. Check for the posterior wall of the throat. It should appear pink and moist without exudate or lesions when healthy. Redness or exudate suggests pharyngitis.

current, high-grade fever (over 39.4° C; 101° F) and absence of cough are more likely to have a bacterial infection (Table 2.9). These are known as the Centor criteria, and a person exhibiting three or all four symptoms should be referred to the doctor for potential antibiotics. However, even if the patient exhibits all of these four 'classic' symptoms, up to 40% will still not have a bacterial infection. To further compound the difficulty of diagnosis, the routine use of throat swabs is not recommended, as asymptomatic carriage of *Streptococcus* affects up to 40% of people, making it impossible to differentiate between infection and carriage. The use of antibiotics in such situations is debatable, but if antibiotics are prescribed, the drug of choice is a 10-day course of phenoxymethylpenicillin with erythromycin or clarithromycin reserved for those with penicillin allergy, in which case a 5-day course of either macrolide antibiotic should be supplied. Doctors are encouraged to adopt 'delayed' prescription strategies to reduce the number of inappropriate antibiotics taken by patients.

Complications arising from 'strep throat' include otitis media (see page 22) and acute sinusitis (see page 22)

Glandular fever (infectious mononucleosis)
Glandular fever is caused by the Epstein–Barr virus and is often called the kissing disease because transmission primarily occurs from saliva. It has a peak incidence in adolescents and young adults. The signs and symptoms of glandular fever can be difficult to distinguish from sore throat because it is characterised by pharyngitis (occasionally with exudates), fever and cervical lymphadenopathy. The person generally suffers from general malaise, which is disproportionate to the symptoms experienced. A macular rash can also occur in a small proportion of patients.

Trauma-related sore throat
Occasionally, patients develop a sore throat from direct irritation of the pharynx. This can be due to substances such as cigarette smoke, a lodged foreign body or from acid reflux.

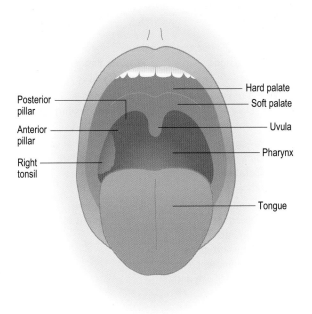

Fig. 2.3 Major structures of the mouth

Clinical features of viral sore throat

Many studies have now shown that it is exceedingly difficult to differentiate viral and bacterial infection on patient history and clinical findings. Patients will present with a sore throat as an isolated symptom or as part of a cluster of symptoms that include rhinorrhoea, cough, malaise, fever, headache and hoarseness (laryngitis). Symptoms are relatively short-lived, with 40% of people being symptom free after 3 days and 85% of people symptom free after 1 week.

Conditions to eliminate

Likely cause

Streptococcal sore throat
Patients who present with pharyngeal or tonsillar exudates, swollen anterior cervical glands, history of, or

Table 2.9						
Features of viral and bacterial sore throat						
	Age	Tonsillar/pharyngeal exudate	Duration	Cervical glands	Cough present	Other symptoms
Viral infection	Any age	Possible, but generally limited	3–7 days	Normal	Common	Low-grade fever, headache
Bacterial infection	School children	Often present and can be substantial	3–7 days	Swollen	Rare	High-grade fever, possible rash

Table 2.10
Examples of medication known to cause agranulocytosis

Captopril
Carbimazole
Cytotoxics
Neuroleptics, e.g., clozapine
Penicillamine
Sulfasalazine
Sulphur-containing antibiotics

Medicine-induced sore throat

A rare complication associated with certain medication is agranulocytosis, which can manifest as a sore throat. The patient will also probably present with signs of infection, including fever and chills. Medicines known to cause this adverse event are listed in Table 2.10.

Laryngeal and tonsillar carcinoma

Both these cancers have a strong link with smoking and excessive alcohol intake, and are more common in men than in women. Sore throat and dysphagia are the common presenting symptoms. In addition, patients with tonsillar cancer often develop referred ear pain. Any person, regardless of age, who presents with dysphagia should be referred.

Fig. 2.4 will help in the differentiation of serious and non-serious conditions in which sore throat is a major presenting complaint.

Evidence base for over-the-counter medication

The majority of sore throats are viral in origin and self-limiting. Medication therefore aims to relieve symptoms and discomfort while the infection runs its course. Lozenge and spray formulations incorporating antibacterial and anaesthetics provide the mainstay of treatment for which there is no shortage on the market. In addition, systemic analgesics and antipyretics will help reduce the pain and fever associated with sore throat.

Local anaesthetics

Lidocaine and benzocaine are included in a number of marketed products. Very few published clinical trials involving products marketed for sore throat have been conducted, yet local anaesthetics have proven efficacy. It therefore appears manufacturers are using trial data on local anaesthetic efficacy for conditions other than sore throats to substantiate their effect.

❗ TRIGGER POINTS indicative of referral: Sore Throat

Symptoms/signs	Possible danger/reason for referral
Duration of more than 2 weeks	Suggests non-acute cause and requires further investigation
Marked tonsillar exudate, accompanied with a high temperature and swollen glands	Possible bacterial cause and may require antibiotics
Adverse drug reaction People taking medicines that can interfere with the immune response (e.g., immunosuppressants, disease-modifying anti-rheumatics)	Requires doctor involvement to monitor
Dysphagia Associated skin rash	Suggests sinister pathology

Antibacterial and antifungal agents

Antibacterial agents include chlorhexidine, tyrothricin, dequalinium chloride and benzalkonium chloride. In vitro testing has shown that many of the proprietary products do have antibacterial activity, and some inhibit *Candida albicans* growth. In vivo tests have also shown antibacterial effects.

The use of antibacterial and antifungal agents should not be routinely recommended since the vast majority of sore throats are caused by viral infections for which they have no action against. As adverse effects are rare and stimulation of saliva from sucking the lozenge may confer symptomatic relief, the use of such products may be justified.

Anti-inflammatories

Benzydamine is available as a spray or mouthwash and one small trial involving benzydamine as a gargle resulted in significantly greater relief of pain compared with placebo (Thomas et al., 2000).

Analgesia

There is good evidence to show that simple systemic analgesia, for example, paracetamol, aspirin and ibuprofen, is effective in reducing the pain associated with sore throat. Thomas et al. (2000) undertook a review of treatments other than antibiotics for sore throats. They identified 22 trials, 13 of which involved NSAIDs (primarily ibuprofen) or paracetamol, and found both NSAIDs and paracetamol

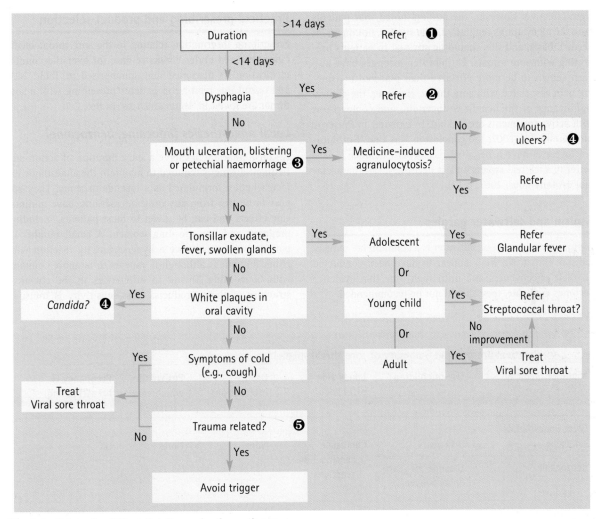

Fig. 2.4   Primer for differential diagnosis of sore throat

❶ Duration longer than 2 weeks
The overwhelming majority of cases resolve spontaneously in this time; it is therefore prudent to refer these cases for further investigation.

❷ Dysphagia
True difficulty in swallowing (i.e., not just caused by pain but by a mechanical blockage) should be referred. Most patients with sore throat will find it less easy to swallow, but this has to be differentiated from actual difficulty in swallowing. Severe inflammation of the throat can cause restriction of the airways and thus hinder breathing. Additionally, rare causes of sore throat also have associated dysphagia symptoms, such as peritonsillar abscess, thyroiditis and oesophageal carcinoma.

❸ Signs of agranulocytosis
A severe reduction in the number of white blood cells can result in neutropenia, which is manifested as fever, sore throat, ulceration and small haemorrhages under the skin.

❹ Mouth ulceration and *Candida* (oral thrush) primers
See Chapter 7 and Figs 7.6 & 7.7 for further differentiation of these conditions.

❺ Trauma related
Simple acts of drinking fluids that are too hot can give rise to ulceration of the pharynx. It is worth asking whether any such factors could have triggered the sore throat.

were effective. However, the authors noted that patients took the medications regularly in the studies, not on an 'as needed' basis, and this should be stressed to patients presenting with sore throats. Flurbiprofen lozenges have also been shown to be more effective than placebo in reducing pain associated with sore throat. However, the clinical significance of the benefit is uncertain, and comparisons with active treatments are lacking. In a review in *Prescrire International* in 2007, the conclusion was that 'flurbiprofen lozenges have a negative risk-benefit balance ... it is better to suck real sweets and, if necessary, take paracetamol' (Anonymous, 2007, p 13).

Aspirin and saltwater gargles

Gargling with aspirin or saltwater is a common lay remedy for sore throat. No trials appear to have been conducted on their effectiveness and until such time that evidence becomes available, they should not be recommended.

Practical prescribing and product selection

Prescribing information relating to the sore throat medicines reviewed under 'Evidence base for over-the-counter medication' is discussed and summarised in Table 2.11, and useful tips relating to patients presenting with a sore throat are given in 'Hints and Tips' in Box 2.3.

Local anaesthetics (lidocaine, benzocaine)

All local anaesthetics have a short duration of action and frequent dosing is required to maintain the anaesthetic effect, whether formulated as a lozenge or spray. They appear to be free from any drug interactions, have minimal side effects and can be given to most patients, including pregnant and breastfeeding women. A small number of patients may experience a hypersensitivity reaction with either ingredient although it appears to be more common with benzocaine. Owing to differences in the chemical structure of these products, cross-sensitivity is unusual,

Table 2.11
Practical prescribing: Summary of sore throat medicines

Name of medicine	Use in children	Likely side effects	Drug interactions of note	Patients in which care exercised	Pregnancy & breastfeeding
Local anaesthetics					
Lidocaine	>12 years	Can cause sensitisation reactions	None	None	OK
Benzocaine	Lozenge >3 years Spray >6 years				
Anti-inflammatories					
Benzydamine	Rinse >12 years Spray >6 years	Oral rinse may cause stinging	None	None	OK, but in pregnancy limit use after 30 weeks
Flurbiprofen	>12 years	None reported	None	Avoid in patients with peptic ulcers	Avoid if possible

HINTS AND TIPS BOX 2.3: SORE THROAT

Stimulation of saliva production	Sucking a lozenge or pastille promotes saliva production, which will lubricate the throat and thus exert a soothing action.
Gargles or lozenges?	Gargles have very short contact time with inflamed mucosa and therefore any effect will be short lived. A lozenge or a pastille is preferable, as contact time will be longer.

and therefore if a patient experiences side effects with one, then the other can be tried. Most products do contain a sugar base, but the amount of sugar is too small to substantially affect blood glucose control and therefore can be recommended to diabetic patients.

Lidocaine spray (Boots Anaesthetic Sore Throat Relief – both 2%, and Covonia Throat Spray – 0.05%)

All are licensed only for adults and children over the age of 12. The dosing for the 2% products are the same: three sprays every 3 hours when needed up to a maximum of six times per day. For Covonia the dose is 3 to 5 sprays between 6 and 10 times a day.

Benzocaine

Unlike lidocaine, benzocaine can be given to children both in lozenge and spray formulations. Lozenges are available and can be given from age 3 and above (Tyrozets 1 lozenge [5 mg] every 3 hours when needed; maximum of 6 in 24 hours); adults can take up to 8 in 24 hours every 2 to 3 hours when needed (e.g., Tyrozets, Boots anaesthetic and antibiotic throat lozenges, Merocaine). Additionally, children over the age of 6 can also use a spray formulation (Ultra Chloraseptic [0.71%] or AAA Spray [1.5%]), for which the dose is one spray every 2 to 3 hours, up to a maximum of 8 doses per day. The adult dose is up to 3 sprays (Ultra Chloraseptic) and 2 sprays (AAA Spray) repeated every 2 to 3 hours.

Anti-inflammatories (benzydamine and flurbiprofen)

Benzydamine (Difflam Sore Throat Rinse, Difflam Spray)

The rinse should be used by adults and children over the age of 12 every 1½ to 3 hours when required. It has no drug interactions of note, can be used by all patient groups and only occasionally does the rinse cause stinging, in which case the rinse can be diluted with water. The manufacturers advise that the product should be stored in the box away from direct sunlight even though the stability of the product is not known to be affected by sunlight.

The dosing for the spray is the same as the rinse (every 1½–3 hours when required), but, unlike the rinse, it can be used in children. For those under the age of 6, the dose is based on mg/kg dosing, for those aged 6 to 12, they should use 4 puffs and adults 4 to 8 puffs.

Flurbiprofen (Strefen)

Strefen lozenges (8.75 mg flurbiprofen) can only be given to adults and children over the age of 12 years. The dose is one lozenge to be sucked every 3 to 6 hours with a maximum of 5 lozenges in 24 hours. They are contraindicated in patients with peptic ulceration and those patients allergic to flurbiprofen, and must be avoided in the last trimester of pregnant patients but are suitable for breastfeeding women.

References
Anonymous. Flurbiprofen: new indication. Lozenges: NSAIDs are not to be taken like sweets! Prescrire Int 2007;16:13.
Thomas M, Del Mar C, Glasziou P. How effective are treatments other than antibiotics for acute sore throat? Br J Gen Pract 2000;50:817–20.

Further reading
Kennedy J. Self care of acute sore throat. SelfCare 2010;2(1):21–4.
Middleton DB. Pharyngitis. Prim Care 1996;23:719–39.
Spurling GKP, Del Mar CB, Dooley L, et al. Delayed antibiotics for respiratory infections. Cochrane Database of Systematic Reviews 2013, Issue 4. Art. No.: CD004417. http://dx.doi.org/10.1002/14651858.CD004417.pub4.
Van Driel ML, De Sutter AIM, Keber N, et al. Different antibiotic treatments for group A streptococcal pharyngitis. Cochrane Database of Systematic Reviews 2010, Issue 10. Art.No.:CD004406. http://dx.doi.org/10.1002/14651858.CD004406.pub2.
Watson N, Nimmo WS, Christian J, et al. Relief of sore throat with the anti-inflammatory throat lozenge flurbiprofen 8.75 mg: a randomised, double-blind, placebo-controlled study of efficacy and safety. Int J Clin Pract 2000;54:490–6.

Website
Sinus Care Center: http://www.sinuscarecenter.com/

Rhinitis

Background

Rhinitis is simply inflammation of the nasal lining. It is characterised by rhinorrhoea, nasal congestion, sneezing and itching. The majority of cases that present in a community pharmacy will be viral infection, colds or allergic rhinitis (AR). Currently there are different classifications of AR. ARIA (Allergic Rhinitis and its Impact on Asthma) guidelines classify AR into intermittent and persistent categories, with both subdivided into mild or moderate–severe disease (Bousquet, 2008). In 2007 the British Society for Allergy and Clinical Immunology published guidelines that differed from ARIA where classification of AR was based on seasonal or perennial types of rhinitis. This text adopts the ARIA criteria. The ARIA classification is based on the timing of the symptoms and is divided into intermittent (occurring on less than 4 days per week and less than 4 weeks at a time) or persistent (occurring on more than 4 days per week and more than 4 weeks at a time). Rhinitis has a significant impact on quality of life, impairing performance at work and school.

Prevalence and epidemiology

AR is a global health problem and has dramatically increased over the last 20 years, with studies suggesting the prevalence has at least doubled in that time. The UK has one of the highest levels of AR in the world, with estimates ranging from 10% to 25% of adults and as many as 40% of children affected. These figures might, however, represent an underestimate, as many people do not consult their doctor and choose to self-medicate. Seasonal intermittent allergic rhinitis (hay fever) commonly affects school-aged children, with 10% to 30% of the adolescent population suffering from the condition. The mean age of onset is 10 years and the incidence peaks between the ages of 13 and 19 years. It is believed that improved living standards and reduced risk of childhood infections might increase susceptibility to hay fever. Allergic rhinitis is a recognised risk factor for the development of asthma.

Aetiology

AR is a mucosal reaction in response to allergen exposure. Initially, the patient must come into contact with an allergen; for intermittent AR this is usually pollen or fungal spores. The allergen lodges within the mucous blanket lining the nasal membranes, and activates immunoglobulin E (IgE) antibodies (formed from previous allergen exposure) on the surface of mast cells. Potent chemical mediators are released, primarily histamine, but also leukotrienes, kinins and prostaglandins, which exert their action via neural and vascular mechanisms. This immediate response to an allergen is known as the early-phase allergic reaction and gives rise to nasal itch, rhinorrhoea, sneezing and nasal congestion. A late-phase reaction then occurs 4 to 12 hours after allergen exposure with nasal congestion as the main symptom.

Also of importance is the phenomenon of nasal priming. Patients, after a period of continuous allergen exposure, can find that they experience the same level of severity in symptoms with lower levels of allergen exposure. Similarly, symptoms will be worse than previously experienced when levels of the allergen are the same. This may explain why patients complain of worsening hay fever symptoms the longer the season goes on. Table 2.12 highlights the main allergens responsible for AR.

Table 2.12 Allergens responsible for rhinitis		
	When	**Causative allergen**
Intermittent allergic rhinitis	February to April	Tree pollens (hazel and alder associated with early symptoms and silver birch in March/April)
	May to August (peak in June and July)	Grass pollen
	September to October	Fungal spores
Persistent allergic rhinitis (e.g., perennial rhinitis)	Year round	House dust mite; animal dander, especially cats

Arriving at a differential diagnosis

Rhinitis is not difficult to diagnose but establishing the underlying cause and categorisation of it requires more skill. Within the community pharmacy setting the majority of patients who present with rhinitis will be suffering from a cold or intermittent AR. Diagnosis is largely dependent on the patient having a family history of atopy, clinical symptoms and when these worsen. Asking symptom-specific questions will help the pharmacist establish a differential diagnosis (Table 2.13), and Table 2.14 highlights those conditions that can be encountered by community pharmacists and their relative incidence.

Clinical features of intermittent AR

The patient will experience a combination or all four of the classical rhinitis symptoms of nasal itch, sneeze (especially paroxysmal), watery rhinorrhoea and nasal congestion. In addition the patient might also suffer from ocular irritation, giving rise to allergic conjunctivitis. The symptoms will occur intermittently (i.e., at times of pollen exposure) and tend to be worse in the morning and evening, as pollen levels peak at this time, as they do when the weather is hot and humid.

Table 2.13
Specific questions to ask the patient: Rhinitis

Question	Relevance
Seasonal variation	Symptoms in the summer months suggest intermittent allergic rhinitis whereas year-round symptoms suggest perennial rhinitis
History of asthma, eczema or intermittent allergic rhinitis in the family	If a first-degree relative suffers from atopy, then intermittent allergic rhinitis is much more likely
Triggers	When pollen counts are high, symptoms of intermittent allergic rhinitis worsen Infective rhinitis and vasomotor rhinitis will be unaffected by pollen count Patients with persistent rhinitis might suffer from worsening symptoms when pollen counts are high, but symptoms should still persist when indoors compared with intermittent rhinitis sufferers who usually see improvement of symptoms when away from pollen

Table 2.14
Causes of allergic rhinitis and their relative incidence in community pharmacy

Incidence	Cause
Most likely	Intermittent allergic rhinitis
Likely	Persistent allergic rhinitis, infective rhinitis
Unlikely	Non-allergic rhinitis, pregnancy, medicines, nasal foreign bodies or blockage

Conditions to eliminate

Likely causes

Persistent AR

Persistent AR is much less common than intermittent AR. As its name suggests, the problem tends to be persistent and does not exhibit seasonality. However, it must be remembered that patients suffering from persistent AR might also be allergic to pollen and experience worsening symptoms in the summer months. Besides not having a seasonal cause, there are a number of other clues to look out for that aid differentiation. Nasal congestion is much more common, which often leads to hyposmia (poor sense of smell) and ocular symptoms are uncommon. Additionally, persistent AR sufferers also tend to sneeze less frequently and experience more episodes of chronic sinusitis. The most common allergen causing persistent AR is the house dust mite but animal dander (particularly from cats, dogs and horses) are common causes of symptoms, and so it is prudent to ask about pets that are kept.

Infective rhinitis

This is normally viral in origin and associated with the common cold. Nasal discharge tends to be more mucopurulent than AR and nasal itching is uncommon. Sneezing tends not to occur in paroxysms and the condition resolves more quickly, whereas AR lasts for as long as the person is exposed to the allergen. Other symptoms, such as cough and sore throat, are much more prominent in infective rhinitis than AR.

Unlikely causes

Non-allergic rhinitis (vasomotor rhinitis or intrinsic rhinitis)

Non-allergic rhinitis is thought to be due to either an overactive parasympathetic nervous system response, or hypoactive sympathetic nervous system response to irritants such as dry air, pollutants, or strong odours. The symptoms can be similar to AR yet an allergy test will be negative. Itching and sneezing are less common and patients might experience worsening nasal symptoms in response to climatic factors, such as a sudden change in temperature.

Rhinitis of pregnancy

It is thought that this occurs because of hormonal changes; however, evidence is lacking (Wallace et al., 2008). It usually starts after the second month of the pregnancy, and resolves spontaneously after childbirth. Nasal congestion is the prominent feature.

Rhinitis medicamentosa and medicine-induced rhinitis

Rhinitis medicamentosa is due to prolonged use of topical decongestants (more than 5–7 days), which causes rebound vasodilatation of the nasal arterioles, leading to further nasal congestion. Although the exact pathophysiology is unclear, it is thought to be due to desensitisation of the alpha-adrenoceptors as a result of constant stimulation. A number of oral medications are implicated in causing rhinitis through other mechanisms, including angiotensin-converting enzyme inhibitors, reserpine, alpha-adrenoceptor antagonists (e.g., terazosin), phosphodiesterase-5 inhibitors (e.g., sildenafil), chlorpromazine, oral contraceptives, aspirin, and other NSAIDs.

Nasal blockage

In the absence of rhinorrhoea, nasal itch and sneezing, it is possible that the problem is mechanical or anatomical. If the blockage is continuous and unilateral, this may relate to a deviated nasal septum in adults. This may develop or be a result of trauma. Referral is needed and surgery is recommended. If the obstruction is bilateral this may relate to nasal polyps in adults. Nasal obstruction is progressive and is often accompanied by hyposmia. Referral is needed for corticosteroids or surgery.

Nasal foreign body

A trapped foreign body in a nostril commonly occurs in young children, often without the parents' knowledge. Within a matter of days of the foreign body being lodged the patient experiences an offensive nasal discharge. Any unilateral discharge, particularly in a child, should be referred for nasal examination, as it is highly likely that a foreign body is responsible.

Fig. 2.5 will aid in differentiating the different types of rhinitis.

⚠ TRIGGER POINTS indicative of referral: Rhinitis

Symptoms/signs	Possible danger/reason for referral
Failed medication Medicine-induced rhinitis	Requires involvement of doctor for further medicine treatment
Nasal obstruction that fails to clear	Suggests polyp
Unilateral discharge, especially in children	Possible trapped foreign body

---

Evidence base for over-the-counter medication

Before medication is started, it is clearly important to try and identify the causative allergen. If this can be achieved, then measures to limit the exposure to the allergen will be beneficial in reducing the symptoms experienced by the patient. This is more easily accomplished in persistent allergic rhinitis than in seasonal intermittent rhinitis.

Allergen avoidance

Avoidance of pollen is almost impossible but if the patient follows a few simple rules then exposure to pollen can be reduced. Patients may choose to stay indoors when pollen counts are high. Windows should be closed (both when in the house and when travelling in cars) and 'wrap around' sunglasses worn. Air conditioning in cars fitted with a pollen filter is also beneficial. Patients should avoid walking in areas with the potential for high pollen exposure (grassy fields, parks and gardens) as well as areas such as city centres, as many intermittent allergy sufferers will have increased sensitivity to other irritants such as car exhaust fumes and cigarette smoke.

The two main causative agents of persistent AR – house dust mite and animal dander – can be more easily avoided. The offending pet can be excluded from certain parts of the house, such as living areas and bedrooms. Acaricidal sprays and strict bedroom cleaning regimes have shown to be of some benefit in reducing rhinitis symptoms (Sheikh et al., 2010). Cleaning regimes should include regular washing of bedding and mattress covers with hot water (to try and kill the mites); replacing carpets with hard wood floors; minimising soft furnishings and avoiding drying clothes on radiators.

Medication

Pharmacists now possess a wide range of therapeutic options to treat AR, allowing the vast majority of sufferers to be appropriately managed in the pharmacy. Management of AR falls broadly into two categories: systemic and topical.

Systemic therapy: Antihistamines

Both sedating and non-sedating antihistamines are clinically effective in reducing the symptoms associated with AR (Sheikh et al., 2009). However, given the sedative effects of first-generation antihistamines, they should not be routinely recommended compared with second-generation, non-sedating antihistamines.

Of the second-generation antihistamines, community pharmacists in the UK currently have a choice between acrivastine, cetirizine or loratadine. All are equally effective and are considered to be non-sedating, although they are not truly non-sedating and do cause different levels of sedation. Loratadine has been shown to have the lowest affinity for histamine receptors in the brain, and a paper published by Mann et al. in 2000 reviewing reported sedation with second-generation antihistamines showed loratadine to be least sedating of the non-sedating antihistamines. In comparison, cetirizine was 3.5 times more

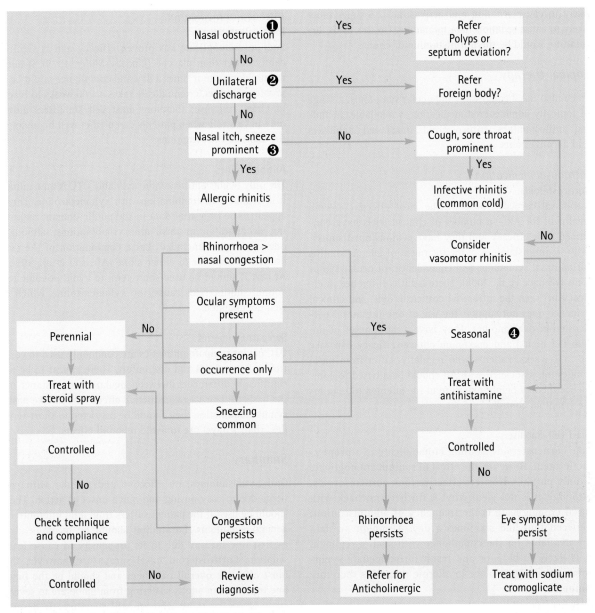

Fig. 2.5 Primer for differential diagnosis of rhinitis

❶ Nasal obstruction
Nasal obstruction differs from nasal congestion in that obstruction refers to a physical blockage of the nasal passage and is normally due to an anatomic fault, whereas congestion refers to the nasal passages being temporarily blocked by nasal secretions that can easily be cleared by nose blowing. Obstruction therefore warrants referral.

❷ Unilateral discharge
Any one-sided nasal discharge must be viewed with suspicion. Accidental lodging of a foreign body by young children is the usual cause.

❸ Nasal itch and sneeze prominent
Nasal itching and sneezing are classically associated with hay fever, although these symptoms are also associated with perennial rhinitis, but to a lesser extent. Sneezing is often said to occur in multiple bouts, which is unlike infective rhinitis. Coughing can occur but is infrequent.

❹ Treatment of vasomotor rhinitis
Because symptoms are similar to hay fever, then it is reasonable to assume that first-line therapy for vasomotor rhinitis would be a systemic antihistamine.

likely to cause sedation and acrivastine, 2.5 times more likely to cause sedation than loratadine. On this basis, loratadine would be the antihistamine of choice.

Topical therapy

To combat nasal congestion and ocular symptoms, a range of topically administered medication is available, including antihistamines, corticosteroids, mast cell stabilisers and decongestants.

Intranasal medication
Corticosteroids

Intranasal corticosteroids are the most effective overall treatment for AR – a number of clinical trials have confirmed their efficacy and they have demonstrated superiority to antihistamines in the treatment of allergic rhinitis for all nasal symptoms, and equivalence for ocular symptoms (Wallace et al., 2008). There is little difference in efficacy between the intranasal corticosteroids, and clinical evidence does not support the use of one intranasal corticosteroid over another. They have a slow onset of action (12 hours) and maximum clinical efficacy can take up to 2 weeks. Patients who regularly suffer from nasal congestion associated with AR should be advised to commence therapy before exposure to the allergen to maximise symptom control.

Mast cell stabilisers

Like corticosteroids, sodium cromoglicate is a prophylactic agent. However, the effect of sodium cromoglicate is only partial – it is less effective than corticosteroids, although it is not clear why. A further drawback with nasal cromoglicate is the frequency of administration; between four and six times a day. Although no data are available for the compliance with such a regimen, it is likely to be poor and result in inadequate symptom control. Their place in allergic rhinitis is therefore limited.

Decongestants

Topical decongestants are effective in the treatment of nasal congestion but are of limited value in treating AR, as prolonged use is associated with rebound congestion; however, they may have a place to treat intermittent symptoms. Their place in therapy is probably best reserved for when nasal congestion needs to be treated quickly and can provide symptom relief while corticosteroid therapy is initiated and has time to begin to exert its action.

Intraocular medication
Mast cell stabilisers

Sodium cromoglicate has proven efficacy and is significantly better than placebo (Lindsay-Miller, 1979). It does require dosing four times a day and compliance might be a problem. Further, cromoglicate takes 4 to 6 weeks to reach maximal response; therefore mast cell stabilisers alone only have a role when patients can predict well in advance the onset of the symptoms.

Antihistamines

The only ocular antihistamine available OTC is antazoline. It is available in combination with xylometazoline. There appear to be little trial data in the public domain regarding decongestant/antihistamine combinations, although one small trial concluded that a combination of the two drugs was superior to either alone (Abelson et al., 1990). At best it should be used short-term to avoid possible rebound conjunctivitis caused by xylometazoline, which is well documented.

Sympathomimetics

OTC ocular sympathomimetics are commonly used to control ocular redness and discomfort. There appear to be no significant differences between ocular decongestants on the basis of their vasoconstrictive effectiveness. Like nasal sympathomimetics, they should be restricted to short-term (less than 7 days) use to avoid rebound effects.

Summary

Oral antihistamines are effective and popular with patients due to easy dosing and quick onset of action. They should be used if the patient suffers from mild intermittent general symptoms. **Loratadine** should be recommended as first-line therapy due to its propensity to cause least sedation. **Corticosteroid nasal sprays** are, however, the **most effective overall** treatment and should be the first-line treatment in adults suffering from moderate to severe cases of AR, or those who are still symptomatic despite regular use of antihistamines.

Practical prescribing and product selection

Prescribing information relating to the rhinitis medicines reviewed in the section 'Evidence base for over-the-counter medication' is presented in Table 2.15 and their relative effect on symptom control is summarised in Table 2.16. Useful tips relating to patients presenting with rhinitis are given in 'Hints and Tips' in Box 2.4.

Table 2.15
Practical prescribing: Summary of rhinitis medicines

Name of medicine	Use in children	Likely side effects	Drug interactions of note	Patients in which care exercised	Pregnancy & breastfeeding
Systemic antihistamines					
Acrivastine	>12 years	Sedation, but rare and least likely with loratadine	None	None	Manufacturers advise avoidance, but safety data have shown them to be safe
Cetirizine	>2 years				
Loratadine	>2 years				
Chlorphenamine	>1 year	Dry mouth, sedation and constipation	Increased sedation with alcohol, opioid analgesics, anxiolytics, hypnotics and antidepressants	Glaucoma, prostate enlargement	Standard references state OK, although some manufacturers advise avoidance
Ocular antihistamines					
Antazoline*	>12 years	Local irritation, bitter taste	Avoid concomitant use with MAOIs and moclobemide due to risk of hypertensive crisis	Avoid in glaucoma	Safety not established, but probably OK
Nasal corticosteroids					
Beclometasone	>18 years	Nasal irritation, bitter taste, headache (fluticasone) nosebleeds	None	Avoid in glaucoma	Manufacturers advise avoidance, but safety data have shown them to be safe
Fluticasone					
Triamcinolone		Headache, nosebleeds, dyspepsia, bronchitis, flu-like symptoms and cough			
Ocular and nasal mast cell stabilisers					
Lodoxamide (ocular)	>4 years	Headache, dizziness, nausea	None	None	A lack of data means the manufacturer advises avoidance

(Continued)

Table 2.15
Practical prescribing: Summary of rhinitis medicines (Continued)

Name of medicine	Use in children	Likely side effects	Drug interactions of note	Patients in which care exercised	Pregnancy & breastfeeding
Sodium cromoglicate ocular	>6 years	Local irritation, blurred vision	None	None	OK
Sodium cromoglicate nasal	>5 years	Nasal irritation. Rare – wheezing and shortness of breath			OK
Ocular sympathomimetics					
Naphazoline	>12 years	Local irritation	Avoid concomitant use with MAOIs and moclobemide due to risk of hypertensive crisis	None	Not adequately studied but not yet shown to be a risk – probably OK

*Only available in combination with naphazoline.

Table 2.16
Efficacy and properties of drug treatments used in allergic rhinitis

Characteristic	Oral antihistamine	Nasal steroid	Nasal decongestant	Nasal cromone
Rhinorrhea	++	+++	-	+
Sneezing	++	+++	-	+
Itching	++	+++	-	+
Blockage	+	+++	++++	+
Eye symptoms	++	++	-	-
Onset of action	1 hr	12 hrs	5–15 min	Variable
Duration	12–24 hrs	12–48 hrs	3–6 hrs	2–6 hrs

-, no effect; +, marginal effect; ++++, substantial effect (under natural exposure conditions).
(Reproduced with permission from Farooque S. Allergic rhinitis: Guide to diagnosis, allergen avoidance and treatment. The Prescriber 2012;5th May:380-39.

HINTS AND TIPS BOX 2.4: RHINITIS

Breakthrough symptoms with one-a-day antihistamines	Patients who suffer breakthrough symptoms using a once daily preparation (loratadine, cetirizine) may benefit from changing to acrivastine, as three-times-a-day dosing may confer better symptom control.
Corticosteroid nasal sprays	These are suspensions and the bottle should be shaken before use. Regular usage is essential for full therapeutic benefit. It should also be explained that maximum relief might not be obtained for several days. However, most begin to act in 3–7 hours.

Systemic antihistamines

Systemic antihistamines selectively inhibit histamine H_1 receptors and suppress many of the vascular effects of histamine. They have rapid onset of action (approximately 30 minutes to 1 hour) and relieve ocular symptoms, rhinorrhoea and nasal irritation, but have less effect on nasal congestion. For maximum effect they are best taken on a regular basis but will have an effect if taken when required. Patient response is variable between the differing antihistamines and more than one type may have to be tried to provide symptom control. They possess very few side effects and can be given safely with other prescribed medication. They can also be prescribed to all patient groups, although manufacturers advise against prescribing to the elderly. First-generation sedating antihistamines are the preferred antihistamines in pregnancy, as the risk of foetal toxicity appears low, with chlorphenamine being the medicine of choice. Of the non-sedating antihistamines, loratadine is the most widely studied, and available data does not indicate an increased risk of teratogenicity, yet manufacturers advise avoidance (presumably on the basis of being outside their product licences). For breastfeeding mothers, non-sedating antihistamines should be avoided, as infant drowsiness has been associated with their use. Expert opinion states cetirizine and loratadine are antihistamines of choice, despite manufacturers advising that they should not be used in this patient group.

Non-sedating antihistamines

Acrivastine (Benadryl Allergy Relief)
Acrivastine is recommended for adults and children over 12 years of age. The dose is one capsule (8 mg) as necessary, up to three times a day. Acrivastine can also be purchased as a combination product (Benadryl Plus), which contains a sympathomimetic (pseudoephedrine). However, if nasal congestion is a problem, corticosteroids should be considered in preference to a decongestant.

Cetirizine (e.g., BecoAllergy, Benadryl One-a-Day and Benadryl Allergy Oral Solution and Liquid Capsules, Piriteze range, Pollenshield, Zirtek range)
Cetirizine is available as either tablets or solution. The dose for adults and children 6 years and over is 10 mg daily and can be given as either 5 mg (5 mL or half a tablet) twice daily or 10 mg (10 mL or one tablet) daily. For children between 2 and 5 years of age, the dose is 2.5 mL (2.5 mg) twice daily. Not all manufacturers have a licence for those children under 6 years of age, so it is important to refer to specific manufacturer literature before making recommendations.

Loratadine (e.g., Clarityn Allergy, Clarityn Rapide)
Loratadine is available as either a tablet or syrup. The dose for individuals over 12 years of age is 10 mg daily. The syrup (1 mg/mL) can be given to children 2 to 12 years old (providing they are over 30 kg) at a dose of 5 mg (5 mL).

Sedating antihistamines

Chlorphenamine (e.g., Piriton Allergy Tablets and Syrup)
This can be given from 1 year upwards (2.5 mL [1 mg] twice daily). The dose for children 2 to 6 years of age is 2.5 mL (1 mg) every 4 to 6 hours, and those children 6 to 12 years of age is 2 mg (5 mL [2 mg] or half a tablet) every 4 to 6 hours. The adult dose is 4 mg every 4 to 6 hours.

Nasal corticosteroids (beclometasone, fluticasone, triamcinolone)

They can be used in most patient groups, although avoidance is recommended in glaucoma. (Glaucoma and/or cataracts have been reported in patients receiving nasal corticosteroids.) In addition, manufacturers recommend that they are not used during pregnancy and breastfeeding due to insufficient evidence to establish safety. However, exposure data do suggest that they are safe. Beclometasone and fluticasone can cause unpleasant taste and smell, as well as nasal and throat irritation. Beclometasone is also reported to cause rashes and urticaria. Fluticasone and triamcinolone also cause headaches and nosebleeds. Dyspepsia, bronchitis, flu-like symptoms and cough have also been reported with triamcinolone. All side effects associated with these three medicines are, however, rare. All products are licensed only for people over the age of 18.

Beclometasone (Beconase Hayfever)

The recommended dose is two sprays into each nostril twice daily (400 µg/day). Once symptoms have improved, it might be possible to decrease the dose to 1 spray twice daily. However, should symptoms recur, patients should revert to the standard dosage.

Fluticasone (Pirinase Hayfever Nasal Spray)

The dose is two sprays into each nostril once daily (200 µg/day), although if symptoms are not controlled, the dose can be increased to twice daily. Like beclometasone, once symptoms are controlled, the patient should use the lowest effective dose.

Triamcinolone (Nasacort Allergy Nasal Spray)

The standard adult dose is two sprays into each nostril (220 µg/day) once daily, which can be reduced to just 1 spray per nostril daily.

Mast cell stabilisers (sodium cromoglicate, lodoxamide)

Sodium cromoglicate and lodoxamide are poorly absorbed, and the amount reaching the systemic circulation is very low. They have no drug interactions and can be given to all patient groups. Clinical experience has shown cromoglicate to be safe in pregnancy, and expert opinion considers sodium cromoglicate to be safe in breastfeeding. Both are prophylactic agents and need to be started at least a week before required; they must be given continuously while exposed to the allergen.

Ocular cromoglicate (e.g., Opticrom Allergy, Optrex Allergy, Murine hayfever relief)

One or two drops should be administered in each eye four times a day. Instillation of the drops can cause a transient blurring of vision.

Lodoxamide (Alomide Allergy)

For adults and children aged 4 years, 1 or 2 drops should be administered in each eye four times a day. Headache, dizziness and nausea have been reported but are uncommon.

Nasal cromoglicate (Rynacrom 4% Nasal Spray)

The dose for adults and children is one spray into each nostril two to four times daily. Nasal irritation is possible, especially during the first few days of use.

Sympathomimetics

For general information about sympathomimetics and product information on nasally administered products, see page 17.

Ocular sympathomimetics

Ocular products either contain a combination of sympathomimetic and antihistamine (antazoline/xylometazoline, Otrivine Antistin) or sympathomimetic alone (e.g., Naphazoline 0.01%). They are useful in reducing redness in the eye but will not treat the underlying pathology that is causing the eye to be red. They should be limited to short-term use to avoid rebound effects. Like all sympathomimetics, they can interact with monoamine oxidase inhibitors (MAOIs) and should not be used by patients receiving such treatment or within 14 days of ceasing therapy.

Otrivine Antistin

Used in adults and children over 12 years, the dose is 1 or 2 drops two or three times a day. Patients with glaucoma should avoid this product due to the potential of the antihistamine component to increase intraocular pressure. Local transient irritation and a bitter taste after application have been reported.

Naphazoline (e.g., Murine Irritation and Redness Relief Eye Drops, Optrex Bloodshot Eyes Eye Drops & Optrex Brightening Eye Drops)

The use of products containing naphazoline is restricted to adults and children over the age of 12 years old. One to 2 drops should be administered into the eye three or four times a day.

Complementary therapies

Butterbur (Petasites hybridus) is promoted as having anti-allergic properties. Two clinical trials have reported favourable outcomes of butterbur in controlling symptoms (Lee et al., 2004; Schapowal, 2002). Both trials found butterbur to be as effective as its comparator drug (cetirizine and fexofenadine, respectively). However, the comparison of butterbur to cetirizine used quality-of-life measures as the main outcome, and the study with fexofenadine was short (1 week) and involved only 16 participants. Another trial found butterbur to be no better than placebo in terms of peak nasal inspiratory flow or nasal symptom scores (Gray et al., 2004). A systematic review of complementary and alternative medicines for rhinitis concluded that the current available evidence does not support the use of complementary (alternative) medicines to treat rhinitis (Passalacqua et al., 2006), and a more recent review also concluded that further data is required (Garbo et al., 2013). Until further larger studies are conducted to assess butterbur's effect, it should not be routinely recommended.

2

References

Abelson M, Paradis A, George M et al. Effects of Vasocon-A in the allergen challenge model of acute allergic conjunctivitis. Arch Ophyhal 1990;108:520-524.

Bousquet J, Khaltaev N, Cruz AA, et al. Allergic Rhinitis and its Impact on Asthma (ARIA) 2008 update (in collaboration with the World Health Organization, GA2LEN and AllerGen). Allergy 2008;63(Suppl 86):S8–160.

Garbo G, Tessema B, Brown, SM. Complementary and Integrative Treatments: Allergy. Otolaryngol Clin North Am 2013;46(3):295–307.

Gray RD, Haggart K, Lee DK, et al. Effects of butterbur treatment in intermittent allergic rhinitis: a placebo-controlled evaluation. Ann Allergy Asthma Immunol 2004; 93(1):56–60.

Lee D, Gray R, Robb F, et al. A placebo-controlled evaluation of butterbur and fexofenadine on objective and subjective outcomes in perennial allergic rhinitis. Clin Exp Allergy 2004;34(4):646–9.

Lee TA, Pickard AS. Meta-analysis of azelastine nasal spray for the treatment of allergic rhinitis. Pharmacotherapy 2007;27(6):852–9.

Lindsay-Miller ACM. Group comparative trial of 2% sodium cromoglycate (Opticrom) with placebo in treatment of seasonal allergic conjunctivitis. Clin Allergy 1979;9:271–5.

Mann RD, Pearce GL, Dunn N, et al. Sedation with 'non-sedating' antihistamines: four prescription-event monitoring studies in general practice. BMJ 2000;320:1184–6.

Passalacqua G, Bousquet PJ, Kai-Hakon C, et al. ARIA Update: 1-Systematic review of complimentary and alternative medicine for rhinitis and asthma. J Allergy Clin Immunol 2006;117:1054–62.

Schapowal A. Randomised controlled trial of butterbur and cetirizine for treating seasonal allergic rhinitis. BMJ 2002; 324:144.

Sheikh A, Hurwitz B, Nurmatov U, et al. House dust mite avoidance measures for perennial allergic rhinitis. Cochrane Database of Systematic Reviews 2010, Issue 7. Art. No.: CD001563. http://dx.doi.org/10.1002/14651858. CD001563.pub3.

Sheikh A, Panesar SS, Dhami S. Hay fever in adolescents and adults. BMJ Clin Evid 2009 [Online]. Available: http://clinicalevidence.com/x/systematic-review/0509/overview.html (Accessed 27 Feb 2015).

Wallace DV, Dykewicz MS, Bernstein DI, et al. The diagnosis and management of rhinitis: an updated practice parameter. J Allergy Clin Immunol 2008;122(2S):1–84.

Further reading

Asher MI, Montefort S, Björkstén B, et al. ISAAC Phase Three Study Group. Worldwide time trends in the prevalence of symptoms of asthma, allergic rhinoconjunctivitis, and eczema in childhood: ISAAC phases one and three repeat multicountry cross-sectional surveys. Lancet 2006;368:733–43.

Farooque S. Allergic rhinitis: Guide to diagnosis, allergen avoidance and treatment. The Prescriber 2012;5th May:380–39.

Hans de Groot, Brand PLP, Fokkens WF, et al. Allergic rhinoconjunctivitis in children. BMJ 2007;335:985–8, http://dx.doi.org/10.1136/bmj.39365.617905.BE.

Jones NS, Carney AS, Davis A. The prevalence of allergic rhinosinusitis: a review. J Laryngol Otol 1998;112:1019–30.

Marshall S. An update on hay fever treatments. Pharm J 2009;282:489–92.

Price D, Bond C, Bouchard J, et al. International Primary Care Respiratory Group (IPCRG) Guidelines: Management of Allergic Rhinitis. Prim Care Respir J 2006;15:58–70.

Saleh HA, Durham SR. Perennial rhinitis. BMJ 2007;335:502–7, http://dx.doi.org/10.1136/bmj.39304.678194.AE

Scadding GK, Durham SR, Mirakian R, et al. BSACI guidelines for the management of rhinosinusitis and nasal polyposis. Clin Exp Allergy 2008;38:260–75.

Skoner DP. Allergic rhinitis: definition, epidemiology, pathophysiology, detection, and diagnosis. J Allergy Clin Immunol 2001;108(Suppl 1):2–8.

Slater JW, Zechnich AD, Haxby DG. Second-generation antihistamines: a comparative review. Drugs 1999;57:31–47.

Websites

Action Against Allergy: www.actionagainstallergy.co.uk
Allergic Rhinitis and its Impact on Asthma (ARIA) resources for pharmacists: http://www.whiar.org/Pharmacy.php
Allergy UK: http://www.allergyuk.org/
The British Society for Allergy and Clinical Immunology: www.bsaci.org

Self-assessment questions

The following questions are intended to supplement the text. Two levels of questions are provided; multiple choice questions and case studies. The multiple choice questions are designed to test factual recall and the case studies allow knowledge to be applied to a practice setting.

Multiple choice questions

2.1 Which of the following conditions causing cough is most prevalent in the immigrant population?

   a. Chronic bronchitis
   b. Asthma
   c. Heart failure
   d. Pneumonia
   e. Tuberculosis

2.2 Which of the following conditions with cough as a major presenting symptom is least likely to produce a productive cough?

   a. Chronic bronchitis
   b. Asthma
   c. Bronchiectasis
   d. Pneumonia
   e. Tuberculosis

2.3 Mrs Jones visits your pharmacy complaining of having a dry cough for the last 7 days. After questioning you decide it is a simple viral infection and recommend simple linctus. If symptoms persisted, after how many further days would referral to the doctor be appropriate?

   a. 3 days
   b. 5 days
   c. 7 days
   d. 10 days
   e. 14 days

2.4 Mr Patel, who is 48 years old, presents with a non-productive cough. Based on epidemiology, what is the most likely cause of the cough?

   a. Acute bronchitis
   b. Upper airways cough syndrome (post-nasal drip)
   c. Asthma
   d. Viral infection
   e. Pneumothorax

2.5 Dyspnoea is a symptom most closely associated with which condition?

   a. Chronic bronchitis
   b. Asthma
   c. Heart failure
   d. Pneumonia
   e. Tuberculosis

2.6 You are recommending treatment for a young women to treat a common cold (primary symptom of nasal congestion). She tells you that she is breastfeeding. What would be the most suitable option?

   a. Vapour inhalation
   b. Steam inhalation
   c. Oral sympathomimetics
   d. Topical sympathomimetics
   e. Antihistamines

2.7 Simon, who is 32 years old, presents with a non-productive cough of 6 days' duration. He has no other symptoms and takes no medication. What would be the most appropriate course of action to take?

   a. Give pholcodine 5 mL qds
   b. Advise only on drinking more fluids
   c. Give dextromethorphan 10 mL qds
   d. Give guafenesin 10 mL qds
   e. Give glycerin lemon and honey 10 mL qds

2.8 Steven Blake, who is 37 years old, visits the pharmacy wanting treatment for his cough. After questioning him, you find out he has a non-productive cough for the last 7 to 10 days. He also states he has had some nasal congestion and has been suffering from occasional shortness of breath. Based on the signs and symptoms listed, what is the most likely diagnosis?

   a. Upper airways cough syndrome (UACS)
   b. Acute bronchitis

c. Chronic bronchitis
d. Pnuemonia
e. Pneumothorax

Questions 2.9 to 2.14 concern the following conditions:

A. Pneumonia
B. Heart Failure
C. TB
D. Chronic bronchitis
E. Laryngotracheobronchitis

Select, from A to E, which of the above conditions

2.9 Is characterised by night sweats

2.10 Has initially a non-productive painful cough that progresses to be productive

2.11 Is closely associated with a history of smoking

2.12 Is associated with a high-grade fever

2.13 Cough is worst in the morning

2.14 Cough has a bark-like quality

Questions 2.15 to 2.17 concern the following medicines:

A. Acrivastine
B. Loratadine
C. Chlorphenamine
D. Cetirizine
E. Antazoline

Select, from A to E, which of the above medicines:

2.15 Causes least sedation

2.16 Is most likely to cause sedation

2.17 Is most suitable for a pregnant women with nasal congestion

Questions 2.18 to 2.20: For each of these questions, *one or more* of the responses is (are) correct. Decide which of the responses is (are) correct. Then choose:

A. If 1, 2 and 3 are correct
B. If 1 and 2 only are correct
C. If 2 and 3 only are correct
D. If 1 only is correct
E. If 3 only is correct

Directions summarised

A	B	C	D	E
a, b and c	a and b only	b and c only	a only	c only

2.18 A patient presents with a productive cough. From the following, which would alert you to make a same-day referral?

a. Patient recently started on Ramipril
b. Cough present for just over 2 weeks
c. Blood is present in the sputum on a regular basis

2.19 A patient presents at your pharmacy with classic hay fever symptoms. You decide an antihistamine would be most suitable; however, the patient is a forklift truck operator. Which antihistamine/s would be most suitable for this patient?

a. Loratadine
b. Acrivastine
c. Chlorphenamine

2.20 A middle-aged man presents with hay fever. The cause is most likely grass pollen. Which of the following allergen avoidance measures would be suitable to suggest?

a. Try to keep windows in the house closed
b. Wear wraparound sunglasses
c. Wash bedlinen frequently

Questions 2.21 to 2.23: These questions consist of a statement in the left-hand column, followed by a statement in the right-hand column. You need to:

● decide whether the first statement is true or false
● decide whether the second statement is true or false

Then choose:

A. If both statements are true, and the second statement is a correct explanation of the first statement
B. If both statements are true, but the second statement is NOT a correct explanation of the first statement
C. If the first statement is true, but the second statement is false
D. If the first statement is false, but the second statement is true
E. If both statements are false

Directions summarised

	1st statement	2nd statement	
A	True	True	2nd explanation is a correct explanation of the first
B	True	True	2nd statement is not a correct explanation of the first
C	True	False	
D	False	True	
E	False	False	

	First Statement	*Second statement*
2.21	Sore throats are usually viral in origin	The most common pathogens are beta-haemolytic *Streptococcus*
2.22	Pneumothorax is associated with elderly women	It occurs due to bacterial invasion of the pleural membranes
2.23	Hay fever symptoms occur because of an IgE-mediated response	Decongestants stop the production of these chemicals

Case study

CASE STUDY 2.1

Mr RT has asked to speak to the pharmacist, as he has a troublesome cough.

a. Discuss the appropriately worded questions you will need to ask Mr RT to determine the seriousness of the cough.

Questions should fall broadly into two groups:

Those that relate to the presenting complaint, for example: nature, duration, onset, periodicity, sputum colour (if applicable), associated symptoms, aggravating/alleviating symptoms.

Those which look at the medical, family and social history of the patient: current medication regimen (recent changes to medication or dosage adjustment), self-medication, general well-being of the patient, smoking status.

Discussion with Mr RT indicates he has a productive cough that appeared a few days ago and the sputum is white. His nose is 'a bit blocked'. He has a headache and he does not have any chest pain. Before you can make a recommendation for the symptoms, you identify he is taking the following medications:

- *Manerix 150 mg bd – he has taken this for over 6 months.*
- *Trusopt tds– he has used this for 2 years*
- *Paracetamol 2 qds prn – for lower back pain*

b. Compare and contrast the different products available to treat Mr RT's symptoms and indicate which you consider would be the most beneficial to him and those that are contraindicated.

Information related to products to treat a productive cough with nasal congestion should be sought. This involves expectorant medication and sympathomimetics. Mr RT's current drug regimen will have to be taken into consideration and checks for interactions and suitability made. For example, Mr RT is taking Manerix, therefore sympathomimetics should be avoided.

A few weeks later Mr RT returns to the pharmacy and complains that he is still having trouble clearing his blocked nose. A friend at work recommended Otrivine Nasal Spray.

c. The use of local decongestants is associated with the phenomenon known as rhinitis medicamentosa. Explain what this is and what advice you would give to Mr RT.

Rhinitis medicamentosa relates to the problem of overly long use of topical sympathomimetics. Prolonged use (normally more than 7 days continuous use) results in vascular engorgement of the nose on withdrawal of the medication. Patients often believe mistakenly that symptoms have returned and begin to use the medication again and thus perpetuate the problem. This cycle of overuse has to be broken and explained to patients so that they understand why they have continued nasal congestion. Strategies to relieve the problem are, if appropriate, a switch to systemically administered decongestants or, if this is not appropriate, then withdrawal of the medication. The patient was counselled that the symptoms will initially worsen, but then that symptoms will gradually resolve. In Mr RT's case he should be advised not to take the nasal spray because of the risk of a drug interaction between the spray and Manerix.

CASE STUDY 2.2

A female patient, who is approximately 30 years old, presents to the pharmacist complaining of a bothersome sore throat. The following information is gained from the patient.

Information gathering	Data generated
Presenting complaint	
What symptoms have you got	Pain when trying to swallow
How long have you had the symptoms	Had for the last 2 days
Any other symptoms	Headache
Additional questions asked	Raised temperature? Don't know True difficulty swallowing – no
Previous history of presenting complaint	Had cough and cold a few months ago
Past medical history	Eczema
Drugs (OTC, Rx, and compliance)	Nothing currently
Allergies	None known
Social history Smoking Alcohol Drugs Employment Relationships	No questions asked in relation to social history
Family history	N/A
Examination	Throat appears normal. No ulceration or pus obviously visible using pen torch. Glands do not feel swollen. Running low fever (38° C [100.4° F])

Using the information gained from questioning and linking this with known epidemiology on sore throat (see Table 2.7), it should be possible to make a differential diagnosis.

Diagnostic pointers with respect to symptom presentation

Below summarises the expected findings for questions when related to the different conditions that can be seen by community pharmacists.

CASE STUDY 2.2 (Continued)

	Age	Tonsillar/ pharyngeal exudate	Duration	Cervical glands	Cough present	Other symptoms
Viral infection	Any age	Possible, but generally limited	3–7 days	Normal	Common	Low-grade fever, headache
Bacterial infection	Schoolchildren	Often present and can be substantial	3–7 days	Swollen	Rare	High-grade fever, possible rash
Thrush	Young and old	No	5–14 days?	Normal	No	No
Glandular fever	Adolescents	Unlikely	>14 days	Swollen	No	Lethargy
Trauma	Any age	Unlikely	Varies, depending on cause	Normal	No	None
Carcinoma	Older people	None	>14 days	Normal?	No?	Dysphagia, ear pain
Medicines	Adults	None	depends	Normal	No	

When this information is applied to the information gained from our patient, we see that her symptoms most closely match viral infection or trauma. As epidemiology states viral infection is the most prevalent cause of sore throat, it seems likely that this is the cause of her symptoms. Trauma appears less likely due to having no systemic symptoms – a supplementary question about precipitating factors should exclude trauma as a cause.

	Age	Tonsillar/ pharyngeal exudate	Duration	Cervical glands swollen	Cough present	Absence of dysphagia	Systemic upset present
Viral infection	✓	✓?	✓	✓	X	✓	✓
Bacterial infection	X	X	✓	X	X?	✓	✓?
Thrush	X	✓	X?	✓	✓	✓	X
Glandular fever	X	✓	X	X	✓	✓	X
Trauma	✓	✓	✓?	✓	✓	✓	X
Carcinoma	X	✓	X	✓	✓	X	X
Medicines	N/A	N/A	N/A	N/A	N/A	N/A	N/A

Danger symptoms/signs (trigger points for referral)

As a final double check, it might be worth making sure the person has none of the 'referral' signs or symptoms. This is the case with this patient.

Adverse drug reaction	X
Associated skin rash	X
Duration of more than 2 weeks	X
Dysphagia	X
Marked tonsillar exudate accompanied with a high temperature and swollen glands	X

CASE STUDY 2.3

Mr JL, an Asian man in his early sixties who is slightly overweight, wants something for his persistent cough. He has tried some OTC products from the supermarket, but they did not work. The following information is gained from the patient.

Information gathering	Data generated
Presenting complaint	
Describe symptoms	Cough with a little bit of phlegm
How long had the symptoms	Weeks. Just has been there in the background. Not really bothered by it but just doesn't seem to want to go. Saw the GP about 6 weeks ago and was given antibiotics. Seemed to help, but the cough came back again
Nature of sputum	Not a lot there really. Seems green/brown
Onset/timing	Not noticed it being better or worse at any time
Other symptoms/ provokes	Generally feel off colour for a while
Additional questions	No blood in sputum that is noticed; no weight loss
Previous history of presenting complaint	Gets coughs and colds periodically but not constantly
Past medical history	GORD, hypothyroidism
Drugs (OTC, Rx, and compliance)	Pantoprazole 1 od Thyroxine 100 µg 1 od
Allergies	KNA
Social history Smoking Alcohol Drugs Employment Relationships	Drinks most nights plus smokes 20–40 a day Currently unemployed
Family history	Lives on own
On examination	N/A

Epidemiology of cough suggests that viral sore throat is the most likely cause of cough in primary care for all ages. However, other conditions are possible and are noted below.

Using the information gained from questioning and linking this with known epidemiology on cough (see Table 2.1), it should be possible to make a differential diagnosis.

Diagnostic pointers with respect to symptom presentation

Below summarises the expected findings for questions when related to the different conditions that can be seen by community pharmacists.

CASE STUDY 2.3 (Continued)

	Acute or chronic	Sputum	Sputum colour	Age	Systemic symptoms	Worse
Viral	Acute	Sometimes	White to green or yellow	Any	Yes	PM
Post-nasal drip	Acute	No	N/A	Adults	No	None
Allergy	Either	No	N/A	Any	No	PM
Acute bronchitis	Acute	Sometimes	White to green or yellowy	Adults	Yes	None
Croup	Acute	No	N/A	Young children	No	PM
Chronic bronchitis	Chronic	Yes	Mucopurulent	>40	No	AM
Asthma	Chronic	Sometimes	Yellow	Any	No	PM
Pneumonia	Acute	Yes	Rust tinged	>50	Yes	PM
Medication	Either	No	N/A	Adults	No	None
Heart failure	Chronic	Yes	Pink tinged	Elderly	No	PM
Bronchiectasis	Chronic	Yes	Mucopurulent	Adults	No	AM & PM
Tuberculosis	Chronic	Yes	Blood present	Any	Yes	None
Cancer	Chronic	Yes	Dark red	>50	No	None
Pneumothorax	Acute	No	N/A	Young adults	No	None
Lung abscess	Chronic	No	N/A	Elderly	Yes	None
Nocardiasis	Chronic	Yes	Mucopurulent	Adults	Yes	None

When this information is applied to the information gained from our patient, we see that the conditions that most closely fit with the man's symptoms are chronic bronchitis, tuberculosis or nocardiasis. Based on epidemiology, nocardiasis seems highly unlikely so is it chronic bronchitis or tuberculosis? The man does smoke heavily and this fits with chronic bronchitis, but he says that he has not had a repeated history of cough. The patient has felt unwell for 'a while' and this suggests systemic involvement. Although rare, tuberculosis appears to be a possibility, and it would seem sensible to refer him to his GP because of the long-standing nature of the symptoms, general malaise and his ethnic background.

CASE STUDY 2.3 (Continued)

	Acute or chronic	Sputum	Sputum colour (productive only)	Age	Systemic symptoms
Viral	X	✓?	X?	✓	✓
Postnasal drip	X	X	N/A	✓	X
Allergy	X?	X	N/A	✓	X
Acute bronchitis	X	✓	X?	✓	✓
Croup	X	X	N/A	X	X
Chronic bronchitis	✓	✓	✓	✓	X
Asthma	✓	✓?	✓?	✓	X
Pneumonia	X	✓	✓?	✓	✓
Medication	X?	X	N/A	N/A	N/A
Heart failure	✓	✓	X	X	X
Bronchiectasis	✓	✓	✓?	✓	X
Tuberculosis	✓	✓	✓?	✓	✓
Carcinoma	✓	✓	✓?	✓	X
Pneumothorax	X	X	N/A	X	X
Lung abscess	✓	X	N/A	✓	✓
Nocardiasis	✓	✓	✓?	✓	✓

Answers

1 = e	2 = b	3 = e	4 = d	5 = c	6 = d	7 = b	8 = b	9 = C	10 = A
11 = D	12 = A	13 = D	14 = E	15 = B	16 = C	17 = C	18 = E	19 = B	20 = B
21 = C	22 = E	23 = C							

Ophthalmology

Background

The eye is one of the most important and complex organs of the body. Vision is taken for granted and only when our sight is threatened do we truly appreciate what we have. Due to its complicated and intricate anatomy, many things can and do go wrong with the eye, and these manifest as ocular symptoms to the patient.

It is the pharmacist's role to differentiate between minor self-limiting and serious sight-threatening conditions. For pharmacists to undertake this role they need to be familiar with the gross anatomy of the eye, be able to take an eye history and perform a simple eye examination.

In addition, pharmacists can play a major role in health promotion towards eye care, especially in those patients who present with repeat medication for degenerative conditions, such as glaucoma. The pharmacist could check patient concordance, ability to administer eye drops and ointments correctly and, potentially, discover any deterioration of the patient's condition.

General overview of eye anatomy

A basic understanding of the main eye structures is useful to help pharmacists assess the nature and severity of the presenting complaint. Fig. 3.1 highlights the principal eye structures.

The eyelids

The eyelids act as protection from excessive light and foreign bodies as well as spread lubricating secretions over the eyeballs. They consist mainly of voluntary muscle with a border of thick connective tissue, known as the tarsal plate. This plate is felt as a ridge when everting the eyelid. Eyelashes also help protect the eye. At the base of the eyelash sebaceous ciliary glands release lubricating fluid. It is these glands that, if infected, can cause styes.

The conjunctiva

This is a transparent, thin continuous mucous membrane that covers the inside of the eyelids (palpebral conjunctiva) and the sclera (bulbar conjunctiva). It acts as a protective layer to the eye. Dilation and congestion of blood vessels of the bulbar conjunctiva cause red eye.

The sclera and cornea

The sclera encircles the eye, apart from a small 'window' at the very front of the eye where the cornea is located. The sclera is often referred to as the 'white' of the eye, and gives shape and rigidity to the eyeball. The transparent cornea allows light to enter the eye and helps converge light onto the retina.

The iris, pupil and ciliary body

The iris is the coloured part of the eye; its main function is to regulate the amount of light entering the eyeball

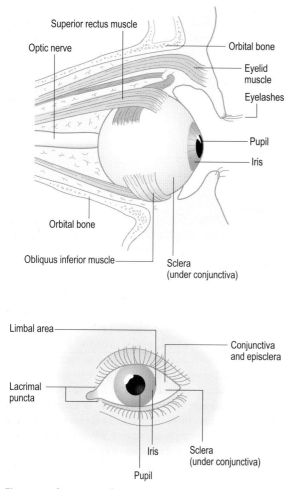

Fig. 3.1 Anatomy of the eye. Above: side view; below: front view.

through the pupil. It is an incomplete circle, with a hole in the middle of the iris, which forms the pupil. The iris attaches to the ciliary body, which serves to hold the lens in place. The ciliary body produces the aqueous, a watery solution that bathes the lens. This is manufactured behind the iris, travels through the posterior chamber and the pupil before draining at the anterior chamber angle (where the iris meets the cornea). If this exit becomes blocked then the intraocular pressure of the eye becomes elevated.

The lens

The lens is responsible for 'fine focusing' light onto the retina. It possesses the ability to vary its focusing power. However, this variable focus power is lost with increasing age as the lens grows harder and less elastic. This is the reason many people require reading glasses as they get older.

The retina

The retina is the light-sensitive layer of the eye and the start of the visual pathway. The functioning of the retina can be compromised by many factors, such as underlying disease states (e.g., age-related macular degeneration), and foreign bodies causing retinal damage and detachment.

History taking and the eye examination

A detailed history should be sought from the patient when attempting to decide on the cause of the presenting complaint. Pay attention to changes in vision, the severity and nature of discomfort, and the presence of discharge. Do not forget to ask about any family history of eye disease (e.g., glaucoma), and the person's previous eye and medication history. Answers to these various questions should enable the pharmacist to build up a picture of the problem and arrive at a differential diagnosis.

The history gained should then be supplemented by performing an eye examination. A great deal of information can be learned from a close inspection of the eye. For example, you can check the size of the pupils, their comparative size and reaction to light, the colour of the sclera, the nature of any discharge and whether there is any eyelid involvement. It is impossible for you to agree with a patient's self-diagnosis or to differentially diagnose any form of conjunctivitis from behind a counter. Pharmacists owe it to their patients to perform a simple eye examination.

The eye examination

Before performing an eye examination, it is important to fully explain to the patient what you are about to do and to gain their consent. There are three basic steps that must be undertaken; the order is unimportant as long as they are all performed:

1. Inspect the eye

2. Check for visual acuity

3. Check pupil reactions

Points 2 and 3 help assess for possible sinister pathology, whereas point 1 should help establish distribution and extent of redness. Before any examination takes place, wash your hands and sit down with the patient so that you are at each other's eye level.

1. Inspect the eye

   To allow a full assessment of the distribution and severity of the affected eye/s, it is necessary to view all aspects of the sclera. This is done by basic manipulation of the eyelids.

   To examine the upper part of the sclera you need to gently pull down the lower lid and ask the patient to look upwards and to both the left and the right.

   To examine the lower part of the sclera you need to gently lift up the upper lid and ask the patient to look downwards and to both the left and the right.

   If only one eye is affected you should perform these procedures on both the good and the bad eye so that you have a comparison between normal and abnormal.

2. Check for visual acuity

   Visual acuity of the patient can be assessed by asking the patient to read small print with the affected eye, while blocking off the good eye. Printed material should be held at a minimum of arm's length and the person asked to read the text.

3. Check pupil size, shape and reactions

   Assess the pupil for size and shape. Pupils should be round and equal in size. Pupil reflexes should be normal in those conditions which are within the remit of community pharmacy management. A light source (a pen torch is adequate) needs to be shone into the eye.

   The patient should look directly at you while you bring in the light source from the side of their face. The light should be shone onto the pupil for less than a second to evoke a pupil reaction. Direct and consensual responses should be checked. Normal reflexes would be expected as are pupil constriction.

Red eye

Background

Conjunctivitis simply means inflammation of the conjunctiva and is characterised by varying degrees of ocular redness, irritation, itching and discharge. Redness of the eye and inflammation of the conjunctiva has been reported as being the most common ophthalmic problem encountered in the Western world.

As conjunctivitis (bacterial, viral and allergic forms) is the most common ocular condition encountered by community pharmacists, this section concentrates on recognising the different types of conjunctivitis and differentially diagnosing these from more serious ocular disorders.

Prevalence and epidemiology

The exact prevalence of conjunctivitis is not known, although statistics for GPs show that eye problems account for up to 5% of their workload, and one small UK community pharmacy-based study found that on average pharmacies saw two cases of red eye per week. Conjunctivitis seems to affect sexes equally and may present in any age of patient, although it is more common in children and the elderly. All three types of conjunctivitis are essentially self-limiting, although viral conjunctivitis can be recurrent and persist for many weeks.

Aetiology

Pathogens that cause bacterial conjunctivitis vary between adults and children. In adults *Staphylococcus* species are most common (over 50% of cases), followed by *Streptococcus pneumoniae* (20%), *Moraxella* species (5%) and *Haemophilus influenzae* (5%). In children, *Streptococcus*, *Moraxella* and *Haemophilus* are most common. The adenovirus is most commonly implicated in viral conjunctivitis and pollen usually causes seasonal allergic conjunctivitis.

Arriving at a differential diagnosis

Red eye is a presenting complaint of both serious and non-serious causes of eye pathology. Community pharmacists must be able to differentiate between those conditions that can be managed and those that need referral. Table 3.1 depicts those conditions which the pharmacist may see.

Redness of the eye can occur alone or present with accompanying symptoms of pain, discomfort, discharge and loss of visual acuity. Along with an examination of the eye, a number of eye-specific questions should always be asked of the patient to establish a differential diagnosis (Table 3.2).

Table 3.1
Causes of red eye and their relative incidence in community pharmacy

Incidence	Cause
Most likely	Bacterial or allergic conjunctivitis
Likely	Viral conjunctivitis, subconjunctival haemorrhage
Unlikely	Episcleritis, scleritis, keratitis, uveitis
Very unlikely	Acute closed-angle glaucoma

? Table 3.2
Specific questions to ask the patient: Red eye

Question	Relevance
Discharge present	Most commonly seen in conjunctivitis. Can vary from watery to mucopurulent, dependent on the type
	Mucopurulent discharge is more suggestive of bacterial conjunctivitis, especially if the eyes are glued together in the absence of itching
Visual changes	Any loss of vision or haloes around objects should be viewed with extreme caution, especially if scleral redness is also present
Pain/discomfort/itch	True pain is generally associated with conditions requiring referral, e.g., scleritis, keratitis, uveitis and acute glaucoma. Pain associated with conjunctivitis is often described as a gritty/foreign body-type pain
Location of redness	Redness concentrated near or around the coloured part of the eye (limbal area) can indicate sinister pathology, for example uveitis. Generalised redness and redness towards the fornices (corner of the eyes) is more indicative of conjunctivitis. Localised scleral redness can indicate scleritis or episcleritis
Duration	Minor eye problems are usually self-limiting and resolve within a few days. Any ocular redness, apart from subconjunctival haemorrhage, and allergic conjunctivitis that lasts more than 1 week requires referral
Photophobia	Photophobia is usually associated with sinister eye pathology, for example, keratitis and uveitis
Other symptoms	Signs and symptoms of an upper respiratory tract infection point towards a viral cause of conjunctivitis
	Vomiting suggests glaucoma

Table 3.3
Symptoms that help distinguish between the different types of conjunctivitis

	Bacterial	Viral	Allergic
Eyes affected	Both, but one eye is often affected first by 24–48 hours	Both	Both
Discharge	Purulent	Watery	Watery
Pain	Gritty feeling	Gritty feeling	Itching
Distribution of redness	Generalised and diffuse	Generalised	Generalised, but greatest in fornices
Associated symptoms	None commonly	Cough and cold symptoms	Rhinitis (may also have family history of atopy)

Clinical features of conjunctivitis

The overwhelming majority of patients presenting to the pharmacy with red eye will have some form of conjunctivitis. Each of the three common types of conjunctivitis has similar but varying symptoms. Each presents with the main symptoms of redness, discharge and discomfort. Table 3.3 and Figs. 3.2, 3.3 and 3.4 highlight the similarities and differences in the classical presentations of the three conditions.

Conditions to eliminate

Likely causes

Subconjunctival haemorrhage
The rupture of a blood vessel under the conjunctiva causes subconjunctival haemorrhage. A segment of, or even the whole eye will appear bright red (Fig. 3.5). It occurs spontaneously but can be precipitated by coughing, straining

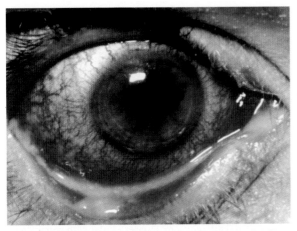

Fig. 3.2 Bacterial conjunctivitis. Reproduced from David A. Palay and Jay H. Krachmer, 2005, *Primary Care Ophthalmology*, 2nd edition, Elsevier Mosby, with permission.

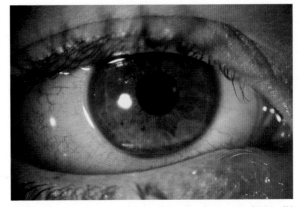

Fig. 3.4 Allergic conjunctivitis. Reproduced from JH Krachmer, MJ Mannis and EJ Holland (eds), 2005, *Cornea: Volume 1 Fundamentals, Diagnosis and Management*, 2nd edition, Elsevier Mosby, with permission.

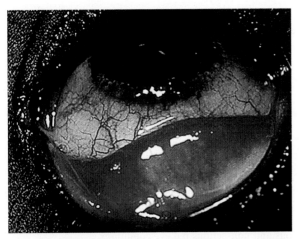

Fig. 3.3 Viral conjunctivitis. Reproduced from Joseph W Sowka OD, Andrew S Gurwood OD and Alan Kabat OD, *Handbook of Ocular Disease Management*, Jobson Publishing, with permission.

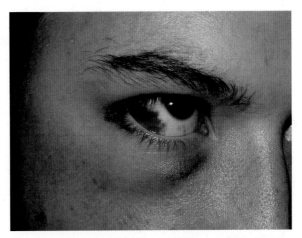

Fig. 3.5 Subconjunctival haemorrhage.

or lifting. The suddenness of symptoms and the brightness of the blood invariably mean patients present very soon after they have noticed the problem. There is no pain and the patient should be reassured that symptoms will resolve in 10 to 14 days without treatment. However, a patient with a history of trauma should be referred to exclude ocular injury.

Unlikely causes

Episcleritis

The episclera lies just beneath the conjunctiva and adjacent to the sclera. If this becomes inflamed the eye appears red, which is segmental, affecting only part of the eye (Fig. 3.6).

The condition affects only one eye in the majority of cases and is usually painless; however, a dull ache might be present. It is more commonly seen in young women and is usually self-limiting, resolving in 2 to 3 weeks, but it can take 6 to 8 weeks before symptoms disappear. Episcleritis is one of those conditions, like subconjunctival haemorrhage, that typically looks worse than it is.

Scleritis

Inflammation of the sclera is much less common than episcleritis. It is often associated with autoimmune diseases. For example, in 20% of cases the patient has rheumatoid arthritis. It presents similarly to episcleritis, but pain (generally severe) is a predominant feature, as is blurred vision. Eye movement can worsen pain. Scleritis also tends to affect older people (mean presentation age is in the early 50s).

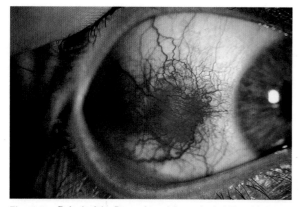

Fig. 3.6 Episcleritis. Reproduced from Jack J Kanski, 2007, *Clinical Ophthalmology: A Systematic Approach,* 6th edition, Butterworth Heinemann, with permission.

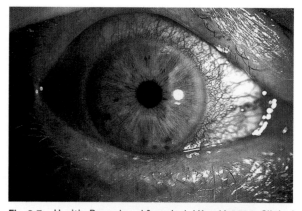

Fig. 3.7 Uveitis. Reproduced from Jack J Kanski, 2006, *Clinical Diagnosis in Ophthalmology,* Elsevier Mosby, with permission.

Discharge is rare or absent in both episcleritis and scleritis.

Keratitis (corneal ulcer)

Inflammation of the cornea often results from recent trauma (e.g., eye abrasion) or administration of long-term steroid drops. Overwear of soft contact lenses has also been implicated in causing keratitis. Pain, which can be very severe, is a prominent feature. The patient usually complains of photophobia, a worsening of redness around the iris (limbal redness) and a watery discharge. Physical examination shows a loss of visual acuity often accompanied with a small pupil. Immediate referral to a medical practitioner is needed as loss of sight is possible if left untreated.

Uveitis (iritis)

Uveitis describes inflammation involving the uveal tract (iris, ciliary body and choroids). It is most commonly seen in individuals between 20 and 50 years of age. The likely cause is an antigen–antibody reaction, which can occur as part of a systemic disease, such as rheumatoid arthritis or ulcerative colitis. Photophobia and pain are prominent features along with redness. Usually, only one eye is affected and the redness is often localised to the limbal area (known as the ciliary flush). On examination the pupil will appear irregularly shaped, constricted or fixed (Fig. 3.7). The patient might also complain of impaired reading vision. Immediate referral to a medical practitioner is needed.

Very unlikely causes

Acute closed-angle glaucoma

There are two main types of glaucoma:

- simple chronic open-angle glaucoma, which does not cause pain

- acute closed-angle glaucoma, which can present with a painful red eye

The latter requires immediate referral to an emergency department. It is due to inadequate drainage of aqueous fluid from the anterior chamber of the eye, which results in a rapid increase in intraocular pressure. The onset can be very quick and characteristically occurs in the evening. Severe unilateral eye pain associated with a headache on the same side as the painful eye is the major presenting symptom. The eye appears red and may be cloudy (Fig. 3.8). Vision is blurred/decreased and the patient might also notice haloes around lights. Vomiting is often experienced due to the rapid rise in intraocular pressure. It classically occurs in older, far-sighted patients. As it is such a painful condition, patients are unlikely to present to the community pharmacist.

Fig. 3.9 can be used to help differentiate between serious and non-serious red eye conditions.

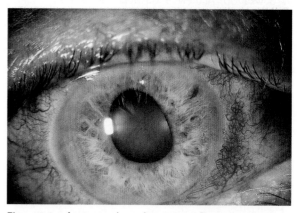

Fig. 3.8 Acute-angle glaucoma. Reproduced from Mark Batterbury, Brad Bowling, Conor Murphy, 2010, Ophthalmology An Illustrated Colour Text, 3rd edition, Elsevier Churchill Livingstone, with permission.

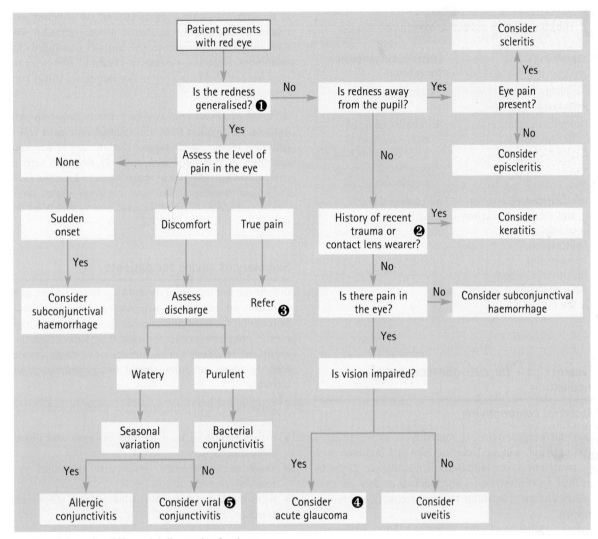

Fig. 3.9 Primer for differential diagnosis of red eye.

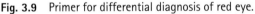

❶ Generalised redness
Most episodes of conjunctivitis will show generalised redness, although the intensity of redness tends to be worse towards the corners of the eye or away from the pupil. Occasionally, severe conjunctivitis can have marked redness throughout the eye; these cases are best referred.

❷ Contact lens wearers
Contact lens wearers are more predisposed to keratitis because the space between the contact lens and cornea can act as an incubator for bacteria and enhance mechanical abrasion. This is especially true if patients sleep with their lenses in, because contact time for abrasion to occur is prolonged.

❸ True pain
It is important to distinguish true pain from ocular irritation. Red eye caused by conjunctivitis causes discomfort,

often described as gritty or a 'foreign body' sensation. It does not normally cause true eye pain. True pain would indicate more serious ocular pathology, such as scleritis, uveitis or keratitis. It is important to encourage the patient to describe the sensation carefully to enable an accurate assessment of the type of pain experienced.

❹ Glaucoma
This is more common in people aged over 50 years and longsighted people. Dim light can precipitate an attack. It is a medical emergency and immediate referral is needed.

❺ Viral conjunctivitis
Associated symptoms of an upper respiratory tract infection might be present (e.g., cough and cold). Viral conjunctivitis often occurs in epidemics and it is not unusual to see a number of cases in a very short space of time.

> **! TRIGGER POINTS indicative of referral: Red eye**
>
> | Symptoms/signs | Possible danger/reason for referral |
> | --- | --- |
> | Clouding of the cornea Associated vomiting | Suggests glaucoma |
> | Redness caused by a foreign body | Requires removal of body – outside remit of community pharmacist. Refer to an optician |
> | Irregular-shaped pupil or abnormal pupil reaction to light Photophobia True eye pain Distortion of vision Redness localised around the pupil | All suggest sinister pathology |

Evidence base for over-the-counter medication

Bacterial conjunctivitis

Bacterial conjunctivitis is regarded as self-limiting – 65% of people will have clinical cure in 2 to 5 days with no treatment – yet antibiotics are routinely given by medical practitioners (and pharmacists) as they are considered clinically desirable to speed recovery and reduce relapse.

Propamidine and dibromopropamidine isethionate have been used for decades to treat conjunctivitis. It is active against a wide range of organisms, including those responsible for bacterial conjunctivitis. However, clinical trials are lacking to substantiate its effectiveness, and a further possible limitation is the licensed dosage regimen (four times a day for drops), which has been reported to be too infrequent to achieve sufficient concentrations to kill or stop the growth of the infecting pathogen.

In the UK, chloramphenicol eye drops (2005) and chloramphenicol ointment (2007) were deregulated. Chloramphenicol has proven efficacy and can be used in all causes of bacterial conjunctivitis, but its routine use has been called into question.

Rose et al. (2005) questioned whether antibiotics were needed in children as no significant difference was seen in the cure rate after 7 days; 86% of the children were clinically cured in the antibiotic group compared with 83% in the placebo group. The authors concluded that antibiotics were not needed in children. However, the most recent Cochrane review (Sheikh et al., 2012) concluded that:

Although acute bacterial conjunctivitis is frequently self-limiting, the findings from this updated systematic review (previous review 2006) suggest that the use of antibiotic eye drops is associated with modestly improved rates of clinical and microbiological remission in comparison to the use of placebo. Use of antibiotic eye drops should therefore be considered to speed the resolution of symptoms and infection.

Summary of advice for patients

Despite the findings from the 2012 Cochrane review, anti-infectives are not always necessary and patients should be told that the condition is generally self-limiting; however, if symptoms persist for more than 5 days then they should be re-assessed and antibiotic eye drops considered. Self-help measures should be recommended and include:

- bathe the eyelids with lukewarm water to remove any discharge
- tissues should be used to wipe the eyes and thrown away immediately
- avoid wearing contact lenses until symptoms have resolved
- wash hands regularly and avoid sharing pillows and towels

Viral conjunctivitis

Currently, there are no specific over-the-counter (OTC) preparations available to treat viral conjunctivitis. Viral causes are highly contagious and the pharmacist should instruct the patient to follow strict hygiene measures (e.g., not sharing towels, washing hands frequently), which will help control the spread of the virus. A patient will remain infectious until the redness and weeping resolves (usually in 10–12 days). Conflicting advice on exclusion from school or work exists. For example, the UK Health Protection Agency state that exclusion from school is unnecessary, whereas the Australian National Health and Medical Research Council recommend exclusion.

Allergic conjunctivitis

Avoidance of the allergen will, in theory, result in control of symptoms. However, total avoidance is almost impossible and the use of prophylactic medication is advocated. The evidence base for ocular mast cell stabilisers and sympathomimetics, and oral antihistamines is discussed in Chapter 2 (page 38).

Practical prescribing and product selection

Prescribing information relating to medication for red eye reviewed in the section 'Evidence base for over-the-counter medication' is discussed and summarised in Table 3.4 and useful tips relating to treatment are given in 'Hints and Tips' in Box 3.1.

Table 3.4
Practical prescribing: Summary of medicines for red eye

Name of medicine	Use in children	Likely side effects	Drug interactions of note	Patients in which care is exercised	Pregnancy & breastfeeding
Allergic conjunctivitis					
Mast cell stabilisers Sodium cromoglicate	>6 years	Local irritation, blurred vision	None	None	OK
Lodoxamide	>4 years	Headache, dizziness, nausea	None	None	OK
Antihistamines Antazoline*	>12 years	Local irritation, bitter taste	Avoid concomitant use with monoamine oxidase inhibitors (MAOIs) and moclobemide due to risk of hypertensive crisis	Avoid in glaucoma	
Sympathomimetics Naphazoline	>12 years	Local irritation	Avoid concomitant use with MAOIs and moclobemide due to risk of hypertensive crisis	None	Not adequately studied but not yet shown to be a risk – probably OK
Bacterial conjunctivitis					
Chloramphenicol	>2 years	Local burning and stinging	None	Avoid if there is a family history of blood and bone marrow problems	In pregnancy ideally avoid OK in breastfeeding
Propamidine and dibromopropamidine isethionate	>12 years	Blurred vision	None	None	OK

*Only available in combination with naphazoline.

HINTS AND TIPS BOX 3.1: EYE DROPS

Children and school	The Health Protection Agency (2000) recommends that children with conjunctivitis do not need to be kept away from schools
Contact lens wearers	Patients who wear soft contact lenses should be advised to stop wearing them while treatment continues and for 48 hours afterwards. This is because preservatives in the eye drops can damage the lenses
Brolene and Golden Eye drops	If the patient is instructed to use the drops every 2 hours rather than four times a day, then the drops will probably be more efficacious. However, this is outside the current product license
Choramphenicol drops	These must be stored in the fridge. If they are put into the eye cold it will be uncomfortable, so patients should be told to remove them from the fridge prior to use to allow them to warm up to room temperature
Administration of eye drops	1. Wash your hands 2. Tilt your head backwards, until you can see the ceiling 3. Pull down the lower eyelid by pinching outwards to form a small pocket, and look upwards 4. Holding the dropper in the other hand, hold it as near as possible to the eyelid without touching it 5. Place one drop inside the lower eyelid, then close your eye 6. Wipe away any excess drops from the eyelid and lashes with the clean tissue 7. Repeat steps 2–6 if more than one drop needs to be administered
Administration of eye ointment	1. Repeat eye drop steps 1 and 2 2. Pull down the lower eyelid 3. Place a thin line of ointment along the inside of the lower eyelid 4. Close your eye, and move the eyeball from side to side 5. Wipe away any excess ointment from the eyelids and lashes using a clean tissue 6. After using ointment, your vision may be blurred but will soon be cleared by blinking

Products for bacterial conjunctivitis

Chloramphenicol (e.g., Golden Eye Antibiotic Drops/Ointment, Optrex Infected Eye Drops/Ointment, Boots Infected Eyes)

Chloramphenicol drops and ointment are licensed for use in children over the age of 2 years. The recommended dosage for the drops is one drop every 2 hours for the first 48 hours, then reducing to four times a day for a maximum of 5 days' treatment. The ointment, if used in conjunction with the drops, should be only applied at night – approximately 1 cm of ointment should be applied to the inside of the eyelid, after which blinking several times will spread the ointment. If used alone, then the ointment should be used three or four times a day. They can be used in most patient groups, although they should be avoided in patients with a family history of blood dyscrasias. In pregnancy and breastfeeding, there is a lack of manufacturer data to recommend their use. Practically, during pregnancy hygiene measures should be adopted and if absolutely necessary they can be used in breastfeeding women.

Propamidine isethionate 0.1% (Brolene and Golden Eye Drops) and Dibromopropamidine isethionate 0.15% (Golden Eye Ointment)

Propamidine and dibromopropamidine isethionate are only licensed for adults and children over the age of 12. The dose for eye drops is one or two drops up to four times daily, whereas the ointment should be applied once or twice daily. If there has been no significant improvement after 2 days, the person should be re-assessed. Blurring of vision on instillation may occur but is transient. The manufacturers state that use in pregnancy has not been established, but there appear to be no reports of teratogenic effects and therefore could be used in pregnancy if deemed appropriate. They are free from drug interactions and can be given to all patient groups, including to women who are breastfeeding.

Products for allergic conjunctivitis

Mast cell stabilisers (sodium cromoglicate, lodoxamide)

Both are prophylactic agents and therefore need to be given continuously while exposed to the allergen. For cromoglicate the dose of one or two drops should be administered in each eye four times a day and can be used in children aged 6 and over. Clinical experience has shown it to be safe in pregnancy and expert opinion considers sodium cromoglicate to be safe in breastfeeding. It has no drug interactions and can be given to all patient groups. Instillation of the drops may cause a transient blurring of vision. Lodoxamide can be used in children aged 4 years and over, and the dosage is one or two drops in each eye four times a day. Headache, dizziness and nausea have been reported but are uncommon. It has no drug interactions and can be given to all patient groups.

Sympathomimetics

These agents can be used to reduce redness of the eye. Products either contain a combination of sympathomimetic and antihistamine (antazoline/xylometazoline, Otrivine Antistin) or sympathomimetic alone (e.g., Naphazoline 0.01%). They are useful in reducing redness in the eye but will not treat the underlying pathology that is causing the eye to be red. They should be limited to short-term use to avoid rebound effects. Like all sympathomimetics they can interact with monoamine oxidase inhibitors (MAOIs) and should not be used by patients receiving such treatment or within 14 days of ceasing therapy.

Otrivine Antistin

Used in adults and children over 12 years, the dosage is one or two drops two or three times a day. Patients with glaucoma should avoid this product due to the potential of the antihistamine component to increase intraocular pressure. Local transient irritation and a bitter taste after application have been reported.

Naphazoline (e.g., Murine Irritation and Redness Relief Eye Drops, Optrex Bloodshot Eyes Eye Drops & Optrex Eye Brightening Drops)

The use of products containing naphazoline is restricted to adults and children over 12 years old. One to two drops should be administered into the eye three or four times a day.

References

Rose PW, Harnden A, Brueggemann AB, et al. Chloramphenicol treatment for acute infective conjunctivitis in children in primary care: a randomised double blind placebo controlled trial. Lancet 2005;366:37–43.

Sheikh A, Hurwitz B, van Schayck CP, et al. Antibiotics versus placebo for acute bacterial conjunctivitis. Cochrane Database of Systematic Reviews 2012, Issue 9. Art. No.: CD001211. http://dx.doi.org/10.1002/14651858.CD001211.pub3.

Further reading

Chen JY, Tey A. GP guide to the diagnosis and management of conjunctivitis. The Prescriber 2014;July/Aug.:22-31.

Drug and Therapeutics Bulletin. Management of acute infective conjunctivitis 2011;49:7. Available at: http://dtb.bmj.com/content/49/7/78.full.pdf (Accessed 7 August 2015).

Everitt HA, Little PS, Smith PW. A randomised controlled trial of management strategies for acute infective conjunctivitis in general practice. BMJ 2006;333:321.

Health Protection Agency, 2010. Guidance on infection control in schools and other childcare settings. Available at: http://www.hpa.org.uk/web/HPAwebFile/HPAweb_C/1194947358374 (Accessed 7 August 2015).

Kanski JJ, Bolton A. Illustrated tutorials in clinical ophthalmology. Oxford: Butterworth-Heinemann; 2001.

Khaw PT, Elkington AR. ABC of eyes. London: BMJ Publishing Group; 1999.

Mohammed N, Smit DP. Basic ophthalmology for the health practitioner: the red eye. S Afr Pharm J 2013;80(7):20-6.

Websites

Eyecare Trust: http://www.eyecaretrust.org.uk/
International Glaucoma Association: http://www.glaucoma-association.com/
The Royal College of Ophthalmologists: www.rcophth.ac.uk
Uveitis Information Group: http://www.uveitis.net/

Eyelid disorders

Background

A number of disorders can afflict the eyelids, ranging from mild dermatitis to malignant tumours. In the context of community pharmacy consultations, the most common presenting conditions will be blepharitis, hordeola (styes) and chalazion (Table 3.5).

Prevalence and epidemiology

Data on the incidence or prevalence of eyelid disorders is limited yet clinical practice suggests that blepharitis and

Table 3.5
Causes of eyelid disorders and their relative incidence in community pharmacy

Incidence	Cause
Most likely	Blepharitis, hordeola
Likely	Contact or irritant dermatitis
Unlikely	Chalazion, ectropion, entropion
Very unlikely	Orbital cellulitis, carcinoma

Table 3.6
Specific questions to ask the patient: The eyelid

Question	Relevance
Duration	A long-standing history of sore eyes is indicative of blepharitis, a chronic, persistent condition, although it can be intermittent with periods of remission
Lid involvement	If the majority of the lid margin is inflamed and red, then this suggests blepharitis. Hordeola tends to show localised lid involvement
Eye involvement	Conjunctivitis is a common complication in blepharitis
Other co-existing conditions	Patients who suffer from blepharitis often have a co-existing skin condition, such as seborrhoeic dermatitis or rosacea

hordeola are frequently mentioned three conditions are frequently encountered. For example, blepharitis has been reported to account for 5% of primary care ophthalmic consultations.

Aetiology

Blepharitis can be classified into three categories that reflect the aetiology of the condition: staphylococcal, seborrhoeic and meibomian gland dysfunction. Further classification of blepharitis is sometimes used based on anatomical location. For example, anterior blepharitis refers to staphylococcal and seborrhoeic causes as they primarily affect the bases of the eyelashes. Posterior blepharitis refers to meibomian gland dysfunction as these are situated on the posterior lid. Patients will, however, show overlapping signs and symptoms that suggest mixed aetiology. Furthermore, it appears that many blepharitis sufferers also have dry eye syndrome, but the exact relationship between the two conditions is unclear.

Styes are caused by bacterial infection (staphylococcal in 90% to 95% of cases) and can either be internal or external. External styes occur on the outside surface of the eyelid and are due to an infected gland, either the Zeis gland (a type of sebaceous gland) or the gland of Moll (a type of sweat gland), both of which are located near the base of the eyelashes. An internal hordeolum is a secondary infection of the meibomian gland in the tarsal plate. Occasionally, internal styes can evolve into a chalazion, a granulomatous inflammation that develops into a painless lump.

Arriving at a differential diagnosis

Blepharitis and hordeola are the most likely presentations and should be relatively straightforward to recognise, so long as a careful history, eye examination and appropriate questioning are undertaken (Table 3.6).

Clinical features of blepharitis

Typically, blepharitis is bilateral with symptoms ranging from irritation, itching and burning of the lid margins. Lid margins may appear red and raw, accompanied with excessive tearing and crusty debris or skin flakes around the eyelashes. Symptoms also tend to be worse in the mornings and patients might complain of eyelids being stuck together (Fig. 3.10). In chronic cases, madarosis (missing lashes) and trichiasis (inturned lash) can occur. This latter symptom

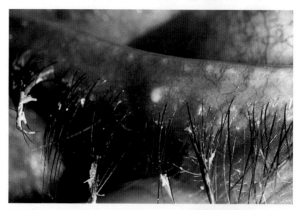

Fig. 3.10 Blepharitis. Reproduced from Jack K Kanski, 2007, *Clinical Ophthalmology: A Systematic Approach*, 6th edition, Butterworth Heinemann, with permission.

can lead to further local irritation and result in conjunctivitis. Seborrhoeic aetiology is likely if greasy crusting of the lashes and oily scale predominates compared with eyelash loss or misdirection, which suggests a staphylococcal cause. Symptoms are often intermittent, with exacerbations and remissions occurring over long periods.

Clinical features of styes

An external stye presents as a swollen upper or lower lid, which will be painful and sensitive to touch. Over time the swelling develops into a pus-filled lesion. The lesion will then either spontaneously shrink and resolve or burst over the next few days (Fig. 3.11). The primary symptoms of an internal stye are as external styes: pain, redness and swelling, although pain is often more severe and pus-filled lesions are not obvious due to inward growth.

Conditions to eliminate

Likely causes

Contact or irritant dermatitis

Many products – especially cosmetics – can be sensitising and result in itching and flaking skin that mimics blepharitis. The patient should be questioned about recent use of such products to allow dermatitis to be eliminated. For further information on dermatitis see Chapter 8, page 263.

Blepharitis unresponsive to therapy

If the patient fails to respond to OTC treatment, or the condition recurs, then it is possible that other causes, such as rosacea, might be responsible for the symptoms. If OTC treatment has failed then medical referral is needed.

Unlikely causes

Chalazion

A chalazion forms when the meibomian gland becomes blocked, and could be confused with a stye. Styes often have a 'head' of pus at the lid margin and will be tender and sore, whereas a chalazion presents as a painless lump. This should be clearly visible if the eyelid is everted. A chalazion is self-limiting, although it might take a few weeks to resolve completely. No treatment is needed unless the patient complains that it is particularly bothersome and is affecting vision. Referral in these circumstances is needed for surgical removal.

Entropion

Entropion is defined as inversion of the eyelid margin. It can occur unilaterally or bilaterally, with the lower eyelid more frequently affected. The in-turning of the eyelid causes the eyelashes to be pushed against the cornea, resulting in ocular irritation and conjunctival redness (Fig. 3.12). It is most often seen in older people. Referral is needed for surgical repair to correct the problem. Taping down the lower lid to draw the eyelid margin away from the eye is sometimes employed as a temporary solution.

Ectropion

Ectropion is the converse to entropion; the eyelid turns outward, exposing the conjunctiva and cornea to the atmosphere (Fig. 3.13). Patients will often present complaining of a continually watering eye. Paradoxically, this can lead to dryness of the eye, as the eye is not receiving adequate lubrication. Ectropion is seen with advancing age and often is noted in people who suffer from Bell's palsy.

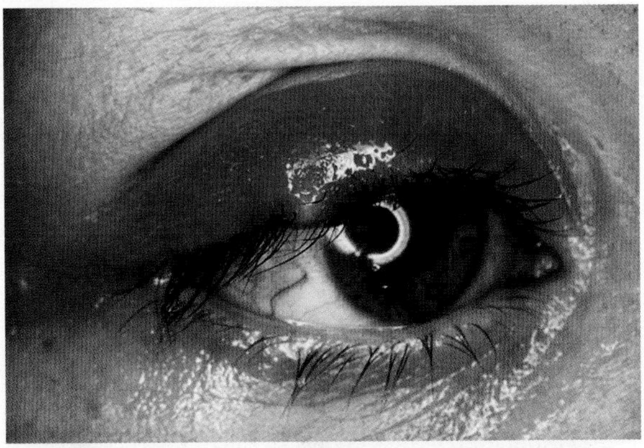

Fig. 3.11 External stye. Reproduced from Jack J Kanski, 2007, *Clinical Ophthalmology: A Systematic Approach*, 6th edition, Butterworth Heinemann, with permission.

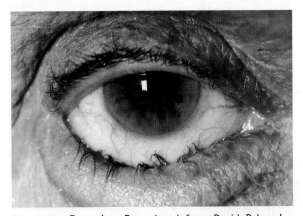

Fig. 3.12 Entropion. Reproduced from David Palay, Jay Krachmer, 2005, *Primary Care Ophthalmology*, 2nd edition, Elsevier Mosby, with permission.

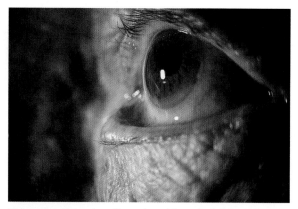

Fig. 3.13 Ectropion. Reproduced from Jack J Kanski, 2007, *Clinical Ophthalmology: A Systematic Approach*, 6th edition, Butterworth Heinemann, with permission.

Very unlikely causes

Orbital cellulitis
Inflammation of the skin surrounding the orbit of the eye is usually a complication from a sinus infection, although in extreme cases of stye the infection can spread to involve the entire lid and even the periorbital tissues. The patient will present with unilateral swollen eyelids, be unwell and might show restricted eye movements. This has to be referred immediately because blindness is a potential complication.

Basal cell carcinoma
This is the commonest form of eyelid malignancy and accounts for over 90% of cases. The lesion is usually nodular

with a reddish hue (due to permanent capillary dilation) and most frequently affects the lower lid margin. No pain or discomfort is present. Long-term exposure to the sun is the main cause. For further information on sun-induced skin damage, see Chapter 8, page 269.

Evidence base for over-the-counter medication

OTC medication is generally not required for blepharitis or styes. No specific products are available and both can respond well to conservative treatment, such as warm compresses.

Practical prescribing and product selection

Blepharitis
The mainstay of treatment for blepharitis is improved lid hygiene. First, the eyelids should be cleaned using a warm compress for 5–10 minutes. A diluted mixture of baby shampoo (1:10) with warm water should then be applied to the eyelids using a cotton bud. This should be done twice a day initially and can be reduced to once a day if symptoms improve. Failure to respond to hygiene measures requires GP referral. As blepharitis can cause dry eye, the prescribing of an ocular lubricant (e.g., hypromellose or carbomers) can be tried, and if there are signs of staphylococcal infection, then topical antibiotics such as fusidic acid gel or even systemic treatment with oxytetracycline should be considered.

Styes
Although styes are caused by bacterial pathogens, the use of antibiotic therapy is not usually needed. Topical application of ocular antibiotics does not result in speedier symptom resolution, but it might prevent a subsequent staphylococcal infection from a lash lower down. A warm compress applied for 5–10 minutes three or four times a day might bring to a head an external stye, and once it bursts the pain will subside and the symptoms will resolve. The use of dibromopropamidine has been advocated in the treatment of styes but is of unproven benefit.

TRIGGER POINTS indicative of referral: Blepharitis and styes

Symptoms/signs	Possible danger/reason for referral
Chalazion that becomes bothersome to the patient	May need surgical intervention; assessment from doctor required
Inward or outward turning of the lower eyelid	Requires medical intervention
Patient with swollen eyelids and associated feelings of being unwell	Suggests orbital cellulitis
Middle-aged/elderly patient with painless nodular lesion on or near eyelid	Suggests sinister pathology, possibly carcinoma

Further reading
Lindsley K, Matsumura S, Hatef E, et al. Interventions for chronic blepharitis. Cochrane Database of Systematic Reviews 2012, Issue 5. Art. No.: CD005556. http://dx.doi.org/10.1002/14651858.CD005556.pub2.
Shields SR. Managing eye disease in primary care. Postgrad Med 2000;108:83–6, 91–6.

Dry eye (keratoconjunctivitis sicca)

Background

Dry eye is a frequent cause of eye irritation, causing varying degrees of discomfort which leads patients to seek medical care. The condition is chronic with no cure.

Prevalence and epidemiology

The exact prevalence of dry eye is unclear due to a lack of consistency in its definition coupled with few population-based studies, which used differing criteria for diagnosis. What is clear, however, is that dry eye syndrome is common. Almost 3% of older adults will develop dry eye each year and its prevalence increases with increasing age. It is also more common in women than men.

Aetiology

Essentially, a reduction in tear volume or alteration in tear composition causes dry eyes. Underproduction of tears can be the result of increased evaporation from the eye, increased tear drainage and a decrease in tear production by the lacrimal gland. Tear composition is complex; the tear film is made up of three distinct layers:

- the innermost mucin layer, which allows tears to adhere to the conjunctival surface
- the middle aqueous layer, containing 90% of the tear thickness
- the outermost lipid layer, which helps slow aqueous layer evaporation

A reduction in any of these layers can lead to dryness, but, frequently, the mucin layer is affected due to a reduction in the mucin-producing goblet cells.

Arriving at a differential diagnosis

There are a number of conditions that can cause dry eye (Table 3.7); however, keratoconjunctivitis sicca (KCS) accounts for the vast majority of dry eye cases.

From a community pharmacist's perspective, many patients will want to buy artificial tears. Good practice would dictate that the pharmacist enquires whether the patient has been instructed from their doctor or optician to buy these products or whether this is a self-diagnosis. If it is a self-diagnosis, the pharmacist should eliminate underlying pathology and ask a number of eye-specific questions to determine whether the self-diagnosis is correct (Table 3.8).

Table 3.7
Causes of dry eye and their relative incidence in community pharmacy

Incidence	Cause
Most likely	Keratoconjunctivitis sicca (KCS)
Likely	Blepharitis, Sjögren's syndrome, medicine-induced dry eye
Unlikely	Ectropion, rosacea
Very unlikely	Bell's palsy

Table 3.8
Specific questions to ask the patient: Dry eye

Question	Relevance
Clarifying questions	Have you had daily, persistent, troublesome dry eyes for more than 3 months? Do you have a recurrent sensation of sand or gravel in the eyes? A positive response to at least one of these questions would indicate dry eye syndrome
Aggravating factors	Dry eye is worsened by dry air, wind, dust and smoke
Associated symptoms	Normally no other symptoms are present in dry eye. If the patient complains of a dry mouth, check for medication that can cause dry mouth. If medication is not implicated, then symptoms could be due to an autoimmune disease
Amount of tears produced	If the patient complains of watery eyes but states that the eyes are dry and sore, check for ectropion

Clinical features of dry eye

Usually affecting both eyes, symptoms reported are eyes that burn, feel tired, itchy, irritated or gritty, with symptoms worsening throughout the day. The conjunctiva is not red unless irritated (e.g., eye rubbing or allergy). Decreased tear production results in irritation and burning.

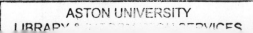
ASTON UNIVERSITY
LIBRARY

Conditions to eliminate

Likely causes

Blepharitis
Chronic disease of eyelashes, eyelids or margins of eyelids can lead to irritation of the conjunctiva. See page 64 for more information on blepharitis.

Sjögren's syndrome
This syndrome has unknown aetiology but is associated with rheumatic conditions. It occurs in the same patient population as keratoconjunctivitis sicca: the elderly and more commonly in women. The patient will have a history of dry eyes but experiences periods of exacerbation and remission. It is also associated with dryness of other mucous membranes, especially the mouth. Criteria for diagnosing and classifying Sjögren's syndrome have been proposed (Vitali et al., 2002).

Medicine-induced dry eye
A number of medicines can exacerbate or produce side effects of dry eyes as a result of decreased tear production (Table 3.9). If medication could be causing dry eyes, then the pharmacist should contact the patient's doctor to discuss possible alternative therapies to alleviate the problem.

Unlikely causes

Ectropion
Sometimes the lower eyelid turns outward. This overexposes the conjunctiva to the atmosphere, leading to eye dryness. For further information see page 65.

Rosacea
Rosacea is a disease of the skin characterised by facial skin findings including erythema, telangiectasia, papules and pustules that mimic acne vulgaris – although many patients also suffer from marginal blepharitis – and keratoconjunctivitis sicca.

Very unlikely causes

Bell's palsy
Bell's palsy is characterised by unilateral facial paralysis, often with sudden onset. A complication of Bell's palsy is that the patient might be unable to close one eye or blink, leading to decreased tear film and dry eye.

> **!** **TRIGGER POINTS indicative of referral: Dry Eye**
>
> | Symptoms/signs | Possible danger/reason for referral |
> | --- | --- |
> | Associated dryness of mouth and other mucous membranes | Sjögren's syndrome? |
> | Outward turning lower eyelid | Requires medical intervention |

Evidence base for over-the-counter medication

Dry eyes are managed by the instillation of artificial tears and lubricating ointments. Products in the UK consist of hypromellose (0.3–1.0%), polyvinyl alcohol, carmellose, carbomer 980, sodium hyaluronate and wool fats.

Despite a lack of published trial data, hypromellose products have been in use for over half a century. They possess film-forming and emollient properties, but unfortunately do not have ideal wetting characteristics, which results in up to hourly administration to provide adequate relief.

This disadvantage of frequent installation has led to the development of other products. Polyvinyl alcohol in a concentration of 1.4% acts as a viscosity enhancer. At this concentration the products have the same surface tension as normal tears, lending them optimal wetting characteristics and hence less frequent dosing, typically four times a day. Similarly to hypromellose, there is a lack of published data confirming their efficacy.

Carbomer has been shown to be more efficacious than placebo and as safe as, but better tolerated, than polyvinyl alcohol. In a comparison study between two proprietary brands, Viscotears and GelTears, both were found to be equally effective, although neither was significantly better than the other (Bron et al., 1998). Sodium hyaluronate has been subject to a number of trials that have shown a reduction in symptom severity. They have also been compared with carbomer products and carboxymethylcellulose, and found to be equally effective.

Table 3.9
Medication that can cause dry eye

Diuretics
Drugs that have an anticholinergic effect – e.g., tricyclic antidepressants (TCAs) antihistamines
Isotretinoin
HRT (particularly oestrogen alone)
Androgen antagonists
Cardiac arrhythmic drugs, beta-blockers
Selective serotonin reuptake inhibitors (SSRIs)

Summary

Despite hypromellose lacking trial evidence, its place in the management of dry eye is well established. In addition, it is very cheap and should therefore be recommended as a first-line treatment. However, other newer products, which possess better wetting characteristics, provide useful alternatives to hypromellose because they can be administered less frequently; these products are more expensive.

Practical prescribing and product selection

Prescribing information relating to medication for dry eye that is reviewed in the section 'Evidence base for over-the-counter medication' is discussed and summarised in Table 3.10, and useful tips on medication are given in 'Hints and Tips' in Box 3.2.

The dosage of all products marketed for dry eye is largely dependent on the patient's need for lubrication, and is therefore given on a when-required basis. None of these products is known to interact with any medicine and they cause minimal and transient side effects.

Hypromellose and carmellose

Hypromellose 0.3% is widely available as a non-proprietary medicine, but it is also available at 0.5% (Isopto Plain) and 1% (Isopto Alkaline); carmellose is available as 0.5% or 1.0% (Celluvisc). All might require hourly or even half-hourly dosing initially, which should reduce as symptoms improve. They are pharmacologically inert and all patient groups should be able to use them safely, including pregnant and breastfeeding women. However, because of a lack of data, some manufacturers err on the side of caution and recommend that it should be avoided.

Polyvinyl alcohol

Three proprietary products are available: Liquifilm Tears Refresh Ophthalmic and Sno Tears. Liquifilm is also available as a preservative-free formulation and can be given to all patient groups.

Carbomer (e.g., Clinitas Gel, GelTears, Liquivisc, Viscotears) *This type.*

Manufacturers recommend that adults and the elderly use one drop three or four times a day or as required, depending on patient need. Due to the products' viscosity properties, carbomer should be used last if other eye drops need to be instilled. Manufacturers advise avoidance in pregnancy and lactation due to insufficient data. Clinical experience, however, has shown carbomer can be used safely in these patient groups.

Table 3.10
Practical prescribing: Summary of medicines for dry eye

Name of medicine	Use in children	Likely side effects	Drug interactions of note	Patients in which care is exercised	Pregnancy & breastfeeding
Hypromellose & carmellose Carbomer 940	Dry eye in children rare; therefore, should be referred	Transient stinging and/ or burning reported. Blurred vision after instillation of carbomer and polyvinyl alcohol	None	None	OK
Polyvinyl alcohol		None reported			
Wool fats ⁄\/					
Hyaluronate					

HINTS AND TIPS BOX 3.2: DRY EYE

Preservatives in eye drops	Many eye drops contain benzalkonium chloride which, itself, can cause eye irritation. If symptoms persists or are worsened by the eye drops, it may be worth trying a preservative-free formulation or single-dose unit preparations

Lubricants

Wool fats (e.g., Lacri-Lube)

These products contain a mixture of white soft paraffin, liquid paraffin and wool fat. They are useful at bedtime when prolonged lubrication is needed, but because they blur vision, they are unsuitable to use during the day. They are pharmacologically inert and can be used in pregnancy and breastfeeding.

Sodium hyaluronate (e.g., Hayabak, Oxyal)

The dose for all products containing sodium hyaluronate is on a when-needed basis.

References

Bron AJ, Daubas P, Siou-Mermet R, et al. Comparison of the efficacy and safety of two eye gels in the treatment of dry eyes: Lacrinorm and Viscotears. Eye 1998;12:839–47.

Vitali C, Bombardieri S, Jonsson R, et al. Classification criteria for Sjogren's syndrome: a revised version of the European criteria proposed by the American-European Consensus Group. Ann Rheum Dis 2002;61:554–8.

Further reading

Brodwall J, Alme G, Gedde-Dahl S, et al. A comparative study of polyacrylic acid [Viscotears] liquid gel versus polyvinylalcohol in the treatment of dry eyes. Acta Ophthalmol Scand 1997;75:457–61.

Johnson ME, Murphy PJ, Boulton M. Carbomer and sodium hyaluronate eyedrops for moderate dry eye treatment. Optometry Vision Sci 2008;85(8):750–7.

Lee JH, Ahn HS, Kim EK, et al. Efficacy of sodium hyaluronate and carboxymethylcellulose in treating mild to moderate dry eye disease. Cornea 2011;30(2):175–9.

Moss SE, Klein R, Klein BEK. Incidence of dry eye in an older population. Arch Ophthalmol 2004;122:369–73.

Sullivan LJ, McCurrach F, Lee S, et al. Efficacy and safety of 0.3% carbomer gel compared to placebo in patients with moderate to severe dry eye syndrome. Ophthalmology 1997;104:1402–8.

Website

Sjögren's Syndrome Foundation: http://www.sjogrens.org/home

Self-assessment questions

The following questions are intended to supplement the text. Two levels of questions are provided; multiple-choice questions and case studies. The multiple-choice questions are designed to test factual recall and the case studies allow knowledge to be applied to a practice setting.

Multiple-choice questions

3.1 A middle-aged woman presents to the pharmacy suffering from a red left eye. The redness appeared quite quickly and she has no other symptoms. Based on this information what is the most likely diagnosis?

a. Bacterial conjunctivitis
b. Allergic conjunctivitis
c. Episcleritis
d. Sub-conjunctival haemorrhage
e. Keratitis

3.2 A man in his late 40s presents to the pharmacy suffering from a red right eye. The redness appeared a day or so ago and he says the feeling is uncomfortable. He says he has not noticed any discharge, but mentions his eye is watering more than usual. Based on this information what is the most likely diagnosis?

a. Scleritis
b. Uveitis
c. Keratitis
d. Viral conjunctivitis
e. Glaucoma

3.3 A woman in her late 30s presents with a red left eye. She says the eye has been red for a little while (at least 2 weeks), but that it has not been bothering her; however, she would like to get rid of the redness before attending a work party. What is the most likely diagnosis?

a. Allergic conjunctivitis
b. Episcleritis
c. Scleritis
d. Blepharitis
e. Sub-conjunctival haemorrhage

3.4 Red eye is a common presenting symptom. Based solely on epidemiology which of the conditions listed below is LEAST likely to be seen in a community pharmacy?

a. Viral conjunctivitis
b. Scleritis
c. Uveitis

d. Sub-conjunctival haemorrhage
e. Episcleritis

3.5 Mr Simmonds, a 54 year old, presents with a red right eye. He has the symptoms for a week or so. He is complaining of photophobia. He takes methotrexate for rheumatoid arthritis. What is the most likely diagnosis?

a. Scleritis
b. Episcleritis
c. Uveitis
d. Glaucoma
e. Keratitis

3.6 Priya Patel, a 27-year-old woman, presents with bilateral red eye of 3 days' duration. She complains also of slight discharge. Visual examination reveals nothing untoward. Your differential diagnosis is conjunctivitis. Which of the following symptoms helps differentiate allergic conjunctivitis from bacterial and viral conjunctivitis?

a. She also has nasal congestion
b. Redness is distributed throughout the conjunctiva
c. She complains of itching eyes
d. Discharge is mucopurulent
e. Symptoms were sudden in onset

3.7 A patient presents with the following symptoms. There is a bright red patch in the eye, which appeared overnight. There is no recent history of trauma to the eye. There is no pain or discomfort, and no discharge from the eye. Vision is normal, and there is no evidence of photophobia. What is the most likely diagnosis for this set of symptoms?

a. Sub-conjunctival haemorrhage
b. Uveitis
c. Episcleritis
d. Keratitis
e. Viral conjunctivitis

3.8 A middle-aged woman presents with a history of a red left eye for the last 24 hours. Which of the following symptoms should alert you to potential sinister pathology?

  a. Discomfort in the eye
  b. Generalised scleral redness
  c. Irregular pupil
  d. Redness located in the fornice
  e. Mucopurulent discharge

Questions 3.9 to 3.13 concern the following conditions:

A. Allergic conjunctivitis
B. Bacterial conjunctivitis
C. Viral conjunctivitis
D. Sub-conjunctival haemorrhage
E. Episcleritis

Select, from A to E, which of the above conditions:

3.9 Shows redness greatest in the fornices.

3.10 Is bilateral and discomfort is described as itching.

3.11 Is usually sudden in onset and unilateral and painless.

3.12 Affects women more than men.

3.13 Is associated with other symptoms such as cough.

Questions 3.14 to 3.16 concern the following symptoms:
A. Swollen and painful upper eyelid
B. Painless lump on the upper eyelid
C. Unilateral swollen eyelid
D. Burning of lid margins
E. In-turning eyelid

Select, from A to E, which of the above symptoms is associated with which condition:

3.14 Stye

3.15 Orbital cellulitis

3.16 Blepharitis

Questions 3.17 to 3.19: For each of these questions, *one or more* of the responses is (are) correct. Decide which of the responses is (are) correct. Then choose:

A. If a, b and c are correct
B. If a and b only are correct
C. If b and c only are correct
D. If a only is correct
E. If c only is correct

Directions summarised

A	B	C	D	E
a, b and c	a and b only	b and c only	a only	c only

3.17 The following statements concern VIRAL conjunctivitis

  a. It usually occurs in epidemics
  b. Both eyes are usually affected
  c. Pain is described as 'gritty'

3.18 Which of the following symptoms would NOT warrant referral to a doctor?

  a. Entropion
  b. Limbal flushing
  c. A hard, red, painless lump under the eyelid

3.19 Which of the following symptoms would automatically warrant referral to a doctor?

  a. True pain within the eye
  b. Irregular pupil
  c. Tunnel vision

3

Questions 3.20 to 3.22: These questions consist of a statement in the left-hand column, followed by a statement in the right-hand column. You need to:

- decide whether the first statement is true or false
- decide whether the second statement is true or false

Then choose:

A. If both statements are true, and the second statement is a correct explanation of the first statement
B. If both statements are true, but the second statement is NOT a correct explanation of the first statement
C. If the first statement is true, but the second statement is false
D. If the first statement is false, but the second statement is true
E. If both statements are false

Directions summarised

	1st statement	2nd statement	
A	True	True	2nd explanation is a correct explanation of the first
B	True	True	2nd statement is not a correct explanation of the first
C	True	False	
D	False	True	
E	False	False	

	First statement	*Second statement*
3.20	Scleritis always presents bilaterally	It is painful
3.21	Conjunctivitis is caused by infection only	Inflammation of the conjunctiva tends to be away from the pupil
3.22	Blepharitis can cause red eye	Skin flaking results in direct conjunctival irritation

Case study

Mrs JR, a 32-year-old-woman, asks you for something to treat her 'sore eyes'. She does not wear contact lenses.

a. **What are your initial thoughts on what the problem could be based solely on the information given?**

Epidemiology of eye problems dictates that Mrs JR is likely to have some form of conjunctivitis or possibly an eyelid/lash problem.

b. **Working from this hypothesis, what would do next?**

Ideally you should look at the eyes to see if there is an obvious cause for the discomfort. A basic inspection (without performing a specific eye examination) should reveal any eyelid/lash problems and scleral redness.

This basic observation reveals no obvious lid or lash involvement but generalised redness in the left eye, which is mirrored in the right eye but not as pronounced.

c. **What are your thoughts now on the differential diagnosis?**

It appears we are dealing with 'red eye' and almost certainly some form of conjunctivitis.

The pharmacy is busy and the consultation room is occupied, meaning you cannot perform a full eye examination. You have to rely on questioning only to arrive at a differential diagnosis.

d. **What questions would you ask Mrs JR to help you differentiate between the different forms of conjunctivitis?**

Discriminatory questions are required that allow you to match the patient's symptoms with the presentations of the various forms of conjunctivitis.

1. **Nature of soreness**
   - Allergic = itch; bacterial and viral = discomfort

2. **If discharge present, what is it like?**
   - Allergic and viral = watery; bacterial = mucopurulent

3. **Is redness particularly worse anywhere in the sclera**
   - Allergy associated with redness in the fornices

   By asking such questions you should be able to build up a picture of the symptoms that should more strongly point to one form of conjunctivitis and, thus, be your differential diagnosis.

CASE STUDY 3.2

A man in his early 30s presents at lunchtime to the pharmacy with a bright red eye. He wants to ease the redness. The following questions are asked, and responses received.

Information gathering	Data generated
On examination	Right eye only and redness fully injected. No visible signs of any capillaries. Visual acuity OK. Pupil reactions normal.
Type/severity of pain	None
Discharge	None
Other symptoms	None
How long had the symptoms	Since mid-morning
Previous history of presenting complaint	No
Past medical history	Takes blood pressure medicines but cannot remember their names
Drugs (OTC, Rx)	Rennies for indigestion now and then
Social history Smoking Alcohol Drugs Employment Relationships	Not relevant in this case to ask
Family history	No history of eye problems in the family (mum and dad)

Using the information gained from questioning and linking this with known epidemiology on red eye (see Table 3.1), it should be possible to make a differential diagnosis.

Diagnostic pointers with regard to symptom presentation

Below summarises the expected findings for questions when related to the different conditions that can be seen by community pharmacists.

CASE STUDY 3.2 (Continued)

	Discharge	Pain	Visual disturbance	Pupil reflex	Eyes affected	Redness
Conjunctivitis – bacterial	Yes, often mucopurulent	Sore, gritty	No	OK	1 or both	Generalised redness
Conjunctivitis – viral	Yes, sometimes watery	Sore, gritty	No	OK	1 or both	Generalised redness
Conjunctivitis – allergic	Yes, watery	Very itchy	No	OK	Both	Worse in fornices
Subconjunctival haemorrhage	No	No	No	OK	Either	Segmental
Episcleritis	No	Little or none	No	OK	1	Segmental
Scleritis	No	Yes	No	OK	1	Segmental
Keratitis	Watery	Yes, severe	Photophobia	Abnormal	1	Around iris
Uveitis	No	Painful	Photophobia	Abnormal	1	Around iris
Glaucoma	No	Yes, severe	Blurred	Abnormal	1	Haloes (vomiting)

When this information is applied to that gained from our patient (below), we see that his symptoms most closely match subconjunctival haemorrhage or episcleritis. By looking at the presenting history subconjunctival haemorrhage is most likely. (Episcleritis is more common in women but not seen as an 'injection' of bright red blood in the eye.) Subconjunctival haemorrhage also has a very sudden onset and fits with the patient's symptoms.

	Discharge absent	Absence of true pain	Visual disturbance	Pupil reflex normal	Eyes affected	Redness
Conjunctivitis – bacterial	✗	✓	✓	✓	✓	✓
Conjunctivitis – viral	✗	✓	✓	✓	✓	✓
Conjunctivitis – allergic	✗	✓	✓	✓	✓	✓
Subconjunctival haemorrhage	✓	✓	✓	✓	✓	✓
Episcleritis	✓	✓	✓	✓	✓	✓
Scleritis	✓	✗	✓	✓	✓	✓
Keratitis	✗	✗	✗	✗	✓	✗
Uveitis	✓	✗	✗	✗	✓	✗
Glaucoma	✓	✗	✗	✗	✓	✗

CASE STUDY 3.3

A mother asks for your advice for her 14-year-old daughter. Emma has a sore and red eye. Questioning reveals that:

- Emma has had the symptoms for 2 to 3 days.
- The redness is located away from the coloured part of the eye.
- There is a slight discharge, although Emma has not noticed much colour in the discharge.
- Her eye feels slightly gritty.
- Her other eye is a little red but not as red as the problem eye.
- She is complaining of slight headaches around her eyes.
- She has taken nothing for the problem and only takes erythromycin for acne from the GP.
- She has not had these types of symptoms before.

a. Using the information in case study 3.2, what do you think is the cause of her symptoms?

Differential diagnosis of bacterial or viral conjunctivitis, but difficult to be definitive, as some of the symptoms overlap between the two conditions.

b. What action are you going to take?

We know that bacterial conjunctivitis will clear without intervention in most cases and viral conjunctivitis is self-limiting, but hygiene measures are important to control the spread of infection. In this case then the person could be told to practice good hygiene measures and, if these fail to control symptoms, then the patient should be offered an antibacterial eye drop.

Answers

1 = d	2 = d	3 = b	4 = c	5 = c	6 = c	7 = a	8 = c	9 = A	10 = A
11 = D	12 = E	13 = C	14 = A	15 = C	16 = D	17 = A	18 = E	19 = A	20 = D
21 = D	22 = A								

Ear conditions

Background

Community pharmacists can offer help to patients with conditions that affect the external and middle ear. However, for full assessment of middle ear problems pharmacists should perform an ear examination using an otoscope. This will currently require most pharmacists to gain further training on their use.

General overview of ear anatomy

The external ear consists of the pinna (Fig. 4.1) and the external auditory meatus (EAM, ear canal). Their function is to collect and transmit sound to the tympanic membrane (eardrum).

The pinna chiefly consists of cartilage and has a firm, elastic consistency. The EAM opens behind the tragus and curves inwards, approximately 3 cm; the inner two-thirds is bony and the outer third cartilaginous. The skin lining the cartilaginous outer portion has a well-developed subcutaneous layer that contains hair follicles, ceruminous and sebaceous glands.

The two portions of the meatus have slightly different directions; the outer cartilaginous portion is upwards and backwards whereas the inner bony portion is forwards and downwards. This is important to know when examining the ear.

History taking and physical examination

A thorough and accurate history coupled with a physical examination of the ear should be undertaken, as certain symptoms can help decide what structure of the ear the problem originates from (Table 4.1) and the likely causes (Table 4.2).

Physical examination

After taking a history of the presenting complaint, the ear should be examined. Before performing an examination explain to the patient what you want to do and gain their consent.

1. First, wash your hands
2. Next, inspect the external ear for redness, swelling and discharge
3. Then, apply pressure to the mastoid area, which is directly behind the pinna (if the area is tender this suggests mastoiditis, a rare complication of otitis media [OM])
4. Next, move the pinna up and down and manipulate the tragus. If either is tender on movement, then this would suggest external ear involvement
5. You should finally examine the EAM. This is best performed using an otoscope
   a. Select correct size speculum for ear canal
   b. Straighten ear canal
      i. Because of the shape of the EAM, when performing an examination the pinna needs to be manipulated to obtain the best view of the ear canal (Fig. 4.2)
   c. Brace hand against face (to accommodate unexpected movement)
   d. Insert otoscope
   e. Visualise eardrum looking for discharge, redness or swelling
   f. Remove otoscope and dispose of speculum in readiness for the next examination

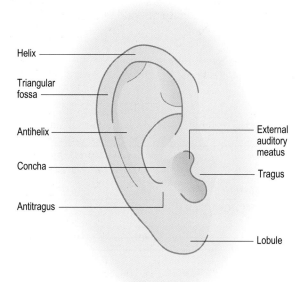

Fig. 4.1 The pinna.

Table 4.1
Ear symptoms and the affected ear structures

Symptom	External ear	Middle ear	Inner ear
Itch	✓		
Pain	✓	✓	
Discharge	✓	✓	
Deafness	✓	✓	✓
Dizziness			✓
Tinnitus			✓

Data from C Acomb, Pharmaceutical Journal, August 1991.

Ear wax impaction

Background

Ear wax is produced in the outer third of the cartilaginous portion of the ear canal by the ceruminous glands. Earwax performs a number of important functions, including mechanical protection of the tympanic membrane, trapping dirt, repelling water and contributing to a slightly acidic medium that has been reported to exert protection against bacterial and fungal infection. Cerumen varies in its composition

Table 4.2
Signs and symptoms of ear pain and possible causes

	Possible causes
Redness and swelling	Perichondritis, haematoma
Discharge	Otitis externa or media. If discharge is mucinous, then it would have originated from middle ear, as EAM has no mucous glands
Pain in mastoid area	Otitis media, mastoiditis
Pain when pressing tragus or moving pinna	Otitis externa

between individuals but can be broadly divided into two types: a 'wet or sticky' type of wax, which is common in children and those of Caucasian and African American ethnicity or 'dry' that is common in Asian populations.

Prevalence and epidemiology

The exact prevalence rates of ear wax impaction is not clear but studies have shown that 2% to 6% of the general population suffer from impacted wax and one Scottish survey of GPs reported an average of nine patients per month (range 5–50 patients) requesting ear wax removal. However, many more patients self-diagnose and medicate without seeking GP assistance, therefore pharmacists have an important role in ensuring that treatment is appropriate. The high number of presentations may be due to patient misconception that ear wax needs to be removed.

A number of patient groups appear to be more prone to ear wax impaction than the general population, for example, patients with congenital anomalies (narrowed ear canal), patients with learning difficulties and those fitted with a hearing aid. The elderly are more susceptible to impaction due to the decrease in cerumen producing glands, resulting in drier and harder ear wax.

Aetiology

The skin of the tympanic membrane is unusual. It is not simply shed as skin is from the rest of the body but is migratory. This is because the auditory canal is the body's only 'dead end' and abrasion of the stratum corneum cannot occur. Skin therefore moves outwards away from the eardrum and out along the ear canal. This means that the ears are largely self-cleaning as the ear canal naturally

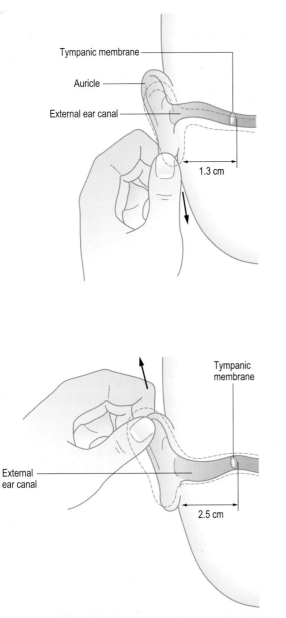

Fig. 4.2 Inspection of the external auditory meatus. Above: in children; below: in adults.

Table 4.3	
Specific questions to ask the patient: Ear wax	
Question	**Relevance**
Course of symptoms	The patient usually has a history of gradual hearing loss with ear wax impaction
Associated symptoms	Dizziness and tinnitus indicates an inner ear problem and should be referred. Ear wax impaction rarely causes tinnitus, vertigo or true pain
History of trauma	Check whether the person has recently tried to clean the ears. This often leads to wax impaction
Use of medicines	If a patient has used an appropriate OTC medication correctly, then this would necessitate referral for further investigation and possibly ear irrigation

problem in the general population. Careful questioning along with inspection of the EAM should mean that wax impaction is readily distinguished from other conditions (Table 4.3).

Clinical features of ear wax impaction

The key features of ear wax impaction are a history of gradual hearing loss (most common symptom), ear discomfort (to variable degrees) and recent attempts to clean ears. Itching, tinnitus and dizziness occur infrequently. Otoscopical examination should reveal excessive wax.

Conditions to eliminate

Trauma of the ear canal

It is common practice for people to use all manners of implements to try and clean the ear canal of wax (e.g., cotton buds, hairgrips and pens). Inspection of the ear canal might reveal laceration of the ear canal and the patient may experience greater conductive deafness because of the wax becoming further impacted. Trauma might also lead to discharge from the ear canal; these cases are probably best referred.

sheds wax from the ear. However, this normal function can be interrupted, usually by misguided attempts to clean ears. Wax therefore becomes trapped, hampering its outward migration.

Arriving at a differential diagnosis

Ear wax is by far the most common external ear problem that pharmacists encounter and is the most common ear

Foreign bodies

Symptoms can mimic ear wax impaction but, over time, discharge and pain is observed. Children are the most likely age group to present with a foreign body in the ear canal and suspected cases need to be referred to a doctor.

> **! TRIGGER POINTS indicative of referral: Ear wax**
>
> | Symptoms/signs | Possible danger/reason for referral |
> |---|---|
> | Dizziness or tinnitus | Suggests inner ear problem; requires further investigation |
> | Pain originating from the middle ear
Fever and general malaise in children | Middle ear infection? |
> | Associated trauma-related conductive deafness
Foreign body in the EAM
OTC medication failure | Requires further investigation by a doctor |

Evidence base for over-the-counter medication

Cerumenolytics have been used for many years to help soften, dislodge and remove impacted ear wax. Two systematic reviews have been published (Burton & Doree, 2009; Hand & Harvey, 2004) to determine whether pharmacological intervention is effective in wax removal. Each had slightly different inclusion criteria, resulting in some trials being included in both but also some trials reviewed in only one of the reviews. All trials reviewed had aspects of poor methodological quality (e.g., lack of clear randomisation and blinding and potential for publication bias as some were company-sponsored trials) and were of relatively small size. The findings from these reviews support the use of oil-based softeners, sodium bicarbonate and sterile water over no treatment at all, but no active treatment proved more superior over any other.

Summary

The evidence from limited trial data suggests simple remedies, such as water, appear to be equally as effective as marketed ear wax products. Additionally, trial data does not clearly point to one particular cerumenolytic having superior efficacy.

Practical prescribing and product selection

Prescribing information relating to ear wax medicines reviewed in the section 'Evidence base for over-the-counter medication' is discussed and summarised in Table 4.4 and useful tips relating to patients presenting with ear wax are given in 'Hints and Tips' in Box 4.1.

Cerumenolytics

Although agents used to soften ear wax have limited evidence of efficacy, they are very safe. They can be given to all patient groups, do not interact with any medicines and can be used in children. They have very few side effects, which if experienced, would appear to be limited to local irritation when first administered. They might, for a short while, increase deafness and the patient should be warned about this possibility.

Table 4.4
Practical prescribing: Summary of medicines for ear wax

Name of medicine	Use in children	Likely side effects	Drug interactions of note	Patients in which care is exercised	Pregnancy & breastfeeding
Oil-based products	No lower age limit stated	None	None	None	OK
Peroxide-based products		Irritation			
Docusate		Irritation			
Sodium bicarbonate		None			
Glycerin	>1 year (Earex Plus)				

HINTS AND TIPS BOX 4.1: EAR WAX

Peanut allergy	Peanut allergy affects approximately 1 in 200 people and patients should be warned about preparations that contain arachis or almond oil
Hypersensitivity reactions to ear drops	Local reactions to the active ingredient or constituents have been reported. If a person has had a previous reaction using ear drops, then care must be exercised
Administration of ear drops	Hold the bottle in your hands for a few minutes before administration to warm the solution. This makes insertion more comfortable
	Lie on a bed with the affected ear pointing towards the ceiling or alternatively tilt your head to one side with the affected ear pointing towards the ceiling
	With one hand straighten the ear canal. Adults pull the pinna up and back and, in children, pull down and back
	Holding the dropper in the other hand, hold it as near as possible to the ear canal without touching it, and place the correct number of drops into the ear canal
	The head should be kept in the same position for several minutes
	Once the head is returned to the normal position, any excess solution should be wiped away with a clean tissue

Oil-based products

Cerumol Ear Drops (Arachis – peanut oil, 57.3%)

The standard dose for adults and children is five drops into the affected ear two or three times a day repeated for up to 3 days. In between administration a plug of cotton wool, moistened with Cerumol or smeared with petroleum jelly, should then be applied to retain the liquid.

Cerumol Olive Oil Drops (olive oil 100%)

For adults and children, two to three drops should be instilled twice a day for up to 7 days. Like Cerumol, a cotton wool plug should be gently placed in the ear to retain the liquid.

Earex (Arachis – peanut oil, almond oil & camphor oil in equal parts)

For adults and children, four drops should be instilled twice a day for up to 4 days. Like Cerumol, a cotton wool plug should be gently placed in the ear to retain the liquid.

Peroxide-based products (Exterol, Earex Advance & Otex range)

For adults and children, five drops should be instilled once or twice daily for at least 3 to 4 days. Unlike Cerumol, the patient should be advised not to plug the ear but retain the drops in the ear for several minutes by keeping the head tilted and then wipe away any surplus. Patients might experience mild, temporary effervescence in the ear as the urea–hydrogen peroxide complex liberates oxygen.

Water-based products (e.g., sodium bicarbonate)

This is only available as a non-proprietary product and should be instilled two to three times a day for up to 3 days.

Docusate (Waxsol, Molcer)

The manufacturers of both products recommend that adults and children use enough ear drops sufficient to fill the affected ear, then place a small plug of cotton wool in the ear and repeat for two consecutive nights.

Glycerin-based products (Earex Plus)

Earex Plus should be used twice daily for 4 days, and it can be given to children over 1 year of age.

References

Burton MJ, Doree C. Ear drops for the removal of ear wax. Cochrane Database of Systematic Reviews 2009, Issue 1. Art. No.: CD004326. http://dx.doi.org/10.1002/14651858.CD004326.pub2.

Hand C, Harvey I. The effectiveness of topical preparations for the treatment of earwax: a systematic review. Br J Gen Prac 2004;54:862–7.

Further reading

Corbridge RJ. Essential ENT Practice. London: Arnold; 1998.
Rodgers R. Hearing loss and wax occlusion in older people. Practice Nursing 2004;15:290–4.

Website

British Tinnitus Association: http://www.tinnitus.org.uk

Otitis externa

Background

Otitis externa refers to generalised inflammation through-out the EAM and is often associated with infection.

Prevalence and epidemiology

The lifetime prevalence of acute otitis externa is 10% and a family doctor will see approximately 16 new cases per year. It occurs in all age groups but is most common in those aged 10 to 14.

It is more common in hot and humid climates and, in Western society, the number of episodes increases in the summer months. People who swim are five times more likely than non-swimmers to develop it, and it is reported to be slightly more common in women than in men.

Aetiology

Primary infection, contact sensitivity or a combination of both causes otitis externa. Changes to microflora result from excessive moisture, leading to skin maceration and skin cerumen breakdown that changes the microflora of the ear canal. Pathogens implicated with acute otitis externa include *Pseudomonas aeruginosa*, *Staphylococcus* spp. and *Streptococcus pyogenes*. Fungal overgrowth with *Aspergillus niger* is also seen especially after prolonged antibiotic treatment.

Certain local or general factors can precipitate otitis externa. Local causes include trauma or discharge from the middle ear and general causes include seborrhoeic dermatitis, psoriasis and skin infections.

Arriving at a differential diagnosis

In common with ear wax impaction, otitis externa is easily recognised, providing a careful history and ear examination has been conducted. However, other otological conditions can present with similar symptoms of pain and discharge (Table 4.5).

It is therefore important to differentiate between otitis externa and conditions that require referral. Table 4.6 highlights some of the questions that should be asked of the patient to establish a differential diagnosis.

Clinical features of otitis externa

Otitis externa is characterised by itching and irritation, which, depending on the severity, can become intense. This

Table 4.5
Causes of ear canal symptoms and their relative incidence in community pharmacy

Incidence	Cause
Most likely	Otitis media
Likely	Otitis externa caused by infection or trauma
Unlikely	Dermatitis (contact, allergic, seborrhoeic or atopic)
Very unlikely	Perichondritis, malignancy

Table 4.6
Specific questions to ask the patient: Otitis externa

Question	Relevance
Symptom presentation	Principal symptom of acute otitis externa is itch/irritation and pain
Discharge	Otitis media is the most common cause of ear discharge and is usually mucopurulent. If discharge is present with otitis externa, then discharge would not be mucopurulent
Systemic symptoms	Otitis externa should not present with any systemic symptoms. Fever and cold symptoms are often present in otitis media. In all forms of dermatitis, systemic symptoms should not be present

provokes the patient to scratch the skin of the EAM, resulting in trauma and pain. Patients might not present until pain becomes a prominent feature. However, there should be a period when irritation is the only symptom apparent. Chewing and manipulation of the tragus and pinna can exacerbate pain. Otorrhoea (ear discharge) follows and the skin of the EAM can become oedematous, leading to conductive hearing loss. On examination the ear canal or external ear, or both, appear red, swollen, or eczematous (Fig. 4.3).

Conditions to eliminate

Likely causes

Acute otitis media
Acute otitis media is most common in children aged 3 to 6 years old and 75% of cases will be seen in children under

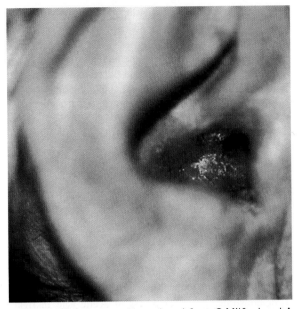

Fig. 4.3 Otitis externa. Reproduced from C Milford and A Rowlands, 1999, Shared Care for ENT, Isis Medical Media Ltd, Martin Dunitz Publishers, with permission of Taylor & Francis Books UK.

the age of 10 years. In older children, ear pain/earache is the predominant feature and tends to be throbbing. In young children this is often manifested as irritability or crying with characteristic ear tugging/rubbing. Systemic symptoms, such as fever and loss of appetite, can also be present. An examination of the ear should reveal a red/ yellow and bulging tympanic membrane with a loss of normal landmarks. Over three quarters of episodes resolve within 3 days without treatment and current UK guidelines do not advocate the routine use of antibiotics. Patients should be managed with analgesia (paracetamol or ibuprofen) unless they are systemically unwell or are under 2 years of age and have discharge. These cases should be referred for consideration of antibiotics (a 5-day course of amoxicillin).

Children may go on to have persistent otitis media. This is either known as chronic suppurative otitis media or otitis media with effusion (glue ear). Suppurative otitis media is characterised with ear discharge (through perforation in the tympanic membrane), lasting more than 2 weeks that is not associated with pain or fever. Glue ear is symptomless, apart from impaired hearing, but can have a negative impact on a child's language and educational development if unresolved.

Unlikely causes

Dermatitis

Allergic, contact, seborrhoeic and atopic forms of dermatitis can occur on the external ear. Itch is a prominent symptom and could be mistaken for otitis externa; however, there should be no ear pain or discharge associated with dermatitis. In addition, in seborrhoeic and atopic forms, skin involvement elsewhere should be obvious.

Very unlikely causes

Perichondritis

In severe cases of otitis externa the inflammation can spread from the outer ear canal to the pinna, resulting in perichondritis (Fig. 4.4). Referral is needed, as systemic antibiotics are required.

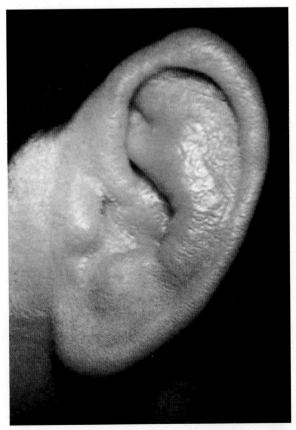

Fig. 4.4 Perichondritis. Courtesy of Joydeep Som, MD. Reproduced from WG Belleza and S Kalman, 2006, Medical Clinics of North America, 2006, Emergencies in the Outpatient Setting: Part 1, Elsevier, with permission.

Trauma

Recent trauma (e.g., blow to the head) can cause an auricular haematoma. This is best known as a cauliflower ear and requires non-urgent referral.

Malignant tumours

Basal and squamous cell carcinomas are typically slow growing and associated with increasing age. Any elderly patient presenting with an ulcerative or crusting lesion needs referral.

> ❗ **TRIGGER POINTS indicative of referral: Otitis externa**
>
> | Symptoms/signs | Possible danger/ reason for referral |
> |---|---|
> | Generalised inflammation of the pinna | Possibly indicates perichondritis |
> | Impaired hearing in children not associated with ear wax | Development of glue ear? |
> | Mucopurulent discharge Systemically unwell | Otitis media? |
> | Slow-growing growths on the pinna in elderly people | Possibly indicate malignancy |

Evidence base for over-the-counter medication

OTC treatment of otitis externa is currently very limited. Inflammation of the EAM would respond to corticosteroids; however, all ear drops/sprays that contain steroids are currently only available on prescription.

This limits OTC options to either oral antihistamines – to try and combat itching and irritation – or analgesia to control pain.

Two small trials comparing the analgesic effect of choline salicylate against aspirin and paracetamol have been conducted. Both trials concluded that choline salicylate reduced pain more quickly than oral analgesia (Hewitt, 1970; Lawrence, 1970).

In addition, acetic acid is available OTC (Earcalm Spray, 2% acetic acid) and is indicated for the treatment of superficial infections of the EAM. The British National Formulary 69 states 'that it may be used to treat mild otitis externa but more severe cases an anti-inflammatory preparation with or without an anti-infective drug is required'. This advice appears to be taken from a 2003 BMJ article (van Balen et al.) that found acetic acid to be far less effective than acetic acid combined with a steroid or a steroid/anti-infective combination. A further review article published in 2008 also found insufficient evidence to demonstrate the effectiveness of acetic acid in treating otitis externa (Hajioff & Mackeith, 2008). However, a Cochrane Review (Kaushik et al., 2010) concluded that acetic acid was as effective as antibiotics and steroids for up to a 1-week treatment. Current UK guidelines (Clinical Knowledge Summaries) therefore advocate its use for symptoms of mild discomfort and/or pruritus where no deafness or discharge is present.

Practical prescribing and product selection

Prescribing information relating to otitis externa medicines reviewed in the section 'Evidence base for over-the-counter medication' is discussed below and summarised in Table 4.7. Pain associated with otitis media can be managed with simple analgesics, such as paracetamol and ibuprofen.

Table 4.7
Practical prescribing: Summary of medicines for otitis externa

Name of medicine	Use in children	Likely side effects	Drug interactions of note	Patients in which care is exercised	Pregnancy & breastfeeding
Choline salicylate	>1 year	None reported	None	None	OK
Acetic acid	>12 years	Transient stinging or burning sensation			

References

Hajioff D, Mackeith S. Otitis Media. BMJ Clinical Evidence
2008;06:510.

Hewitt HR. Clinical evaluation of choline salicylate ear drops.
The Practitioner 1970;204:438–40.

Kaushik V, Malik T, Saeed SR. Interventions for acute otitis
externa. Cochrane Database of Systematic Reviews
2010, Issue 1. Art. No.: CD004740. http://dx.doi.
org/10.1002/14651858.CD004740.pub2.

Lawrence N. A comparison of analgesic therapies for the relief
of acute otalgia. Br J Clin Pract 1970;24:478–9.

van Balen FA, Smit WM, Zuithoff NP, et al. Clinical efficacy
of three common treatments in acute otitis externa
in primary care: randomised controlled trial. BMJ
2003;327:1201–5.

Further reading

Milford C, Rowlands A. Shared Care for ENT. Oxford: Isis
Medical Media Ltd; 1999.

Rosenfeld RM, Brown L, Cannon CR, et al. Clinical practice
guideline: acute otitis externa. Otolaryngol Head Neck
Surg 2006;134:S4–S23.

Choline salicylate (Earex Plus – choline salicylate 43.22%, glycerol 12.62%)

Choline salicylate can be given to adults and children over the age of 1 year. The EAM should be completely filled with drops and then plugged with cotton wool soaked with the ear drops. This should be repeated every 3 to 4 hours.

Acetic acid (Earcalm Spray)

This can be given to adults and children aged 12 and over. The dosage is one spray (60 mg) into the affected ear at least three times a day. The maximum dosage frequency is one spray every 2 to 3 hours. Treatment should be continued until 2 days after symptoms have disappeared but, if symptoms do not improve or worsen within 48 hours, the patient should be referred to a medical practitioner. The spray should not be used for more than 7 days.

4

Self-assessment questions

The following questions are intended to supplement the text. Two levels of questions are provided: multiple choice questions and case studies. The multiple choice questions are designed to test factual recall and the case studies allow knowledge to be applied to a practice setting.

Multiple choice questions

4.1 Which of the listed products has the most evidence of efficacy in treating ear wax?

    a. Oil-based products (e.g., Cerumol)
    b. Peroxide-based products (e.g., Otex)
    c. Water-based products (e.g., sodium bicarbonate)
    d. Saline
    e. All products are comparable

4.2 From the list of symptoms below, which are most closely associated with outer ear problems?

    a. Itch and pain
    b. Pain and discharge
    c. Discharge and deafness
    d. Deafness and dizziness
    e. Dizziness and tinnitus

4.3 Tenderness associated with manipulation of the tragus suggests what?

    a. Middle ear problem
    b. Inner ear problem
    c. Outer ear problem
    d. Perichondritis
    e. Mastoiditis

4.4 Which of the listed patient groups is most susceptible to suffer from ear wax impaction?

    a. Young children
    b. Young adults
    c. Middle-aged adults
    d. The elderly
    e. All groups are equally susceptible

4.5 A patient presents with a left ear problem. Which of the following symptoms would most strongly suggest a referral to the GP?

    a. Redness in the outer ear
    b. Pain
    c. Hearing loss
    d. Mucopurulent discharge
    e. Swollen ear canal

4.6 Mrs Brown brings in her 8-year-old son who has been complaining of ear pain that he has had for the last 24 hours. He is generally well and otoscopical investigation reveals a red/yellow and bulging tympanic membrane. What course of action are you going to take?

    a. Tell Mrs Brown her son has otitis media, and the symptoms will resolve on their own. No further action is required.
    b. Tell Mrs Brown her son has otitis media, and the symptoms will resolve on their own. The pain can be managed with simple analgesia.
    c. Tell Mrs Brown her son has otitis media and the symptoms will resolve on their own. However, it would be best to get him checked out by the GP.
    d. Tell Mrs Brown her son has otitis media, and the symptoms will NOT resolve on their own. He needs antibiotics and must see the doctor.
    e. Tell Mrs Brown her son has otitis media, and the symptoms will resolve on their own. The pain can be managed with ear drops.

4.7 Manufacturers of ear wax products recommend plugging the ear with cotton wool except for:

    a. Cerumol
    b. Earex
    c. Earex Advance
    d. Molcer
    e. Waxsol

4.8 Which patient group is most susceptible to otitis externa?

    a. Infants
    b. Children under 5 years old
    c. Elderly
    d. Teenagers
    e. People in their thirties

Questions 4.9 to 4.14 concern the following signs and symptoms:

A.   Itch
B.   Discharge

C. Deafness
D. Ear tugging
E. Swollen pinna
F. Lesions slow to heal
G. Tinnitus
H. Dizziness

Select from A to E, which of the above is most associated with the following statements:

4.9 Otitis media

4.10 Ear wax

4.11 Perichondritis

4.12 Otitis externa

4.13 Ménière's disease

4.14 Malignancy

Questions 4.15 to 4.17: For each of these questions *one or more* of the responses is (are) correct. Decide which of the responses is (are) correct. Then choose:

A. If a, b and c are correct
B. If a and b only are correct
C. If b and c only are correct
D. If a only is correct
E. If c only is correct

Directions summarised

A	B	C	D	E
a, b and c	a and b only	b and c only	a only	c only

4.15 Which of the following signs or symptoms would warrant referral to a doctor?

a. Tinnitus
b. Bulging tympanic membrane
c. Conductive deafness

4.16 Which of the following symptoms are suggestive of otitis media in young children:

a. Irritability
b. Throbbing ear pain
c. Deafness

4.17 Malaise or fever is seen in:

a. Otitis externa
b. Labyrinthitis (otitis interna)
c. Otitis media

Questions 4.18 to 4.20: These questions consist of a statement in the left-hand column, followed by a statement in the right-hand column. You need to:

● decide whether the first statement is true or false
● decide whether the second statement is true or false

Then choose:

A. If both statements are true, and the second statement is a correct explanation of the first statement
B. If both statements are true, but the second statement is NOT a correct explanation of the first statement
C. If the first statement is true, but the second statement is false
D. If the first statement is false, but the second statement is true
E. If both statements are false

Directions summarised

	1st statement	2nd statement	
A	True	True	2nd explanation is a correct explanation of the first
B	True	True	2nd statement is not a correct explanation of the first
C	True	False	
D	False	True	
E	False	False	

	First statement	*Second statement*
4.18	Ear wax removal is generally not necessary	If ear wax products are used and ineffective, then ear irrigation can be tried
4.19	Acetic acid is effective for otitis externa	It works by killing bacteria
4.20	Simple analgesia is recommended for otitis media	Antibiotics are now no longer recommended

Case study

CASE STUDY 4.1

Mr SW has asked to speak to the pharmacist as his ear is bothering him.

a. Discuss the appropriately worded questions you will need to ask Mr SW to determine the diagnosis of his symptoms.

   Questions to establish a differential diagnosis:
   Nature of symptoms
   Progression of symptoms (check the order in which the symptoms are presented)
   Any precipitating factors
   Questions to help confirm the diagnosis
   Previous history of symptoms
   Questions to help establish the severity of symptoms
   Whether the symptoms are getting better, worse or staying about the same
   Degree of discomfort
   If medication has already been tried

   Symptoms reveal Mr SW has a loss of hearing in his left ear. Symptoms started a few days ago and his hearing is now worse. He describes it as if he has been swimming and got water in his ear. He is unaware of why he has the symptoms; he has not had these symptoms before; symptoms are just a bit bothersome, as he is struggling to hear conversations properly at work, especially in meetings. He has tried no medication.

b. Based on this description what would be your differential diagnosis?

Ear wax

1. You ask if it is OK to look in his ear with an otoscope to confirm your differential diagnosis.

   c. How would a physical examination help confirm or refute your diagnosis?

2. You would be expecting to see visible ear wax impaction and, if the eardrum was observable, this should be normal and show no redness, bulging or loss of landmarks.

4

CASE STUDY 4.2

Mrs PR asks to speak to the pharmacist about her 7-year-old son Luke. She wants some Calpol to treat his earache.

a. How do you respond?

The pharmacist needs to determine the cause of the pain and establish the severity of the earache.

b. Based on the age of the child what would be your initial thoughts on a differential diagnosis?

Otitis media (OM) immediately springs to mind. It is a very common complaint in this age group and earache is a predominant symptom.

c. Basing your initial thoughts on a diagnosis of otitis media, what questions would you ask to help confirm these thoughts?

Are there any associated symptoms?

- It would be likely they will be irritable and off-colour if (OM).

Description of the pain

- Pain is usually described as throbbing

You find out that the earache has been present for a day or so and Luke is more irritable than normal. Mrs PR says he has a temperature, but she has not actually taken it. Apart from this, Luke has no other symptoms. However, he has had this problem about a year ago and was given Calpol then and it seemed to have helped.

d. What course of action are you going to take?

It appears Luke has a middle ear infection. Examination of the tympanic membrane would confirm this and, if possible, should be carried out in the pharmacy. Instigation of Calpol seems reasonable, and Mrs PR could buy some for Luke. If symptoms do not subside in the next 24 h, then referral to the doctor would be appropriate.

Answers

| 1 = e | 2 = a | 3 = c | 4 = d | 5 = d | 6 = b | 7 = c | 8 = d | 9 = D | 10 = C |
| 11 = E | 12 = A | 13 = G | 14 = F | 15 = B | 16 = D | 17 = E | 18 = B | 19 = C | 20 = C |

Central nervous system

Age <12 referel
Prignancy referel   give paracetamol

Cluster worsen at night
Cancer - headach   worsen at Morning.
If then is nausa and vomiting ⟶ need to Concern !!

In this chapter

Background

The number of patient requests for advice and/or products to treat headache and insomnia make up a smaller proportion of pharmacist's workload than other conditions such as coughs and colds yet sales for analgesics and hypnotics are extremely high (£360 million for oral adult analgesia and £45 million for sleep aids in 2014). The vast majority of patients will present with benign and non-serious conditions and only in very few cases will sinister pathology be responsible.

General overview of CNS anatomy

The central nervous system (CNS) comprises the brain and spinal cord. Its major function is to process and integrate information arriving from sensory pathways and communicate an appropriate response back via afferent pathways. CNS anatomy is complex and outside the scope of this book. The reader is referred to any good anatomical text for a comprehensive description of CNS anatomy.

History taking

A differential diagnosis for all CNS conditions will be made solely from questions asked of the patient. It is especially important that a social and work-related history is sought alongside questions asking about the patient's presenting symptoms because pressure and stress are implicated in the cause of conditions such as headache and insomnia.

Headache

Background

Headache is not a disease state or condition but rather a symptom, of which there are many causes. Headache can be the major presenting complaint, for example in migraine, cluster and tension-type headache, or one of many symptoms, for example in an upper respiratory tract infection. Table 5.1 highlights those conditions that may be seen in a community pharmacy in which headache is one of the major presenting symptoms.

Headache classification

If the pharmacist is to advise on appropriate treatment and referral, then it is essential to make an accurate diagnosis. However, with so many disorders having headache as a symptom, pharmacists should endeavour to follow an agreed classification system. The International Headache Society (IHS) classification is now almost universally accepted (Table 5.2). The system first distinguishes between primary and secondary headache disorders. This is useful to the community pharmacist, as any **secondary headache disorder is symptomatic of an underlying cause and would normally require referral**. In the IHS system, primary headaches are classified on symptom profiles,

Table 5.1
Causes of headache and their relative incidence in community pharmacy

Incidence	Cause
Most likely	Tension-type headache
Likely	Migraine, sinusitis, eye strain
Unlikely	Cluster headache, medication-overuse headache, temporal arteritis, trigeminal neuralgia, depression
Very unlikely	Glaucoma, meningitis, subarachnoid haemorrhage, raised intracranial pressure

relying on careful questioning, coupled with epidemiological data on the distribution a particular headache disorder has within the population.

Prevalence and epidemiology

The exact prevalence of headache is not precisely known. However, virtually everyone will have suffered from a headache at sometime; it is probably the most common pain syndrome experienced by people. It has been estimated that up to 80–90% of the population will experience one or more headaches per year.

Tension-type headache has been reported to affect between 30% and 80% of people in Western countries. Migraine affects approximately 15–20% of women and

Table 5.2
The International Headache Society classification of headache

Primary headaches	**1.** Migraine, including:
	  1.1 Migraine without aura
	  1.2 Migraine with aura
	2. Tension-type headache, including:
	  2.1 Infrequent episodic tension-type headache
	  2.2 Frequent episodic tension-type headache
	  2.3 Chronic tension-type headache
		3. Cluster headache and other trigeminal autonomic cephalalgias, including:
		  3.1 Cluster headache
		4. Other primary headaches

Secondary headaches	**5.** Headache attributed to head and/or neck trauma, including:
	  5.2 Chronic post-traumatic headache
	6. Headache attributed to cranial or cervical vascular disorder, including:
	  6.2.2 Headache attributed to subarachnoid haemorrhage
	  6.4.1 Headache attributed to giant cell arteritis
	7. Headache attributed to non-vascular intracranial disorder, including:
	  7.1.1 Headache attributed to idiopathic intracranial hypertension
	  7.4 Headache attributed to intracranial neoplasm
	8. Headache attributed to a substance or its withdrawal, including:
	  8.1.3 Carbon monoxide-induced headache
	  8.1.4 Alcohol-induced headache
		8.2 Medication-overuse headache
		  8.2.1 Ergotamine-overuse headache
		  8.2.2 Triptan-overuse headache
		  8.2.3 Analgesic-overuse headache
		9. Headache attributed to infection, including:
		  9.1 Headache attributed to intracranial infection
		10. Headache attributed to disorder of homoeostasis
		11. Headache or facial pain, attributed to disorder of cranium, neck, eyes, ears, nose, sinuses, teeth, mouth or other facial or cranial structures including:
		  11.2.1 Cervicogenic headache
		  11.3.1 Headache attributed to acute glaucoma
		12. Headache attributed to psychiatric disorder

Neuralgias and other headaches	**13.** Cranial neuralgias, central and primary facial pain and other headaches including: 13.1 Trigeminal neuralgia	**14.** Other headache, cranial neuralgia, central or primary facial pain

Source: Adapted by the British Association of Headache (BASH) from the International Headache Society Classification Subcommittee, The International Classification of Headache Disorders, 3rd ed. Cephalalgia 2013, Blackwell Publishing, reproduced with permission.

is approximately two to three times more common than in men. Prevalence peaks between 30 to 40 years of age. Conversely, cluster headache, which is also most prevalent in the 30–40-year-old age group, is five to six times more common in men.

Aetiology

Considering headache affects almost everyone, the mechanisms that bring about headache are still poorly understood. Pain control systems modulate headaches of all types, independent of the cause. However, the exact aetiology of tension-type headache and migraine are still to be fully elucidated. Tension-type headache is commonly referred to as muscle contraction headache, as electromyography has shown pericranial muscle contraction, which was often exacerbated by stress. However, similar muscle contraction is noted in migraine sufferers, and this theory has now fallen out of favour. Consequently, no current theory for tension-type headache is unanimously endorsed, but recent studies suggest a neurobiological basis.

Traditionally, migraine was thought to be a result of abnormal dilation of cerebral blood vessels but this vascular theory cannot explain all migraine symptoms. The use of $5\text{-}HT_1$ agonists to reduce and stop migraine attacks suggests some neurochemical pathophysiology. Migraine is therefore probably a combination of vascular and neurochemical changes – the neurovascular hypothesis. Migraine also appears to have a genetic component with about 70% of patients having a first-degree relative with a history of migraine.

Arriving at a differential diagnosis

Given that headache is extremely common, and most patients will self-medicate, any patient requesting advice should ideally be questioned by the pharmacist, as it is likely that the headache has either not responded to OTC medication or is troublesome enough for the patient to seek advice. Arrival at an accurate diagnosis will rely exclusively on questioning; therefore a number of headache-specific questions should be asked (Table 5.3).

Table 5.3
Specific questions to ask the patient: Headache

Question	Relevance
Onset of headache	In early childhood or as a young adult, primary headache is most likely. After 50 years of age the likelihood of a secondary cause is much greater
	Headache that follows head trauma might indicate post-concussive headache or intracranial pathology
Frequency and timing	Headache associated with the menstrual cycle or at certain times, e.g., weekend or holidays, suggests migraine
	Headaches that occur in clusters at the same time of day/night suggest cluster headache
	Headaches that occur on most days with the same pattern suggests tension-type headache
Location of pain (see Fig. 5.1)	Cluster headache is nearly always unilateral in frontal and ocular areas (can also be felt in temporal areas)
	Migraine headache is unilateral in 70% of patients but can change from side to side from attack to attack
	Tension-type headache is often bilateral, either in frontal or occipital areas, and described as a tight band
	Very localised pain suggests an organic cause
Severity of pain	Pain is a subjective, personal experience and there are therefore no objective measures. Using a numeric pain intensity scale should allow you to assess the level of pain the person is experiencing: 0 represents no pain and 10 the worst pain possible
	Dull and band-like suggests tension-type headache
	Severe to intense ache or throbbing suggests haemorrhage or aneurysm
	Piercing, boring, searing eye pain suggests cluster headache
	Moderate to severe throbbing pain that often starts as dull ache suggests migraine

(Continued)

Table 5.3 Specific questions to ask the patient: Headache (Continued)	
Question	**Relevance**
Triggers	Pain that worsens on exertion, coughing and bending suggests a tumour
	Food (in 10% of sufferers), menstruation and relaxation after stress are indicative of migraine
	Lying down makes cluster headache worse
Attack duration	Typically migraine attacks last between a few hours and 3 days
	Tension-type headaches last between a few hours and several days, e.g., a week or more
	Cluster headache will only normally last 2–3 hours
Associated symptoms	Headache and fever at same time imply an infectious cause
	Nausea suggests migraine or more sinister pathology, e.g., subarachnoid haemorrhage and space-occupying lesions
	Scalp tenderness is associated with temporal arteritis

In addition to these symptom-specific questions, the pharmacist should also enquire about the person's social history because social factors – mainly stress – play a significant role in headache. Ask about the person's work and family status to determine whether the person is suffering from greater levels of stress than normal.

Clinical features of headache

In a community pharmacy the overwhelming majority of patients (80–90%) will present with tension-type headache. A further 10% will have migraine. Very few will have other primary headache disorders, and fewer still will have a secondary headache disorder (see Table 5.1).

Tension-type headache

Tension-type headaches can be classed as either episodic or chronic. Episodic tension-type headache can be further subdivided into infrequent and frequent forms. Most patients will present to the pharmacist with the infrequent episodic form – that is, they occur less than once per month. Headaches last from 30 minutes to up to 7 days in duration and often the patient will have a history of recent headaches. They might have tried OTC medication without complete symptom resolution or say that the headaches are becoming more frequent. Pain is bifrontal or bioccipital, generalised and non-throbbing (Fig. 5.1). The patient might

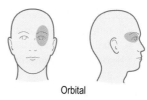
Frontal — Tension or migraine

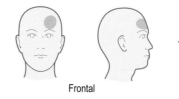
Orbital — Cluster, glaucoma, sinusitis

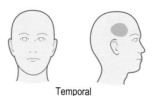
Occipital — Subarachnoid haemorrhage, tension

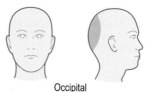
Temporal — Migraine, temporal arteritis

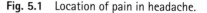

Fig. 5.1 Location of pain in headache.

describe the pain as a tightness or a weight pressing down on their head. The pain is gradual in onset and tends to worsen progressively throughout the day. Pain is normally mild to moderate and not aggravated by movement, although it is often worse under pressure or stress. Nausea and vomiting are not associated with tension-type headache and it rarely causes photo or phonophobia. Overall, the headache has a limited impact on the individual.

Patients who have frequent episodic tension-type headaches suffer more frequent headaches (more than monthly episodes) and over time these can develop into chronic tension-type headache. Headaches occur for more than 15 days per month and might be daily and last for at least 3 months. These types of headaches can severely affect the patient's quality of life and should not be managed by the community pharmacist.

Migraine

There are an estimated 5 million migraine sufferers in the UK, half of whom have not been diagnosed by their doctor. The peak onset for a person to have their first attack is in adolescence or as a young adult (mean age of onset for men is 14; for women it is 18 years of age). Migraines are rare over the age of 50 and anyone in this age group presenting for the first time with migraine-like symptoms should be referred to the doctor to eliminate secondary causes of headache. If this is not their first attack they will normally have a history of recurrent and episodic attacks of headache. Attacks last anywhere between 4 and 72 hours. The average length of an attack is 24 hours. Migraines are three times as common in women than in men. The IHS classification recognises several subtypes of migraine, but the two major subtypes are migraine with aura (classical migraine) and migraine without aura (common migraine). A migraine attack can be divided into three phases:

- Phase one: Premonitory phase, which can occur hours or possibly a couple of days before the headache. The patient might complain of a change in mood or notice a change in behaviour. Feelings of well-being, yawning, poor concentration and food cravings have been reported. These prodromal features are highly individual but are relatively consistent to each patient. Identification of 'triggers' is sometimes possible (Table 5.4)
- Phase two: Headache with or without aura

Table 5.4
Triggers and strategies to reduce migraine attacks

Trigger	Strategy
Stress	Maintain regular sleep pattern Perform regular exercise Modify work environment Do relaxation techniques, e.g., yoga
Diet Any food can be a potential trigger but food that is implicated includes: Cheese Citrus fruit Chocolate	Maintain a food diary. If an attack occurs within 6 h of food ingestion and is reproducible, it is likely that it is a trigger for migraine Eat regularly and do not skip meals Note: Detecting triggers is complicated because they appear to be cumulative, jointly contributing to a 'threshold' above which attacks are initiated.

- Phase three: Resolution phase, as the headache subsides, the patient can feel lethargic, tired and drained before recovery, which might take several hours.

Headache with aura (classic migraine)

This accounts for less than 25% of migraine cases. The aura, which is fully reversible, develops over 5 to 20 min and can last for up to 1 h. It can either be visual (accounts for about 90% of auras experienced) or neurological. Visual auras can take many guises, such as scotomas (blind spots), fortification spectra (zig-zag lines) or flashing and flickering lights. Neurological auras (pins and needles) typically start in the hand, migrating up the arm before jumping to the face and lips. Within 60 min of the aura ending the headache usually occurs. Pain is unilateral, throbbing and moderate to severe. Sometimes the pain becomes more generalised and diffuse. Physical activity and movement tends to intensify the pain. Nausea affects almost all patients but less than a third will vomit. Photophobia and phonophobia often mean patients will seek out a dark, quiet room to relieve their symptoms. The patient might also suffer from fatigue, find concentrating difficult and be irritable.

Headache without aura (common migraine)

The remaining 75% of sufferers do not experience an aura but do suffer from all other symptoms as described above.

Other likely causes of headache

Eye strain

People who perform prolonged close work, for example VDU operators, can suffer from frontal-aching headache. In the first instance patients should be referred to an optician for a routine eye check.

Sinusitis

The pain tends to be relatively localised, usually orbital, unilateral and dull. For further information on the signs and symptoms of sinusitis see page 22. A course of decongestants could be tried, but if treatment failure occurs, referral to the doctor for possible antibiotic therapy would be appropriate.

Unlikely causes

Cluster headache

Cluster headache is predominantly a condition that affects men over the age of 30. Typically the headache occurs at the same time each day with abrupt onset and lasts between 10 minutes and 3 hours, with 50% of patients experiencing night-time symptoms. Patients are awoken 2 to 3 h after falling asleep with very intense unilateral orbital-boring pain. Additionally, conjunctival redness, lacrimation and nasal congestion (which laterally becomes watery) are observed on the pain side of the head. Facial flushing and sweating is common. Patients tend to be restless and irritable and often 'pace the floor'.

The condition is characterised by periods of acute attacks, typically lasting a number of weeks to a few months with sufferers experiencing between one and three attacks per day. This is then followed by periods of remission, which can last months or years. During acute phases, alcohol can trigger an attack. Nausea is usually absent and a family history uncommon.

Referral is required, as sumatriptan, the drug of choice to treat acute attacks, does not have an OTC license for cluster headache. Verapamil is also used as a prophylactic agent.

Medication-overuse headache

Patients with long-standing symptoms of headache who regularly use medicines to treat pain can develop medication-overuse headache. Pain receptors (nociceptors) instead of being 'switched off' when analgesics are taken are in fact 'switched on'. The consequence is a cycle where patients take more and more painkillers that are stronger and stronger to control the pain. Patients will experience daily or near daily headaches that are described as dull and nagging. Obviously in these cases a medication history is essential and should prompt the pharmacist to refer the patient to the doctor. Treatment is to stop all analgesia for a number of weeks and requires careful planning. Symptoms usually resolve within 2 months of withdrawing medication.

Temporal arteritis

The temporal arteries that run vertically up the sides of the head, just in front of the ears, can become inflamed. When this happens, they are tender to touch and might be visibly thickened. Unilateral pain is experienced, and the person generally feels unwell with fever, myalgia and general malaise. Scalp tenderness is also possible, especially when combing the hair. It is most commonly seen in the elderly, especially in women. Prompt treatment with oral corticosteroids is required, as the retinal artery can become compromised, leading to blindness. Urgent referral is needed.

Trigeminal neuralgia

Pain follows the course of either the second (maxillary; supplying the cheeks) or third (mandibular; supplying the chin, lower lip and lower cheek) division of the nerve, leading to pain experienced in the cheek, jaws, lips or gums. Pain is short lived, usually lasting only a couple of minutes but is severe and lancing and is almost always unilateral. It is three times more common in women than in men.

Depression

A symptom of depression can be tension-type headaches. However, other more prominent symptoms should be present. The DSM-5 criteria are often used to aid a diagnosis of depression. The pharmacist should check for a loss of interest or pleasure in activities, fatigue, inability to concentrate, loss of appetite, weight loss, sleep disturbances and constipation. If the patient exhibits some of these characteristics (especially loss of interest in doing things and feeling down/hopeless) then referral to the doctor is necessary. Recent changes to the patient's social circumstances, for example loss of job, might also support your differential diagnosis.

Very unlikely causes

Glaucoma

Patients experience a frontal/orbital headache with severe pain in the eye. The eye appears red and is painful. Vision is blurred and the cornea can look cloudy. In addition, the patient might notice haloes around the vision. For further information on glaucoma see page 58.

Meningitis

Severe generalised headache associated with fever (although neonates may not have fever), an obviously ill patient, neck stiffness, and nausea/vomiting and latterly a non-blanching purpuric rash are classically associated with meningitis. However, not all patients will exhibit all symptoms, and any child that has difficulty in placing their chin on their chest and is running a temperature above 38.9° C (102° F), should be referred urgently.

Subarachnoid haemorrhage

The patient will experience very intense and severe pain, located in the occipital region. Nausea and vomiting are often present and a decreased lack of consciousness is prominent. Patients often describe the headache as the worse headache they have ever had. It is extremely unlikely that a patient would present in the pharmacy with such symptoms but if one did then immediate referral would be needed.

Conditions causing raised intracranial pressure

Space-occupying lesions (brain tumour, haematoma and abscess) can give rise to varied headache symptoms, ranging from severe chronic pain to intermittent moderate pain. Pain can be localised or diffuse and tends to be more severe in the morning with a gradual improvement over the next few hours. Coughing, sneezing, bending and lying down can worsen the pain. Nausea and vomiting are common. After a prolonged period of time neurological symptoms, such as drowsiness, confusion, lack of concentration, difficulty with speech and paraesthesia, start to become evident.

Any patient with a recent history (lasting 2–3 months) of head trauma, headache of long-standing duration or insidious worsening of symptoms, especially associated with decreased consciousness and vomiting, must be referred urgently for fuller evaluation.

Fig. 5.2 (and summary table in Case Study 5.1) will help in the differentiation of serious and non-serious causes of headache.

TRIGGER POINTS indicative of referral: Headache

Symptoms/signs	Possible danger/reason for referral
Headache in children under 12 years old who have a stiff neck, high temperature or skin rash	Meningitis?
Headache occurs after recent (1–3 months) trauma or injury	Haematoma?
Nausea and/or vomiting in the absence of migraine symptoms	All can suggest sinister pathology and require further investigation
Neurological symptoms, if migraine is excluded, especially change in consciousness	
New or severe headache in patients over age 50	
Progressive worsening of headache symptoms over time	
Very sudden and/or severe onset of headache	
Headache unresponsive to analgesics	Simple analgesia is effective; if this has not worked the patient's symptoms require further investigation. Suspect medication-overuse headache.
Headache that has lasted for more than 2 weeks	Most acute (or uncomplicated) cases will last less than 2 weeks. Further investigation required

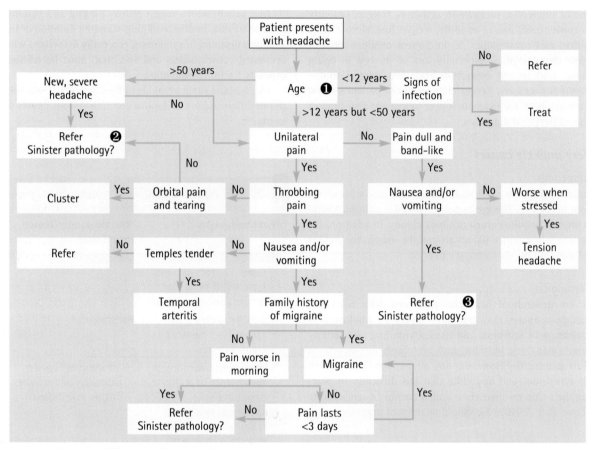

Fig. 5.2 Primer for differential diagnosis of headache.

❶ Age

Caution should be exercised in children who present with headache. Although the majority of headaches will not have an organic cause, children under 12 are probably best referred if they show no signs of a systemic infection (e.g., fever, malaise).

❷ Referral for suspected sinister pathology

With increasing age it is more likely that a sinister cause of headache is responsible for the symptoms, especially if the patient has not experienced similar headache symptoms before. Mass lesions (tumours and haematoma) and temporal arteritis should be considered.

❸ Referral for suspected sinister pathology

Nausea and vomiting in the absence of migraine-like symptoms should be treated seriously. Mass lesions and subarachnoid haemorrhage need to be eliminated.

Evidence base for over-the-counter medication

Simple analgesia (paracetamol, aspirin and ibuprofen) has shown clinical benefit in relieving migraine attacks. A recent Cochrane review (Derry & Moore, 2013) found that a single oral dose of paracetamol 1000 mg was effective in relieving moderate to severe migraine symptoms, compared with placebo. Approximately 20% of patients will be pain free in 2 hours (reduced from moderate to severe) and approximately 60% of patients can expect a reduction in the severity of pain from moderate/severe to mild pain by 2 hours. (Note that the addition of metoclopramide saw an efficacy equivalent to a dose of 100 mg sumatriptan – such products are available OTC in other countries, e.g., Australia.) A further Cochrane review (Rabbie et al., 2013) investigating ibuprofen's effect on migraine concluded that it was an effective treatment and the 400-mg dose was superior to the 200-mg dose.

For episodic tension-type headache, a systematic review by Verhagen et al. (2006) investigated the comparative efficacy of simple analgesics. The authors concluded that all simple analgesics had similar efficacy (measured as >50% pain relief).

Combinations of simple analgesics with codeine are available (page 287) and promoted for 'strong pain relief'. However, there is doubt whether the amount of codeine in these preparations is sufficient to provide any additional pain relief. In addition, codeine requires conversion to morphine by cytochrome P450 2D6 to exert its analgesic effects. There is genetic variability in this metabolism, with up to 30% of the population being poor metabolisers and in whom codeine has little or no analgesic effect. Further, there is growing evidence of problems with the overuse of these products resulting from dependence on the codeine components (Frei et al., 2010). In response to the ongoing concerns about codeine-containing products, the MHRA, in 2009, issued new guidance to restrict codeine-containing products for the short-term (3 days) treatment of acute, moderate pain which is not relieved by paracetamol, ibuprofen or aspirin alone. In 2013 the MHRA issued further guidance that codeine should not be given to children under the age of 12

In summary, simple analgesia should be tried as first-line options for the relief of pain in migraine and tension-type headache.

Complementary therapies

Feverfew (*Tanacetum parthenium*) is a medicinal herb used for the treatment of fever, headaches and digestive problems. It is available in a number of commercially produced herbal products to prevent migraine (e.g., Migraherb migraine relief capsules). A Cochrane Review identified six randomised, double-blind trials ($n=561$), comparing feverfew extract or powdered feverfew to placebo in the prevention of migraine (Wider et al., 2015). This updated review included one additional study, which was larger than previous studies ($n=218$). This study's findings reported that feverfew reduced migraine frequency by 1.9 attacks from 4.8 to 2.9 and placebo reduced the frequency by 1.3 from to 4.8 to 3.5 per month, resulting in a difference in effect between feverfew and placebo of 0.6 attacks per month. In conclusion, due to this new evidence, the authors concluded that, although this large trial points to a positive effect, there is still not enough evidence to routinely recommend feverfew.

Additionally, four UK products are specifically marketed to aid in the relief of pain and/or nausea associated with migraine: Migraleve, Midrid, Buccastem M and Imigran Recovery. The evidence for these products is reviewed.

Migraleve

Migraleve is available as either Migraleve Pink tablets, which contain a paracetamol/codeine combination (500/8 mg) plus buclizine 6.25 mg or Migraleve Yellow tablets, which contain only the analgesic combination. A number of trials have investigated Migraleve Pink tablets against placebo, buclizine and ergotamine products in an attempt to establish clinical effectiveness.

A review of two trials in which Migraleve was compared against buclizine (Jorgensen, 1974) and placebo (Scopa et al., 1974) showed Migraleve was as effective as buclizine and superior to placebo in reducing severity of migraine attacks. However, patient numbers were small ($n=21$ and 20, respectively) and statistical significance was not reported. Migraleve has also been compared with ergotamine-containing products; the standard drug at the time the trial was conducted. Results from a GP research group (Anon, 1973) concluded that Migraleve was equally as effective as Migril in treating migraine. However, results should be viewed with caution because the trial suffered from poor design, lacked randomisation, placebo or proper blinding. A further trial (Carasso & Yehuda, 1984) also reported beneficial effects of Migraleve. The most recent trial (Adam, 1987) was well designed, being double-blind, randomised and placebo controlled. The author concluded that, compared with placebo, Migraleve did significantly reduce the severity of attacks significantly but not their total duration.

Midrid

Midrid capsules contain isometheptene mucate 65 mg and paracetamol 325 mg. A number of trials have investigated the effect of Midrid on reducing the severity of migraine attacks. Trials date back to 1948, although it was not until the 1970s that soundly designed trials were performed. Two studies (Diamond, 1975, 1976) using similar methodology investigated isometheptene versus placebo and paracetamol. Both were double-blind, placebo controlled and had identical inclusion criteria. The 1975 trial concluded that isometheptene was superior in relieving headache severity compared with placebo, although the dose of isometheptene used was double to that found in Midrid. The 1976 trial also concluded that isometheptene was significantly superior to placebo and appeared to be better than paracetamol alone, but this did not reach statistical significance. A further trial (Behan, 1978) compared Midrid against placebo and ergotamine. Fifty patients who suffered four or more migraine attacks per month were recruited to the study. Diary cards were completed for six attacks in which patients rated relief from headache on a 4-point rating scale. The author concluded that Midrid was as effective as ergotamine and that both were more beneficial than placebo, although it is unclear whether this was statistically significant.

Summary

Limited trial data for both products suggest that they might be more effective than placebo. They could be recommended, but it is not known which product is most efficacious. However, with the deregulation of sumatriptan in 2006, their place in therapy is now questionable.

Prochlorperazine (Buccastem M)

Prochlorperazine has been found to be a potent antiemetic in a number of conditions, including migraine. It works by blocking dopamine receptors found in the chemoreceptor trigger zone. It is administered via the buccal mucosa and therefore patients will need to be counselled on correct administration.

Sumatriptan

Sumatriptan was the first 'triptan' to be marketed in the UK and, subsequently, deregulated to OTC status. Triptans are $5-HT_1$ agonists and stimulate $5-HT_{1B}$ and $5-HT_{1D}$ receptors. Triptans cause constriction of the cranial blood vessels, stop the release of inflammatory neurotransmitters at the trigeminal nerve synapses and reduce pain signal transmission. As a class of medicines they have been extensively researched. Most trials with sumatriptan (and other triptans) use end point data of a 2-hour pain-free response, headache relief and functional disability. In all end points sumatriptan 100 mg was significantly superior to placebo. At the lower 50 mg, OTC dose evidence of efficacy is less strong than 100 mg but is still effective (Derry et al., 2012).

Practical prescribing and product selection

Prescribing information relating to specific products used to treat migraine in the section 'Evidence base for over-the-counter medication' is discussed and summarised in Table 5.5 and useful tips relating to patients presenting with migraine are given in 'Hints and Tips' in Box 5.1.

Migraleve

The dose for adults and children over 15 years old is two Migraleve Pink tablets when the attack is imminent or has begun. If further treatment is required, one or two Migraleve Yellow tablets can be taken every 4 hours. The dose for children aged between 12 and 14 years old is half that of the adult dose. The maximum adult dose is eight tablets (two Migraleve Pink and six Migraleve Yellow) in 24 hours and for children aged between 12 and 14 years of age, the maximum dose is four tablets (one Migraleve Pink and three Migraleve Yellow) in 24 hours.

The buclizine component of Migraleve Pink tablets can cause drowsiness and antimuscarinic effects, whereas the codeine content might result in patients experiencing constipation. Buclizine and codeine can interact with POM and OTC medication, especially those that cause sedation. The combined effect is to potentiate sedation and it is important to warn the patient of this. It appears that Migraleve is safe in pregnancy but because of the codeine component, it is best avoided in the third trimester. It is also generally safe in breastfeeding, but drowsiness in the baby is possible. However, recent MHRA advice (2013) now states codeine should not be given during breastfeeding. (https://www.gov.uk/drug-safety-update/codeine-for-analgesia-restricted-use-in-children-because-of-reports-of-morphine-toxicity).

Midrid

Midrid is licensed for use only in adults. The dosage is two capsules at the start of an attack, followed by one capsule every hour until relief is obtained. A maximum of five capsules can be taken in a 12-h period. It is a sympathomimetic agent and like decongestants, it interacts with monoamine oxidase inhibitors (MAOIs), which might lead to fatal hypertensive crisis, and it can affect diabetes and hypertension control (see page 25). Side effects reported with Midrid include transient rashes and other allergic reactions. Midrid is best avoided in both pregnancy and breastfeeding due to lack of data.

Buccastem M

Buccastem M is indicated for previously diagnosed migraine sufferers aged 18 years and over who experience nausea and vomiting. The dosage is one or two tablets twice daily. Side effects include drowsiness, dizziness, dry mouth, insomnia, agitation and mild skin reactions. Because it crosses the blood-brain barrier, it will potentiate the effect of other CNS depressants and interact with alcohol. Prochlorperazine has been safely used in pregnancy, although the manufacturer advises avoidance unless absolutely necessary. Minimal prochlorperazine passes into the breast milk and could be used.

Sumatriptan (e.g., Imigran Recovery, Migraitan)

Patients over the age of 18, but younger than 65, should take a single tablet (50 mg) as soon as possible after the onset of the headache. If the headache clears and then recurs, a second tablet can be taken, provided there was a response to the first tablet and more than 2 hours have elapsed between the first and second tablet. No more than 100 mg can be taken during any 24-hour period. If there is no response to the first tablet, a second tablet should not be taken for the same attack. Sumatriptan is associated with a well-recognised side effect profile with the most common adverse events (classified as occurring in 1–10% of patients) being dizziness, drowsiness, tingling, feeling warm, flushed or weak, sensation of heaviness in any part

Table 5.5
Practical prescribing: Summary of medicines for migraine

Name of medicine	Use in children	Likely side effects	Drug interactions of note	Patients in which care is exercised	Pregnancy & breastfeeding
Migraleve	>12 years	Dry mouth, sedation and constipation	Increased sedation with alcohol, opioid analgesics, anxiolytics, hypnotics and antidepressants	Glaucoma, prostate enlargement	Pregnancy – Avoid in 3rd trimester Breastfeeding – OK but infant drowsiness reported
Midrid	>12 years	Dizziness, rash	Avoid concomitant use with MAOIs and moclobemide due to risk of hypertensive crisis. Avoid in patients taking beta-blockers and TCAs	Control of hypertension and diabetes may be affected, but a short treatment course is unlikely to be clinically important	Avoid
Buccastem M	>18 years	Drowsiness	Increased sedation with alcohol, opioid analgesics, anxiolytics, hypnotics and antidepressants	Patients with Parkinson's disease, epilepsy and glaucoma	Manufacturers advise avoidance, but it has been used safely in both pregnancy and breastfeeding
Imigran Recovery	>18 years	Dizziness; drowsiness; tingling feeling; warm, flushed or weak and sensation of heaviness in any part of the body; pressure in the throat, neck, chest and arms or legs; shortness of breath	MAOIs, ergotamine	Avoid in people with a previous MI, IHD, TIA, peripheral vascular disease, cardiac arrhythmias, hypertension; history of seizures; hepatic and renal impairment; atypical migraines	Avoid, but data do suggest it can be used safely. Only use if absolutely necessary

IHD, ischaemic heart disease; MAOI, monoamine oxidase inhibitor; MI, myocardial infarction; TCA, tricyclic antidepressant; TIA, transient ischaemic attack.

HINTS AND TIPS BOX 5.1: MIGRAINE

Analgesia	Recommend a soluble or orodispersible formulation to maximise absorption before it is inhibited by gastric stasis
Administration of buccal tablets	1. Place the tablet either between the upper lip and gum, above the front teeth, or between the cheek and upper gum 2. Allow the tablet to dissolve slowly. The tablet will soften and form a gel-like substance after 1–2 hours 3. The tablet will take between 3–5 hours to completely dissolve. If food or drinks are to be consumed during this time, place the tablet between the upper lip and gum, above the front teeth 4. The tablets should not be chewed, crushed or swallowed 5. Touching the tablet with the tongue or drinking fluids can cause the tablet to dissolve faster

of the body, shortness of breath, and pressure in the throat, neck, chest and arms or legs. Triptans are associated with rare cases of cardiac disorders and therefore to allow wider availability via OTC sales, the warnings associated with prescription use have become contraindications; those patients ineligible for OTC use are:

- a previous myocardial infraction, ischaemic heart disease, peripheral vascular disease, cardiac arrhythmias and history of transient ischaemic attack and stroke
- known hypertension
- history of seizures
- hepatic and renal impairment
- atypical migraines
- concomitant administration of MAOIs and ergotamine, or other 5-HT$_1$ receptor agonists.

To facilitate pharmacists in the appropriate supply of sumatriptan, migraine questionnaires can be used (http://www.imigranrecovery.co.uk/migraine_questionnaire.html). These should prove useful as sumatriptan supply is associated with various product license restrictions, which might be difficult to remember.

The manufacturer advocates avoidance in pregnancy and breastfeeding; however, data in the Summary of Products Characteristics states it has been used safely in the first trimester of pregnancy, and breastfeeding can be continued providing 12 hours have elapsed since taking the dose. Given that triptans are not given continuously and that the drug has poor bioavability (14%), the amount of sumatriptan that reaches the infant's circulation is expected to be very low (less than 1%).

References

Adam El. A treatment for the acute migraine attack. J Int Med Res 1987;15:71–5.

Anon. Reports from the general practitioner clinical research group. Migraine treated with an antihistamine-analgesic combination. The Practitioner 1973;211:357–61.

Behan PO. Isometheptene compound in the treatment of vascular headache. The Practitioner 1978;221:937–9.

Carasso RL, Yehuda S. The prevention and treatment of migraine with an analgesic combination. Br J Clin Pract 1984;38:25–7.

Derry CJ, Derry S, Moore RA. Sumatriptan (oral route of administration) for acute migraine attacks in adults. Cochrane Database of Systematic Reviews 2012, Issue 2. Art. No.: CD008615. http://dx.doi.org/10.1002/14651858.CD008615.pub2.

Derry S, Moore RA. Paracetamol (acetaminophen) with or without an antiemetic for acute migraine headaches in adults. Cochrane Database of Systematic Reviews 2013, Issue 4. Art. No.: CD008040. http://dx.doi.org/10.1002/14651858.CD008040.pub3.

Diamond S, Medina JL. Isometheptene – A non-ergot drug in the treatment of migraine. Headache 1975;15:211–13.

Diamond S. Treatment of migraine with isometheptene, acetaminophen, and dichloralphenazone combination: A double-blind, crossover trial. Headache 1976;16:282–7.

Frei MY, Nielsen S, Dobbin MD, et al. Serious morbidity associated with misuse of over-the-counter codeine-ibuprofen analgesics: a series of 27 cases. Med J Aust 2010;193(5):294.

Jorgensen PB, Weightman D, Foster JB. Comparison of migraleve and buclizine in prophylaxis of migraine. Curr Ther Res Clin Exp 1974;16(12):1276–80.

Rabbie R, Derry S, Moore RA. Ibuprofen with or without an antiemetic for acute migraine headaches in adults. Cochrane Database of Systematic Reviews 2013, Issue 4. Art. No.: CD008039. http://dx.doi.org/10.1002/14651858.CD008039.pub3.

Scopa J, Jorgensen PB, Foster JB. Migraleve in the prophylaxis of migraine. Curr Ther Res Clin Exp 1974;16(12):1270–5.

Verhagen AP, Damen L, Berger MY, et al. Is any one analgesic superior for episodic tension-type headache? J Fam Pract 2006:55;1064–72.

Wider B, Pittler MH, Ernst E. Feverfew for preventing migraine. Cochrane Database of Systematic Reviews 2015, Issue 4. Art. No.: CD002286. http://dx.doi.org/10.1002/14651858.CD002286.pub3.

Further reading

Coutin IB, Glass SF. Recognizing uncommon headache syndromes. Am Fam Physician 1996;54:2247–52.

Ferrari MD, Goadsby PJ, Roon KI, et al. Triptans (serotonin, 5-HT1B/1D agonists) in migraine: detailed results and methods of a meta-analysis of 53 trials. Cephalalgia 2002;22:633–58.

Goadsby PJ. Recent advances in the diagnosis and management of migraine. Br Med J 2006;332:25–9.

Kennedy J. Self-care of frequent headache. SelfCare 2010;1(4):145–8

Merrington DM. Comments on Migraleve trial reports. Curr Ther Res Clin Exp 1975;18:222–5.

National Clinical Guideline Centre. Headaches. Diagnosis and management of headaches in young people and adults (full NICE guideline). Clinical guideline 150. National Institute for Health and Care Excellence, 2012. www.nice.org.uk

Headache Classification Committee of the International Headache Society (IHS). The International Classification of Headache Disorders, 3rd edition. Cephalalgia 2013; 33(9): 629–808.

Websites

The migraine Trust: http://migrainetrust.org
Migraine Action Association: http://www.migraine.org.uk/
International Headache Society: http://www.ihs-headache.org/
Migraine in primary care advisors (MIPCA): www.mipca.org.uk
Organisation for the understanding of cluster headaches (OUCH-UK): http://www.ouchuk.org
National Headache Foundation: http://www.headaches.org/

Insomnia

Background

The length of sleep people need varies but typically people aged between 20 and 45 require 7 to 8 hours per day, although 10% of people can function on less than 5 hours of sleep per night. Sleep requirements also decrease with increasing age and people over 70 commonly have 6 hours of sleep per day. Insomnia is classified by its duration: transient (a few days), short-term (up to 4 weeks) or chronic (greater than 4 weeks).

It is likely that everyone at some point will experience insomnia, as it can arise from many different causes (Fig. 5.3), but for most people the problem will be of nuisance value, affecting next-day alertness. The pharmacist can manage most patients with transient or short-term insomnia; however, cases of chronic insomnia are best referred to the doctor, as there is usually an underlying cause.

Prevalence and epidemiology

Approximately 20–40% of adults report occasional sleep difficulty (Morphy et al., 2007; Cunnington et al., 2013; Wilsmore et al., 2013) and half of them consider it to be significant. It is twice as common in women than in men and prevalence increases (in both sexes) with increasing age. It is reported that only 5–10% of patients go on to develop chronic insomnia, although chronic insomnia is more common in the elderly, affecting approximately 20% of people over 65 years of age.

Aetiology

Sleep is essential to allow the body to repair and restore brain and body tissues. The mechanisms controlling sleep are complex and not yet fully understood but reflect disturbances of arousal- and/or sleep-promoting systems in the brain. Their relative activities determine the degree of alertness during wakefulness and depth and quality of sleep. Insomnia may be caused by any factor, which increases activity in arousal systems or decreases activity in sleep systems.

Arriving at a differential diagnosis

The key to arriving at a differential diagnosis is to take a detailed sleep history. Asking symptom-specific questions will help the pharmacist determine the most likely cause of the person's insomnia (Table 5.6). Two key features of insomnia need to be determined: the type of insomnia and how it affects the person. Transient insomnia is often caused by a change of routine, for example, time zone changes or a change to shift patterns, excessive noise, sleeping in a new environment (e.g., hotel) or extremes of temperature. Short-term insomnia is usually related to acute stress such as sitting exams, bereavement, loss of job, forthcoming marriage or house move. Asking the patient to tell you what they are thinking about before they fall asleep and when they awake will give you a clue to the cause of the insomnia.

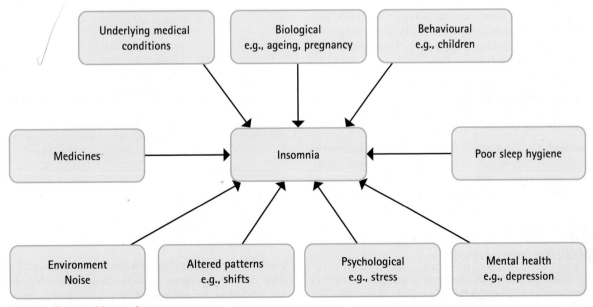

Fig. 5.3 Causes of insomnia.

Table 5.6
Specific questions to ask the patient: Insomnia

Question	Relevance
Pattern of sleep	An emotional disturbance (predominantly anxiety) is commonly associated in patients who find it difficult to fall asleep; patterns that include patients who fall asleep but wake early and cannot fall asleep again, or who are then restless, are sometimes associated with depression
Daily routine	Has there been any change to the work routine – changes to shift patterns, additional workload, resulting in longer working hours and greater daytime fatigue
	Too much exercise or intellectual arousal before going to bed can make sleep more difficult
Underlying medical conditions	Medical conditions likely to cause insomnia are gastro-oesophageal reflux disease (GORD) pregnancy, pruritic skin conditions, asthma, Parkinson's disease, painful conditions (osteoarthritis), hyperthyroidism (night sweats), menopausal symptoms (hot flushes) and depression.
Recent travel	Time zone changes will affect the person's normal sleep pattern and it can take a number of days to re-establish normality
Daytime sleeping	Elderly people might 'nap' throughout the day, which results in less sleep needed in the evening, making patients believe they have insomnia

Often it can be difficult to determine the cause of insomnia, and getting the patient to keep a sleep diary (retiring and waking times, time taken to fall asleep, etc.) is sometimes beneficial, as it allows an objective measure of the person's habits compared with their subjective perceptions.

Clinical features of insomnia

Insomnia is a subjective complaint of poor sleep in terms of its quality and duration. Patients will complain of difficulty in falling asleep, staying asleep or lack of refreshment by sleep. Sometimes patients will experience daytime fatigue but not generally sleepiness. This tiredness can lead to poor performance at work.

Conditions to eliminate

Insomnia in children

Bedwetting is the most common sleep arousal disorder in children. If this is not the cause, then insomnia invariably stems from a behavioural problem, such as fear of the dark, insecurity or nightmares. Children should not be given sleep aids but referred to their doctor for further evaluation, as the underlying cause needs to be addressed.

Medicine-induced insomnia

Medication can cause all three types of insomnia (Table 5.7). The stimulant effects of caffeine (contained in chocolate, tea, coffee and cola drinks) should not be underestimated. Drinking four or more cups of coffee can cause insomnia in the average

Table 5.7
Medication that may cause insomnia

Stimulants	Caffeine, theophylline, sympathomimetics amines (e.g., pseudoephedrine), MAOIs – especially in early treatment
Antiepileptics	Carbamazepine, phenytoin
Alcohol	Low to moderate amounts can promote sleep but when taken in excess or over a long period, it can disturb sleep
Beta-blockers	Can cause nightmares, especially propranolol. Limit by swapping to a beta-blocker that does not readily cross the blood-brain barrier
SSRIs	Especially fluoxetine
Diuretics	Ensure doses not taken after midday to stop the need to urinate at night
Griseofulvin	

MAOIs, monoamine oxidase inhibitors; SSRIs, selective serotonin reuptake inhibitors.

healthy adult. It is therefore advisable to instruct patients to avoid caffeine-containing products 6 hours before bedtime. Abruptly stopping some medications can also lead to insomnia. This is particularly seen with the long-term use of sedative drugs, such as benzodiazepines and tricyclic antidepressants.

Underlying medical conditions

Many medical conditions may precipitate insomnia (see Table 5.6). It is therefore necessary to establish a medical history from the patient. A key role for the pharmacist in these situations is to ensure that the underlying condition is being treated optimally and to check that the medication regimen is appropriate. If improvements to prescribing could be made then the prescriber should be contacted to discuss possible changes to the patient's medication.

Depression

It is well known that between one-third and two-thirds of patients suffering from chronic insomnia will have a recognisable psychiatric illness, most commonly depression. Many of these patients do not seek medical help and will self-medicate. The patient will complain of having difficulty staying asleep and suffer from early morning waking. The

pharmacist should look for other symptoms of depression such as fatigue, loss of interest and appetite, feelings of guilt, low self-esteem, difficulty in concentrating and constipation.

Fig. 5.4 will help in the differential diagnosis of the different types of insomnia.

Evidence base for over-the-counter medication

Many cases of transient and short-term insomnia should be managed initially by non-pharmacological measures. If these fail to rectify the problem then short-term use of sedating antihistamines may be tried.

Sleep hygiene

Once a diagnosis of insomnia has been reached, underlying causes ruled out and any misconceptions about normal sleep addressed, then educating patients about behaviour and practice which affects sleep should be tackled (Table 5.8).

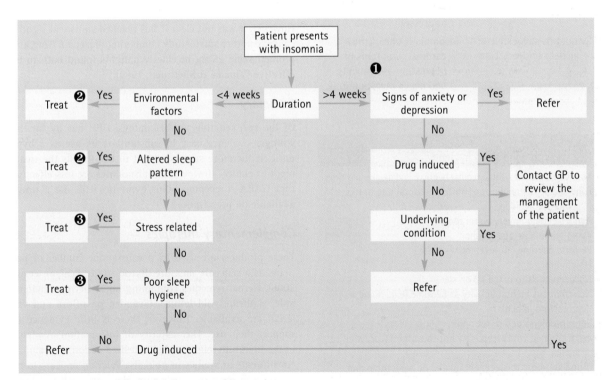

Fig. 5.4 Primer for differential diagnosis of insomnia.

❶ No cases of insomnia lasting longer than 4 weeks should be treated with OTC medication. If a previously undiagnosed medical condition is suspected, most often anxiety or depression or if insomnia has been possibly caused by the patient's pre-existing condition/medicines, then the GP should be consulted and treatment options discussed/suggested.

❷ Patients should not take antihistamines for more than 7 to 10 continuous days as tolerance to their effect can develop.

❸ In the first instance, strategies to manage the patient's insomnia should be suggested rather than issuing medication.

! **TRIGGER POINTS indicative of referral: Insomnia**

Symptoms/signs/ populations	Possible danger/reason for referral
Duration >4 weeks Children under 12 years old	Outside the remit of community pharmacists. Likely to be associated with underlying non-transient causes and requires investigation
Insomnia for which no cause can be ascertained	Sleeping aids are for short-term, usually reactive, causes which should be easily identifiable (e.g., jet lag, shift work, etc.)
Previously undiagnosed medical conditions	A number of medicines and medical conditions cause insomnia, and the cause needs to be addressed
Symptoms suggestive of anxiety or depression	Insomnia is one of the cardinal symptoms of depression and anxiety and needs investigation

Table 5.8
Key steps to good sleep hygiene

Maintain a routine, with a regular bedtime and awakening time
Food snacks, alcoholic- and caffeine-containing drinks should be avoided
Avoid sleeping in very warm rooms
Avoid stimulants and alcohol
Perform daytime, not evening, exercise
No daytime naps
No sleeping in to catch up on sleep
No strenuous mental activity at bedtime (e.g., doing a crossword in bed)
Solve problems before retiring
Associate bed with sleep – try not to watch TV or listen to music
If unable to get to sleep, get up and do something and return to bed when sleepy

Medication

The sedating antihistamines diphenhydramine (DPH) and promethazine are the mainstays of OTC pharmacological treatment.

Diphenhydramine

A substantial body of evidence exists to support the clinical effectiveness of DPH as a sleep aid. At doses of 50 mg DPH has been shown to be consistently superior to placebo in inducing sleep, and as effective as 60 mg of sodium pentobarbital (Rickels et al., 1984; Teutsch et al., 1975) and 15 mg of temazepam (Meuleman et al., 1987). Doses higher than 50 mg DPH do not produce statistically superior clinical effect and night-time doses should therefore not exceed this amount. It appears to be most effective at shortening sleep-onset time.

Promethazine

Promethazine is widely accepted to cause sedation when used for its licensed indications; however, there are few trials that have investigated its use as a hypnotic. A study by Adam and Oswald (1986) recruited 12 healthy volunteers who took placebo or promethazine 20 or 40 mg in a blinded fashion. The authors concluded that both doses of promethazine increased the length of sleep, and sleep disturbances were reduced compared with placebo. However, it was not clear if this reached statistical significance. Another small study comparing diazepam 5 mg and promethazine 25 mg in elderly patients found both to be effective (Viukari & Miettinen, 1984).

Summary

Of the two sedating antihistamines, DPH has by far the stronger evidence base to substantiate its use as a hypnotic. It therefore seems prudent to use this as the treatment of choice. However, antihistamines are less effective than GABA-A receptor-acting hypnotics (e.g., the 'z' drugs available on prescription).

Complementary therapies

These products are used by a substantial number of patients as a self-care measure (Byrne, 2006; Pearson et al., 2006). Herbal remedies containing hops, German chamomile, skullcap, wild lettuce, lavender, passiflora and valerian are available. However, there is little evidence to support their use. The majority of information available in the literature relates to hypothesised action of chemical constituents or studies in animals. Valerian appears to be the only product in which more than one trial has been conducted on humans. One systematic review (Stevinson & Ernst, 2000) found some evidence of efficacy in long-term studies (14–28 nights of therapy) but inconclusive evidence in the short-term (1–4 nights of therapy). In addition, the trials were often of short duration, used volunteers or patients with different criteria, and were usually methodologically poor. A number of branded products, containing combinations of herbal ingredients, are available OTC (e.g., Kalms range, Nytol herbal tablets, Potters Nodoff, Niteherb).

Melatonin

Melatonin is advocated for sleep disturbance, particularly associated with jet lag. A Cochrane review (Herxheimer & Petrie, 2002) found melatonin to be effective in reducing jet lag. The timing of the dose is critical. It has to be taken at bedtime after darkness has fallen on the first day of travel, then again in the same way on the second, and any subsequent day, of travel. Once at the final destination, it should be taken for the following few days at the same time.

Practical prescribing and product selection

Prescribing information relating to medicines for insomnia in the section 'Evidence base for over-the-counter medication' is discussed and summarised in Table 5.9 and useful tips relating to patients presenting with insomnia are given in 'Hints and Tips' in Box 5.2.

Antihistamines that are used for insomnia are first-generation antihistamines and interact with other sedating medication, resulting in potentiation of sedation. Additionally, they possess antimuscarinic side effects, which commonly lead to dry mouth and possibly to constipation. It is these antimuscarinic properties that mean patients with glaucoma, and prostate enlargement should ideally avoid their use, as it could lead to increased intraocular pressure and precipitation of urinary retention.

Diphenhydramine (e.g., Nytol, Nightcalm)

Diphenhydramine is licensed only for adults and children over 16 years of age. The dose is 50 mg (either two tablets [Nytol] or one tablet [Nytol one-a-night]) and it should be taken 20 min before going to bed.

Promethazine

Proprietary brands of promethazine on sale to the public include Sominex (20 mg) and Phenergan (10 mg or 25 mg). Adults and children over 16 years of age should take one tablet an hour before bedtime.

Table 5.9
Practical prescribing: Summary of medicines for insomnia

Name of medicine	Use in children	Likely side effects	Drug interactions of note	Patients in which care is exercised	Pregnancy & breastfeeding
Diphenhydramine	>16 years	Dry mouth, sedation and grogginess next day	Increased sedation with alcohol, opioid analgesics, anxiolytics, hypnotics and antidepressants	Glaucoma, prostate enlargement	Some manufacturers advise avoidance
Promethazine					In breastfeeding occasional use OK, but discontinue if baby becomes drowsy

HINTS AND TIPS BOX 5.2: INSOMNIA

Antihistamines	Tolerance can develop with continuous use
Patients who self-treat for depression	St John's wort (hypericum) is used by many patients to treat depression. There is a growing body of evidence that it is more effective than placebo for mild depression and is comparable in effect to tricyclic antidepressants. However, pharmacists should not recommend it routinely. If depression is suspected then the patient should be referred for further assessment. St John's wort also interacts with other medicines including warfarin, SSRIs, antiepileptics, digoxin, ciclosporin, theophylline and contraceptives

References

Adam K, Oswald I. The hypnotic effects of an antihistamine: promethazine. Br J Clin Pharmacol 1986;22:715–17.

Byrne J. Insomnia in older people: current approaches to treatment. The Prescriber 2006;17:54–6.

Cunnington D, Junge MF, Fernando AT. Insomnia: prevalence, consequences and effective treatment. Med J Aust 2013;199(8):36–40.

Herxheimer A, Petrie KJ. Melatonin for the prevention and treatment of jet lag. Cochrane Database of Systematic Reviews 2002, Issue 2. Art. No.: CD001520. http://dx.doi.org/10.1002/14651858.CD001520.

Meuleman JR, Nelson RC, Clark RL. Evaluation of temazepam and diphenhydramine as hypnotics in a nursing-home population. Drug Intell Clin Pharm 1987;21:716–20.

Morphy H, Dunn, KM, Boardman HF, et al. Epidemiology of insomnia: a longitudinal study in a UK population. Sleep 2007;30(3):274–280.

Pearson NJ, Johnson LL, Nahin RL. Insomnia, trouble sleeping, and complementary and alternative medicine: Analysis of the 2002 national health interview survey data. Arch Intern Med 2006;166(16):1775–82.

Rickels K, Morris RJ, Newman H, et al. Diphenhydramine in insomniac family practice patients: a double-blind study. J Clin Pharmacol 1983;23:234–42.

Stevinson C, Ernst E. Valerian for insomnia: a systematic review of randomized clinical trials. Sleep Med 2000;1:91–9.

Teutsch G, Mahler D L, Brown CR, et al. Hypnotic efficacy of diphenhydramine, methapyrilene and pentobarbital. Clin Pharmacol Ther 1975;17:195–201.

Viukari M, Miettinen P. Diazepam, promethazine and propiomazine as hypnotics in elderly inpatients. Neuropsychobiology 1984;12(2–3):134–7.

Wilsmore BR, Grunstein RR, Fransen M et al. Sleep habits, insomnia, and daytime sleepiness in a large and healthy community-based sample of New Zealanders. J Clin Sleep Med 2013;9(6):559.

Further reading

Buscemi N, Vandermeer B, Hooton N, et al. The efficacy and safety of exogenous melatonin for primary sleep disorders: A meta-analysis. J Gen Intern Med 2005;20:1151–8.

Gillin JC, Byerley WF. The diagnosis and management of insomnia. N Engl J Med 1990;322:239–48.

Mellinger GD, Balter MB, Uhlenhuth EH. Insomnia and its treatment. Prevalence and correlates. Arch Gen Psychiatry 1985;42:225–32.

NICE Guidance. Depression in adults. Available at: http://guidance.nice.org.uk/CG90

Sproule BA, Busto UE, Buckle C, et al. The use of non-prescription sleep products in the elderly. Int Geriatr Psychiatry 1999;10:851–7.

Website

National Sleep Foundation: http://www.sleepfoundation.org/

Nausea and vomiting

Background

Nausea is an unpleasant sensation, which may be a precursor to the forceful expulsion of gastric contents (vomiting). They are common symptoms of many disorders, especially gastrointestinal conditions. However, infection, acute alcohol ingestion, anxiety, severe pain, labyrinth and cardiovascular causes can also produce nausea and vomiting.

Deregulation of domperidone and prochlorperazine meant that community pharmacists could more effectively manage nausea and vomiting. Until their deregulation, treatment choices were limited to anticholinergics and first-generation antihistamines, used as prophylactic agents for the prevention of motion sickness. Unfortunately in 2014 domperidone was reclassified back to prescription-only status over fears over its potential cardiac side effects.

This now means UK pharmacists only have prochlorperazine to use to combat nausea and vomiting associated with migraine. Despite this, it is still important for pharmacists to assess patient symptoms and make appropriate referrals to the doctor.

Prevalence

Population based data show that vomiting occurs once a month in 2–3% of the general population.

Aetiology

Nausea occurs because activity in the vomiting centre (located in the medulla oblongata) increases. Information received from the receptor cells in the walls of the gastrointestinal tract and parts of the nervous system reach a 'threshold value' that induces the vomiting reflex. Additionally, further input is received at the vomiting centre from an area known as the chemoreceptor trigger zone. This is highly sensitive to certain circulating chemicals, for example, substances released by damaged tissues as a result of bacterial infection.

Arriving at a differential diagnosis

Nausea and/or vomiting rarely occur in isolation. Other symptoms are usually present and should therefore allow for a differential diagnosis to be made. Most cases will have a gastrointestinal origin, with viral gastroenteritis and food poisoning being the most common acute cause in all age groups. However, questioning the

(?) Table 5.10
Specific questions to ask the patient: Nausea and vomiting

Question	Relevance
Presence of abdominal pain	Certain abdominal conditions, e.g., appendicitis, cholecystitis and cholelithiasis, can also cause nausea and vomiting. However, for all three conditions abdominal pain would be the presenting symptom and not nausea and vomiting. The severity of the pain alone would trigger referral
Timing of nausea and vomiting	Early morning vomiting is often associated with pregnancy or excess alcohol intake If vomiting occurs immediately after food, this suggests gastritis, and if vomiting begins after 1 or more hours after eating food, then peptic ulcers are possible
Signs of infection	Acute cases of gastroenteritis will normally have other associated symptoms such as diarrhoea, fever and abdominal discomfort If infection is due to food contamination, then other people are often affected at the same time

patient about associated symptoms should be made, as other causes of nausea and vomiting need to be eliminated (Table 5.10).

Clinical features associated with gastroenteritis

Gastroenteritis is characterised by acute onset, vomiting and/or diarrhoea and systemic illness (e.g., fever). Most cases, regardless of infecting pathogen, resolve in a few days and rarely last more than 10 days. In children under 5 years old over 60% of cases are viral in origin with the rotavirus and small round structured virus most commonly identified. Vomiting usually precedes diarrhoea by several hours. Bacterial gastroenteritis presents with similar symptoms, although fever is usually a more prominent feature.

Conditions to eliminate

Gastritis

Gastritis is often alcohol- or medicine-induced and can present as acute or chronic nausea and vomiting. Epigastric pain is usually present. For further information on gastritis see page 165.

Nausea and vomiting associated with headaches

Vomiting and especially nausea are common symptoms in patients who suffer from migraines. However, other causes of headache, such as raised intracranial pressure, can also cause nausea and vomiting. For further information on nausea and vomiting associated with headaches see page 96.

Nausea and vomiting in neonates (up to 1 month old)

Vomiting in neonates should always be referred because it suggests some form of congenital disorder, for example Hirschsprung's disease.

Nausea and vomiting in infants (1 month to 1 year old)

In the first year of life the most common causes of nausea and vomiting are feeding problems, gastrointestinal and urinary tract infection. Vomiting in infants needs to be differentiated from regurgitation. Regurgitation is an effortless backflow of small amounts of liquid and food between meals or at feed times; vomiting is the forceful expulsion of gastric contents. The infant will usually have a fever and be generally unwell if vomiting is associated with infection. If projectile vomiting occurs in an infant under 3 months of age, then pyloric stenosis should be considered. Due to the higher risk of dehydration in this age group, it is prudent to refer to a doctor if symptoms persist for more than 24 hours.

Nausea and vomiting in children (1 year to 12 years old)

Children under 12 years old who experience nausea and vomiting will usually have gastroenteritis, fever or otitis media. In most instances the conditions are self-limiting, and medication designed to reduce pain and temperature (analgesia) and replace fluid (oral rehydration therapy) will help resolve symptoms.

Pregnancy

Pregnancy should always be considered in women of childbearing age if nausea and vomiting occur in the absence of other symptoms. Sickness affects >50% of women and tends to be worse in the early morning and peaks at 9 weeks' gestation.

Excess alcohol consumption

The patient should always be asked about recent alcohol intake, as excess quantities are associated with nausea and early morning vomiting.

Medicine-induced nausea and vomiting

Many medications can cause nausea and vomiting. Frequently implicated medicines are cytotoxics, opiates, iron, antibiotics, NSAIDs, potassium supplements, selective serotonin reuptake inhibitors (SSRIs), nicotine gum (ingestion of nicotine rather than buccal absorption), theophylline and digoxin toxicity. If medication is suspected then the pharmacist should contact the prescriber to discuss alternative treatment options.

Middle ear diseases

Any middle ear disturbance or imbalance may produce nausea and vomiting. Tinnitus, dizziness and vertigo are suggestive of Ménière's disease.

Product selection

If dehydration is suspected the patient should replace fluids. Oral rehydration solutions should be offered. For further information on these products see page 176.

! TRIGGER POINTS indicative of referral: Nausea and vomiting

Symptoms/signs/ populations	Possible danger/reason for referral
Suspected pregnancy	Offer pregnancy test
Vomiting in children under 1 year old lasting longer than 24 hours	Risk of dehydration
Children who fail to respond to OTC treatment	
Unexplained nausea and vomiting in any age group	Identifiable causes account for the vast majority of presentations. Unknown causes should be viewed with caution
Moderate to severe abdominal pain	Requires further and fuller investigation

Prochlorperazine

Prochlorperazine (Table 5.11) is licensed for the relief of nausea and vomiting associated with migraine. It has potent antiemetic properties in a number of conditions, including migraine. For dosing and counselling on Buccastem M please refer to page 102.

Further reading

Bekhti A, Rutgeerts L. Domperidone in the treatment of functional dyspepsia in patients with delayed gastric emptying. Postgrad Med J 1979;55:S30–32.

Dollery C. Therapeutic drugs, 2nd edition. Edinburgh: Churchill Livingstone, 1999.

Table 5.11
Practical prescribing: Summary of medicines for nausea and vomiting

Name of medicine	Use in children	Likely side effects	Drug interactions of note	Patients in which care is exercised	Pregnancy & breastfeeding
Prochlorperazine	>18 years	Drowsiness	Increased sedation with alcohol, opioid analgesics, anxiolytics, hypnotics and antidepressants	Patients with Parkinson's disease, epilepsy and glaucoma	Manufacturers advise avoidance, but it has been used safely in both pregnancy and breastfeeding

Self-assessment questions

The following questions are intended to supplement the text. Two levels of questions are provided: multiple choice questions and case studies. The multiple choice questions are designed to test factual recall, and the case studies allow knowledge to be applied to a practice setting.

Multiple choice questions

5.1 A 32-year-old woman presents to the pharmacy one Monday afternoon complaining of a headache. Based on epidemiology alone, what would be the most likely cause of the headache?

    a. Migraine
    b. Eye-strain
    c. Tension-type headache
    d. Sinusitis
    e. Cluster headache

5.2 A 41-year-old man wants some advice about a headache he has. He reveals that the pain is towards the back of his head. Knowing this information, what headache conditions cannot be ruled out based on location?

    a. Migraine
    b. Temporal arteritis
    c. Sub-arachnoid haemorrhage
    d. Sinusitis
    e. Cluster headache

5.3 When differentiating headaches from one another, it is useful to consider other symptoms to aid diagnosis, with some symptoms warranting referral. From the list of symptoms below, which would indicate referral with a patient suffering headache?

    a. Flashing or flickering lights
    b. Pins and needles in the arms
    c. Scalp tenderness
    d. Symptoms that improve as the day progresses
    e. Symptoms that last longer than 1 week

5.4 Headache is the main presenting symptom in migraine sufferers. From the following descriptions, which one best describes the headache symptoms of migraine?

    a. Pain which is unilateral and lancing
    b. Pain which is unilateral, orbital and boring
    c. Pain which is unilateral, frontal and dull
    d. Pain which is unilateral, orbital and severe
    e. Pain which is unilateral and throbbing

5.5 A 41-year-old man wants some advice about a headache he has. He tells you that he has had the symptoms for a couple days. The headache is at the front of his head and it feels like a dull throb. Which of the questions listed below would be most discriminatory in assessing if it were a migraine or a tension-type headache?

    a. How severe is the pain?
    b. What medicines do they take?
    c. What medicines have they tried to ease the pain?
    d. Where is the pain?
    e. Do they feel sick?

5.6 Which sign or symptom warrants referral?

    a. Headache lasting 7 to 10 days
    b. Headache described as vice-like
    c. Headache associated with the workplace environment
    d. Headache in children under 12 years old with no sign of infection
    e. Headache associated with cough and cold symptoms

5.7 Chronic insomnia is associated with:

    a. Change to shift patterns
    b. Acute stressful situations
    c. Foreign travel
    d. Excessive caffeine intake
    e. None of the above

5.8 Which complementary therapy/medicine has the most evidence to support its use in treating insomnia?

    a. Acupuncture
    b. Lavender
    c. Chamomile
    d. Valerian
    e. Reflexology

Questions 5.9 to 5.14 concern the following conditions:

    A. Sinusitis
    B. Cluster headache
    C. Migraine

D. Temporal arteritis
E. Meningitis
F. Tension-type headache
G. Sub-arachnoid haemorrhage
H. Medication-overuse headache
I. Glaucoma

Select, from A to I, which of the above conditions is most appropriate with the following statements:

5.9 Is more common in men

5.10 Is almost exclusively seen with advancing age

5.11 Onset tends to be in early adulthood

5.12 Is more common in women

5.13 Is frequently seen in elderly women

5.14 Is associated with childhood

Questions 5.15 to 5.17: For each of these questions *one or more* of the responses is (are) correct. Decide which of the responses is (are) correct. Then choose:

A. If a, b and c are correct
B. If a and b only are correct
C. If b and c only are correct
D. If a only is correct
E. If c only is correct

Directions summarised

A	B	C	D	E
a, b and c	a and b only	b and c only	a only	c only

5.15 Which of the following statements about migraine are true?

a. Symptoms are usually unilateral
b. Nausea is experienced by most people
c. Acute attacks usually resolve in about 3 days

5.16 Which statements are appropriate when discussing sleep hygiene with patients?

a. Sleep in cool rooms
b. Avoid evening exercise
c. Avoid doing mental exercises near bedtime

5.17 A patient has nausea and vomiting. Which statement would alert you to referring the patient:

a. Symptoms of less than 24 hours in an adult
b. Mild generalised epigastric pain
c. Dizziness

Questions 5.18 to 5.20: These questions consist of a statement in the left-hand column, followed by a statement in the right-hand column. You need to:

● decide whether the first statement is true or false
● decide whether the second statement is true or false

Then choose:

A. If both statements are true and the second statement is a correct explanation of the first statement
B. If both statements are true but the second statement is NOT a correct explanation of the first statement
C. If the first statement is true but the second statement is false
D. If the first statement is false but the second statement is true
E. If both statements are false

Directions summarised

	1st statement	2nd statement	
A	True	True	2nd explanation is a correct explanation of the first
B	True	True	2nd statement is not a correct explanation of the first
C	True	False	
D	False	True	
E	False	False	

	First statement	*Second statement*
5.18	Nausea is a common symptom in the first trimester of pregnancy	The exact mechanism that induces nausea is uncertain
5.19	Gastroenteritis is bacterial in origin	Fever is rare in gastroenteritis
5.20	Oral rehydration therapy is recommended for treating symptoms of gastroenteritis	Dehydration is the most important complication associated with gastroenteritis

Case study

CASE STUDY 5.1

Mr AM, a male in his early 30s, presents in the pharmacy at lunchtime complaining of headaches. The following questions are asked, and responses received.

Information gathering	Data generated
What symptoms/describe the symptoms	General aching feeling all over the head
How long has he/she had the symptoms	Had for the last week
Other symptoms	No problems with lights, etc. No sickness. No recent trauma
Where exactly	As above
Any time worse/better	Seems to get worse as day goes on
Severity of pain (1–10)	4
Frequency of pain	Most of the time
Eye test; recent trauma	Eyes OK, no need for glasses; No
Previous history of presenting complaint	None
Past medical history	None
Drugs (OTC, Rx, and compliance)	None
Allergies	Penicillin
Social history Smoking Alcohol Employment Relationships	Non-smoker, drinks red wine (a couple of glasses each night). Works in marketing. Married with 2 young children. Job OK, but busy with new promotion
Family history	Not known
On examination	Not applicable

Diagnostic pointers with regard to symptom presentation

Below summarises the expected findings for questions when related to the different conditions that can be seen by community pharmacists.

CASE STUDY 5.1 (Continued)

	Duration	Timing & nature	Location	Severity (pain score from 0–10)*	Precipitating factors	Who is affected?
Tension-type headache	Can last days	Symptoms worsen as day progresses. Non-throbbing pain	Bilateral & most often at back of head	2–5	Stress due to changes in work or home environment	All age groups and both sexes equally affected
Migraine	Average attack lasts 24 hours	Associated with menstrual cycle and weekends. Throbbing pain & nausea. Dislike of bright lights and loud noise	Usually unilateral	4–7	Food (in 10% of sufferers) & family history	3 times more common in women. Rare in children.
Cluster headache	1–3 hours	Attacks occur at same time of day. Intense, boring pain	Unilateral	>7	Alcohol	3–5 times more common in men
Sinusitis	Days	Dull ache that starts off being unilateral	Frontal	2–6	Valsalva movements	Adults
Eye strain	Days	Aching	Frontal	2–5	Close vision work	All ages
Temporal arteritis	Hours to days	Variable	Unilateral around temples	3–6	None	Elderly
Trigeminal neuralgia	Minutes	Lancing pain at any time	Face	>7	None	Adults
Depression	Days to months	Non-throbbing pain	Generalised	2–5	Social factors	Adults
Glaucoma	Hours	Often in the evening and sudden onset	Unilateral and orbital	>7	Darkness	Older adults
Meningitis	Hours to days	Associated with systemic infection	Generalised	>7	None	Children
Subarachnoid haemorrhage	Minutes to hours	Variable	Occipital	>7	None	Adults
Raised intracranial pressure	Days to months	Worse in the mornings	Variable	>4/5	None	Older adults

CASE STUDY 5.1 (Continued)

When this information is applied to that gained from our patient (below) we see that his symptoms most closely match tension-type headache, which may (or may not) be triggered by extra pressure at work. Depression is also a possibility, although less likely. It might be worth checking symptoms relating to the DSM-V classification to eliminate depression.

	Duration	Timing & nature	Location	Severity (pain score from 0–10)	Precipitating factors	Who is affected?
Tension	✓	✓	✓	✓	✓	✓
Migraine	✗	✗	✗	✓	✗	✓?
Cluster	✗	✗	✗	✗	?	✓
Sinusitis	✓	✓?	✗	✓	✗	✓
Eye strain	✓	✓	✗	✓	✗	✓
Temporal arteritis	✓	✓?	✗	✓	n/a	✗
Trigeminal neuralgia	✗	✗	✗	✗	n/a	✓
Depression	✓	✓?	✓	✓	✓?	✓
Glaucoma	✗	✗	✗	✗	✗	✗
Meningitis	✗	✗	✓	✗	n/a	✗
Subarachnoid haemorrhage	✗	✗	✗	✗	n/a	✓
Raised intracranial pressure	✓	✗	✓	✓	n/a	✗

Danger symptoms/signs (trigger points for referral)

As a final double check it might be worth making sure the person has none of the 'referral signs or symptoms'; this is the case with this patient.

CASE STUDY 5.2

Mrs PC, a 36-year-old woman, asks you for something to treat her headache. On questioning you find out the following:

- The pain is located mainly behind left eye and at the front of head but also at the back of head
- Mrs PC is experiencing aching, no sickness or visual disturbances
- She has had the headache for about 5 days
- There is no recent history of head trauma
- The pain worsens as day progresses
- She has not had this type of headache before
- Work at the moment is busy because of a conference she is organising
- She has tried paracetamol, which helps for a while but the pain comes back after a few hours
- She takes nothing from GP, except the minipill

a. Using the information on epidemiology and data on signs and symptoms of each condition from Case Study 5.1, what is the likely differential diagnosis?

Tension-type headache, probably as a result of additional stress at work while organising the conference.

b. From the above responses, which symptoms allowed you to rule out other conditions?

- *Age (36): Most likely causes are tension-type and migraine headaches based solely on age.*
- *Sex (female): Women experience more migraines than men and less cluster headache; therefore migraine is a possibility.*
- *Duration (5 days): Most migraines do not last beyond 72 hours. Cluster headache duration is even less. More sinister causes of headache tend to last longer than 5 days; therefore tension-type headache is likely.*

- *Location (behind eye and back of head): The pain seems fairly generalised, which is indicative of tension-type headache.*
- *Nature of pain (ache): Again, tension-type headaches are often described as non-throbbing. Pain does not appear to be severe, which means sinister pathology is less likely.*
- *Associated symptoms (none): No nausea or vomiting. This tends to exclude migraine and conditions causing raised intracranial pressure.*
- *Medication (paracetamol): This appears to work but does not really help in establishing the cause of the headache.*
- *New headache (yes): The patient has not suffered from this type of headache before, a fact that might be suggestive of a more serious cause of headache. Further questioning is needed to make a judgement on whether referral would be appropriate.*
- *Lifestyle (work is busy): Stress is a contributing factor of tension-type headache. It appears the patient is suffering from more stress than normal and that could be a cause of the headache.*
- *Medication from GP (minipill): Unlikely to cause the headache, but further questions should be asked of the patient about how long she has been taking the medication. Most ADRs normally coincide with new medication or an alteration to the dosage regimen.*
- *Recent trauma (none): This tends to exclude headache caused by space-occupying lesions. It is worth remembering that symptoms manifest themselves once pressure is exerted on adjacent structures to a haematoma, tumour or abscess. It might therefore take longer than several weeks for the patient to notice symptoms. As a result, always ask about trauma over the last 6 to 12 weeks.*
- *Periodicity (worse as day goes on): This is suggestive of tension-type headache. It therefore appears that the majority of questions point to tension-type headache as the most likely cause of headache.*

CASE STUDY 5.3

Mr FD, A 67-year-old man, asks you for a strong painkiller for his headache. He has had the headache for a few days, but it does not seem to be going away. After talking with the man, you find out the following:

- *The headache is located in the frontal area and is unilateral*
- *He describes the pain as throbbing*
- *He has never had a headache like this before*
- *He has not suffered from migraines in the past*
- *There are no symptoms of nausea or vomiting*
- *There are no associated symptoms of upper respiratory tract infection*
- *He is retired and has a non-stressful lifestyle*
- *He has tried paracetamol but without much success*
- *He takes atenolol for hypertension*

a. Using the information on epidemiology and data on signs and symptoms of each condition from Case Study 5.1, what is the likely differential diagnosis?

It appears that tension-type headache and migraine can be ruled out. Cluster headache is a possibility, but the type of pain and location is not right. This suggests the headache might be a secondary type of headache, requiring referral. Sinusitis is a secondary cause of headache, but the patient shows no recent symptoms of URTI. From the remaining secondary causes of headache, it appears the symptoms most closely match temporal arteritis.

b. **What extra questions could you have asked to support this conclusion?**

Enquire about tenderness in the temple region or if the scalp was tender to touch.

CASE STUDY 5.4

The wife of a 54-year-old man enters the pharmacy and asks for Imigran Recovery; she has seen it advertised in the paper and her husband seems to have all the symptoms.

Information gathering	Data generated
Presenting complaint (possible questions)	
Describe symptoms	Very painful headache. Worst towards the back of the head; feels nauseous and vomited twice, but vomiting seems to have subsided
How long has he/she had the symptoms?	12 hours
Severity of pain	Very painful (7–8 out of 10)
Nature of the pain	Just said it is very painful
Other symptoms/provokes	Cannot do anything. Painful even to do 'normal' things like shower, dress, etc.
Eye test; recent trauma	Not had eye test for a year, but eyes OK; No recent trauma
Any symptoms before headache?	No
Additional questions	Nothing seems to ease the pain
Previous history of presenting complaint	None

Information gathering	Data generated
Past medical history	Hypercholesterolaemia
Drugs (OTC, Rx and compliance)	Simvastatin 40 mg 1 on
	Ezetrol 10 mg 1 od
	Uses antihistamines OTC during spring/summer
Allergies	Not asked – not relevant in this case
Relevant social history	Executive for a marketing firm – busy job
Family history	None for presenting complaint
On examination	His wife states that he generally looks tired, and pain is aggravated by light

a. Given the information the woman has given you, is her husband a suitable candidate for Imigran Recovery?

Imigran Recovery is not indicated in this instance because it is the first presentation of symptoms and he has heart disease.

b. If the patient was suitable for Imigran Recovery, given his symptoms, would you sell them to his wife?

No. Symptoms are not fully consistent with migraine. Severity, location and lack of previous history suggest it is not migraine. Symptoms are suggestive of sinister pathology.

Answers

1 = c	2 = c	3 = c	4 = e	5 = e	6 = d	7 = e	8 = d	9 = B	10 = I
11 = C	12 = C	13 = D	14 = E	15 = A	16 = A	17 = E	18 = B	19 = E	20 = B

Women's health

Background

Women have unique healthcare needs ranging from pregnancy to menstrual disorders. Many of these conditions are outside the remit of the community pharmacist and specialist care is needed. However, a small number of conditions can be adequately treated with over-the-counter (OTC) remedies. This chapter explores such conditions and attempts to outline when referral should be made.

General overview of the female reproductive and urological anatomy

The female reproductive anatomy comprises both internal and external genital organs. The external genital organs include the mons pubis, labia majora and minora, Bartholin glands and clitoris. Their role is to allow sperm to enter the vagina, to protect the internal genital organs and provide sexual pleasure. The internal genital organs comprise the vagina, uterus, fallopian tubes and ovaries. The vagina is approximately 4 to 5 cm long, and is a muscular, tube-like organ. It is lined by a mucous membrane, and is kept moist by fluids produced by the lining and the cervix, which is found at the opening of the uterus. The main function of the uterus is to sustain a developing fetus. It is a muscular, pear-shaped organ, lined with two layers of cells called the endometrium. The outer layer of the endometrium, called the functional layer, changes in response to oestrogen and progesterone as part of the menstrual cycle. Oestrogen secretion in the follicular phase (first half) of the menstrual cycle causes the endometrium to proliferate and thicken. The increase in progesterone during the luteal phase (second half) causes the endometrium to move into a secretory phase, which is designed to make the endometrium more receptive to implanting an embryo. If fertilisation and implantation of the embryo do not occur the lining of the endometrium is shed during menses. Ovulation, when the release of an oocyte ready for potential fertilisation takes place, involves the ovaries and the fallopian tubes. The oocyte is released from the de Graff's follicles in the ovary after a surge in levels of follicle stimulating hormone (FSH) and luteinizing hormone (LH) secreted from the pituitary. The released oocyte travels down the fallopian tubes towards the uterus, where if it is fertilised it will implant.

The female urological anatomy is the same as in men in that it comprises kidneys, ureters, a bladder and a urethra. However, the proximity of these to the female reproductive organs means that a woman often suffers more urological problems, particularly caused by pressure during pregnancy and damage during childbirth. In addition, the female urethra is much shorter (approximately 5 cm) compared with males (approximately 20 cm). This makes it much easier for bacteria, such as from the rectum, to travel to the bladder, leading to cystitis.

History taking

As with all conditions that present in the community pharmacy, it is essential to take an accurate history from the patient. However, the patient might feel uncomfortable or embarrassed about discussing symptoms, especially in a busy pharmacy. Male pharmacists may find that this level of embarrassment is heightened both from the patient's and pharmacist's perspectives. It is essential that the patient is made to feel at ease. The use of consultation rooms should be considered to provide adequate privacy.

Cystitis

Background

Cystitis literally means inflammation of the bladder, although, in practice cystitis refers to inflammation of urethra and bladder. In men cystitis is uncommon because of the longer urethra, which provides a greater barrier to bacteria entering the bladder; fluid from the prostate gland also confers some antibacterial property. This is especially so in men under the age of 50. After 50 years of age urinary tract infections in men become more common due to prostate enlargement.

Prevalence and epidemiology

Urinary tract infections (UTI) are one of most common infections treated in general medical practice and will affect up to 15% of women each year. Patients aged between 15 and 34 account for the majority of cases seen within a primary care setting, and it is estimated that up to 50% of all women will experience at least one episode of cystitis in their lifetime, half of whom will have further attacks. Certain factors do increase the risk of a UTI. For instance, in young women, frequent or recent sexual activity and previous episodes of cystitis; the use of diaphragms or spermicidal agents; advancing age; and diabetes (can indicate poor diabetic control). Additionally, cystitis affects 1% to 4% of pregnant women (Le et al., 2004).

Recurrent cystitis (usually defined as three episodes in the past 12 months or two episodes in the past 6 months) is relatively common, even though no identifiable risk factors are present.

Aetiology

Infection is caused, in the majority of cases, by the patient's own bowel flora that ascend the urethra from the perineal and perianal areas. Bacteria are thus transferred to the bladder where they proliferate. The most common bacterial organisms implicated in cystitis are *Escherichia coli* (>80% of cases), *Staphylococcus* (up to 10%) and *Proteus*. However, several studies have shown that up to 50% of women do not have positive urine cultures according to traditional criteria (>10^5 bacteria per mL of urine), although they do have signs and symptoms of infection. These patients with 'low count bacteriuria' are classed as having a urinary tract infection.

Arriving at a differential diagnosis

The majority of patients who present in the community pharmacy will have acute uncomplicated cystitis (Table 6.1) and will have made a self-diagnosis. The pharmacist's aims are, therefore, to confirm a patient self-diagnosis, rule out upper urinary tract infection (pyelonephritis) and identify patients who are at risk of complications as a result of cystitis. Asking symptom-specific questions will help the pharmacist establish a differential diagnosis (Table 6.2).

Clinical features of acute uncomplicated cystitis

Cystitis is characterised by pain when passing urine and causes frequency, urgency, nocturia and haematuria. The diagnostic probability of cystitis is over 90% if patients exhibit dysuria and frequency without vaginal discharge or irritation. In addition, the patient might report only passing small amounts of urine, with pain worsening at the

Table 6.1
Causes of cystitis symptoms and their relative incidence in community pharmacy

Incidence	Cause
Most likely	Acute uncomplicated cystitis
Likely	Pyelonephritis
Unlikely	Sexually transmitted disease, oestrogen deficiency
Very unlikely	Medicine-induced cystitis, vaginitis

?

Table 6.2
Specific questions to ask the patient: Cystitis

Question	Relevance
Duration	Symptoms that have lasted longer than 5–7 days should be referred because of the risk that the person might develop pyelonephritis
Age of the patient	Cystitis is unusual in children and should be viewed with caution. This might be a sign of a structural urinary tract abnormality. Referral is needed Elderly female patients (>70 years) have a higher rate of complications associated with cystitis and are, therefore, best referred
Presence of fever	Referral is needed if the person presents with fever associated with dysuria, frequency and urgency, as fever is a sensitive indicator of an upper urinary tract infection
Vaginal discharge	If a patient reports vaginal discharge then the likely diagnosis is not cystitis but a vaginal infection
Location of pain	Pain experienced in the loin area suggests an upper urinary tract infection

end of voiding urine. Symptoms usually start suddenly. Suprapubic discomfort not associated with passing urine might also be present but is not common. Haematuria, although common, should be viewed with caution because it might indicate stones or a tumour. Such cases are best referred.

Conditions to eliminate

Likely conditions

Pyelonephritis
The most frequent complication of cystitis is when the invading pathogen involves the ureter or kidney by ascending from the bladder to these higher anatomical structures. The patient will show signs of systemic infection such as fever, chills, flank or loin pain and possibly nausea and vomiting. Pain relief can be offered, but a medical referral is needed to confirm the diagnosis; exclude pelvic inflammatory disease and issue appropriate treatment (7-day course of ciprofloxacin 500 mg twice daily).

Unlikely causes

Sexually transmitted diseases
Sexually transmitted diseases (STDs) can be caused by a number of pathogens, for example *Chlamydia trachomatis* and *Neisseria gonorrhoea*. Symptoms are similar to acute uncomplicated cystitis but they tend to be more gradual in onset and last for a longer period of time. In addition pyuria (pus in the urine) is usually present. Although STDs are an unlikely cause in older adults, they should be considered more likely in young adults (18–25) in whom the prevalence of conditions, such as gonorrhoea and chlamydia, is increasing.

Oestrogen deficiency (atrophic vaginitis)
Postmenopausal women experience thinning of the endometrial lining as a result of a reduction in the levels of circulating oestrogen in the blood. This increases the likelihood of irritation or trauma, leading to cystitis symptoms. If the symptoms are caused by intercourse, symptomatic relief can be gained with a lubricating product. Referral for possible topical oestrogen therapy would be appropriate if the symptoms recur.

Very unlikely causes

Medicine-induced cystitis
Non-steroidal anti-inflammatory agents (NSAIDs, especially tiaprofenic acid), allopurinol, danazol and cyclophosphamide have been shown to cause cystitis.

Vaginitis
Vaginitis exhibits similar symptoms to cystitis, in that dysuria, nocturia and frequency are common. It can be caused by direct irritation (e.g., use of vaginal sprays and toiletries). All patients should be questioned about an associated vaginal discharge. The presence of vaginal discharge is highly suggestive of vaginitis.

Fig. 6.1 will aid the differentiation of cystitis from other conditions.

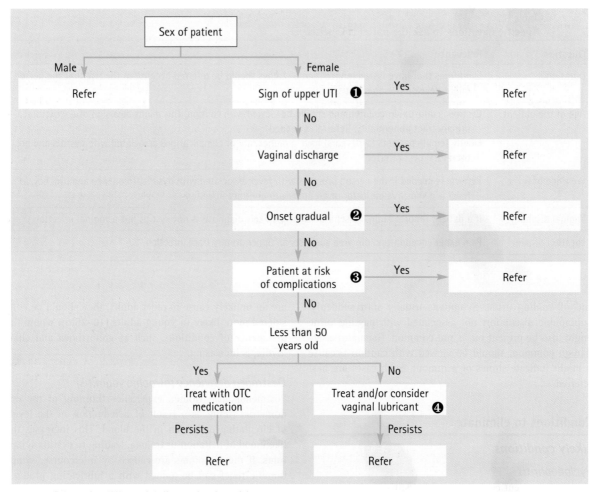

Fig. 6.1 Primer for differential diagnosis of cystitis.

❶ **Involvement of the higher urinary tract structures**
Symptoms such as fever, flank pain, nausea and vomiting suggest conditions such as pyelonephritis.

❷ **Gradual onset**
STDs should be considered in patients whose symptoms are not sudden.

❸ **At-risk patients**
Patients at risk of developing upper urinary tract infection (UTI) include those with diabetes, pregnant women, the

immunocompromised, the elderly and those patients in whom symptoms have been present for more than 5 to 7 days.

❹ **Patients over 50 years old**
Oestrogen deficiency might account for the patient's symptoms, resulting in local atrophy of the vagina.

6

! TRIGGER POINTS indicative of referral: Cystitis

Symptoms/signs	Possible danger/reason for referral
Children under 16 years of age	Difficult to distinguish between upper and lower urinary tract infections in children and, if recurrent, may indicate an abnormality in the urinary tract
Patients with diabetes	More likely to develop complications from a UTI
Duration longer than 7 days	Does not suggest an uncomplicated UTI
Haematuria	Blood may indicate a stone or a tumour
Vaginal discharge	May indicate vaginitis
Immunocompromised	More likely to develop complications from a UTI
Patients with associated fever and flank pain	Suggestive of a complicated UTI and/or pyelonephritis
Pregnancy	Pressure on the urinary tract caused by a baby makes management of UTIs more difficult and can increase the risk of pyelonephritis
Women older than 70 years of age	More susceptible to complicated UTIs and pyelonephritis. Also symptoms may be indicative of atrophic vaginitis

Evidence base for over-the-counter medication

Alkalinising agents

Current OTC treatment is limited to products that contain alkalinising agents, namely sodium citrate, sodium bicarbonate and potassium citrate. (Previous applications to reclassify trimethoprim and nitrofurantoin in the UK have been made but were withdrawn. Trimethoprim is, however, available OTC in some countries, e.g., New Zealand.) Alkalinising agents are used to return the urine pH back to normal, thus relieving symptoms of dysuria. However, they have little trial data to support their use. Only one trial by Spooner (1984) could be found to support their efficacy. Spooner concluded that, when treated with a 2-day course of Cymalon, 80% of patients with cystitis for whom there was no clear clinical evidence of bacterial infection did gain symptomatic relief.

Cranberry juice

Cranberry juice is a popular alternative remedy to treat and prevent urinary tract infections, although few clinical trials have been performed to substantiate or refute its clinical effectiveness. A Cochrane review (Jepson et al., 2012) identified 10 studies comparing cranberry juice or cranberry tablets to placebo. The review found cranberry products significantly reduced the incidence of UTIs at 12 months, particularly in women who suffer recurrent infections. However, dropout rates in the trials were high, suggesting many patients may not be able to tolerate cranberry juice long term. The authors concluded that there was evidence that cranberry juice did offer some protection against recurrence of urinary tract infections in women that suffer symptomatic UTIs. However, it is still unclear what amount and concentration needs to be consumed, or how long patients should take it for.

The same authors also reviewed the use of cranberry juice in the treatment of existing UTIs (Jepson et al., 1998, updated in 2010). However, they were unable to find any randomised controlled trials (RCTs) that met their criteria. The authors concluded that there was no good evidence yet to support the use of cranberry juice for the treatment of UTIs.

Studies involving cranberry juice were not associated with any serious adverse events, but widespread use of cranberry juice has resulted in the identification of a possible interaction with warfarin, although evidence is currently conflicting (Jepson et al., 2012). Until evidence is conclusive it would seem prudent that patients on warfarin should be advised not to take products containing cranberry.

Practical prescribing and product selection

Prescribing information relating to cystitis medicines reviewed in the section 'Evidence base for over-the-counter medication' is discussed and summarised in Table 6.3, and useful tips relating to patients presenting with cystitis are given in 'Hints and Tips' in Box 6.1.

Alkalinising agents

All marketed products are presented as a 2-day treatment course. The majority are presented as sachets (Effercitrate are dissolvable tablets), and the dosage is one sachet to be taken three times a day, although potassium citrate can be bought as a ready-made solution (the dosage is 10 mL three times a day, diluted well with water) They possess very few side effects and can be given safely with other prescribed medication, although, in theory, products containing potassium should be avoided in patients taking angiotensin-converting enzyme (ACE) inhibitors, potassium-sparing diuretics and spironolactone. However, in practice it is highly unlikely that

Table 6.3
Practical prescribing: Summary of medicines for cystitis

Name of medicine	Use in children	Likely side effects	Drug interactions of note	Patients in which care is exercised	Pregnancy & breastfeeding
Potassium citrate					
Effercitrate	>6 year*	Gastric irritation	None	Patients taking ACE inhibitors, potassium-sparing diuretics and spironolactone	OK
Cystopurin	>6 years*	None			
Sodium citrate					
Cymalon	Not recommended	None reported	None	Patients with heart disease, hypertension or renal impairment	OK
Canesten Oasis					

ACE, angiotensin converting enzyme.
*Children should not be treated for UTI by pharmacists as unusual in this age group.

HINTS AND TIPS BOX 6.1: CYSTITIS

Fluid intake	Patients should be advised to drink about 5 L of fluid during every 24-h period. This will help promote bladder voiding, which is thought to help 'flush' bacteria out of the bladder
Product taste	The taste of potassium citrate mixture is unpleasant. Patients should be advised to dilute the mixture with water to make the taste more palatable

a 2-day course of an alkalinising agent will be of any clinical consequence. They can also be prescribed to most patient groups and can be given in pregnancy, although most manufacturers advise against prescribing in pregnancy, presumably on the basis that pregnant women have a higher incidence of complications resulting from cystitis. The manufacturers of Effercitrate and Cystopurin state they can be used in children, but good practice would dictate that children under 16 should be referred to a medical practitioner.

References

Jepson RG, Williams G, Craig JC. Cranberries for preventing urinary tract infections. Cochrane Database of Systematic Reviews 2012, Issue 10. Art. No.: CD001321. http://dx.doi.org/10.1002/14651858.CD001321.pub5.

Jepson RG, Mihaljevic L, Craig JC. Cranberries for treating urinary tract infections. Cochrane Database of Systematic Reviews 1998, Issue 4. Art. No.: CD001322. http://dx.doi.org/10.1002/14651858.CD001322.

Le J, Briggs GG, McKeown A, et al. Urinary tract infections during pregnancy. Ann Pharmacother 2004;38(10):1692–701.

Spooner JB. Alkalinisation in the management of cystitis. J Int Med Res 1984;12:30–4.

Further reading

Bent S, Nallamothu BK, Simel DL, et al. Does this woman have an acute uncomplicated urinary tract infection? JAMA 2002;287:2701–10.

Car J. Urinary tract infections in women: diagnosis and management in primary care. Br Med J 2006;332:94–7.

Website

Cystitis and overactive bladder foundation: http://www.cobfoundation.org

Vaginal discharge

Background

Patients of any age can experience vaginal discharge. The three most common causes of vaginal discharge are bacterial vaginosis (most common), vulvovaginal candidiasis

Table 6.4
Causes of vaginal discharge and their relative incidence in community pharmacy

Incidence	Cause
Most likely	Bacterial vaginosis
Likely	Thrush (medicine-induced thrush)
Unlikely	Trichomoniasis, atrophic vaginitis, cystitis

viscosity. Normal secretions have no odour. The epithelium of the vagina contains glycogen, which is broken down by enzymes and bacteria (most notably lactobacilli) into acids. This maintains the low vaginal pH, creating an environment inhospitable to pathogens. The glycogen concentration is controlled by oestrogen production; therefore any changes in oestrogen levels will result in either increased or decreased glycogen concentrations. If oestrogen levels decrease glycogen concentration also decreases, giving rise to an increased vaginal pH and making the vagina more susceptible to opportunistic infection, such as *Candida albicans;* 95% of thrush cases are caused by *C. albicans.* The remaining cases are caused by *C. glabrata*, although symptoms are indistinguishable.

(thrush) and trichomoniasis (Table 6.4). As thrush is the only condition that can be treated OTC, the text concentrates on differentiating this from other conditions.

Prevalence and epidemiology

It has been reported that sexually active women have a 75% chance of experiencing at least one episode of thrush during their childbearing years, and half of these will have more than one episode. Most cases are acute attacks, but some women will develop recurrent thrush, defined as four or more attacks each year. The condition is uncommon in prepubertal girls, unless they have been receiving antibiotics. In adolescents it is the second most common cause of vaginal discharge after bacterial vaginosis.

Aetiology of thrush

The vagina naturally produces a watery discharge (physiological discharge), the amount and character of which varies depending on many factors, such as ovulation, pregnancy and concurrent medication. At the time of ovulation the discharge is greater in quantity and of higher

Arriving at a differential diagnosis

Many patients will present with a self-diagnosis, and the pharmacists' role will often be to confirm a self-diagnosis of thrush. This is very important, as studies have shown that misdiagnosis by patients is common (Ferris et al., 2002) and can have important consequences because other conditions can lead to greater health concerns. For example, bacterial vaginosis has been linked with pelvic inflammatory disease (PID) and the preterm delivery of low-birth-weight infants, and *C. trachomatis* can cause infertility. Symptoms of pruritus, burning and discharge are possible in all three common causes of vaginal discharge; therefore no one symptom can be relied upon with 100% certainty to differentiate between thrush, bacterial vaginosis and trichomoniasis. However, certain symptom clusters are strongly suggestive of a particular diagnosis. Asking symptom-specific questions will help the pharmacist establish a differential diagnosis (Table 6.5).

Table 6.5
Specific questions to ask the patient: Vaginal discharge

Question	Relevance
Discharge	Any discharge with a strong odour should be referred. Bacterial vaginosis and trichomoniasis are associated with a fishy odour. Discharge in bacterial vaginosis tends to be grey-white and trichomoniasis green-yellow. By contrast, discharge associated with thrush is often described as 'curd-like' or 'cottage cheese-like' with little or no odour. Note physiological discharge is clear and odourless but can cause slight staining of underwear
Age	Thrush can occur in any age group, unlike bacterial vaginosis and trichomoniasis, which are rare in premenarchal girls. In addition, trichomoniasis is also rare in women aged over 60
Pruritus	Vaginal itching tends to be most prominent in thrush compared with bacterial vaginosis and trichomoniasis where itch is slight or absent
Onset	In thrush the onset of symptoms is sudden, whereas in bacterial vaginosis and trichomoniasis onset tends to be less sudden

Clinical features of thrush

The dominant feature of thrush is vulval itching. This is often accompanied with discharge (in up to 20% of patients). The discharge has little or no odour and is curd-like. Symptoms are generally acute in onset.

Conditions to eliminate

Bacterial vaginosis

This is the most common cause of vaginal discharge seen in a community pharmacy setting; it must be eliminated as a cause of symptoms, as treatment requires antibiotics (metronidazole 400 mg twice daily for 5–7 days). The exact cause of bacterial vaginosis is unknown but results from an overgrowth of anaerobic bacteria and reduction in lactobacilli concentration. *Gardnerella vaginalis* is often implicated. Approximately half of patients will experience a thin, white discharge with a strong fishy odour. Odour is worse after sexual intercourse and may worsen during menses. Itching and soreness are not usually present. Certain risk factors include change in sexual partner, multiple sexual partners, low social class and race (more common in African and African American women). It may remit and relapse for several months.

Unlikely causes

Trichomoniasis

Trichomoniasis, a protozoan infection, is primarily transmitted through sexual intercourse. It is uncommon compared with bacterial vaginosis and thrush. Up to 50% of patients are asymptomatic. If symptoms are experienced a profuse, frothy, greenish-yellow and fishy-smelling discharge, accompanied by vulvar itching and soreness, is typical. Other symptoms can include vaginal spotting, dysuria and urgency. Referral for metronidazole (400 mg bd for 5–7 days) is required.

Cystitis

Dysuria can affect up to one in three women with vaginal infection. However, the patient will often be able to sense that it is an external discomfort, rather than an internal discomfort, located in the urethra or bladder, that occurs with urinary tract infections. Other symptoms such as nocturia and urgency will be more prominent if cystitis is suspected.

Atrophic vaginitis

Symptoms consistent with thrush in postmenopausal women, especially vaginal itching and burning, may be due to atrophic vaginitis. However, clinically significant atrophic vaginitis is uncommon in postmenopausal women, and should be referred to rule out malignancy.

There are also several factors that predispose women to thrush and require consideration before initiating treatment.

Medicine-induced thrush

Broad-spectrum antibiotics, corticosteroids, immunosuppressants and medication affecting the oestrogen status of the patient (oral contraceptives, hormone replacement therapy, tamoxifen and raloxifene) can predispose women to thrush. It is, therefore, not unusual to see a patient prescribed an antibiotic and treatment for thrush at the same time.

Diabetes

Patients with poorly controlled diabetes (type 1 or 2) are more likely to suffer from thrush because hyperglycaemia can enhance production of protein surface receptors on *C. albicans* organisms. This hinders phagocytosis by neutrophils, thus making thrush more difficult to eliminate.

Pregnancy

Hormonal changes during pregnancy will alter the vaginal environment and have been reported to make eradication of *Candida* more difficult. Topical agents are safe and effective in pregnancy, but OTC-licensed indications are not allowed to be sold to pregnant women and, therefore, these patients must be referred to the doctor.

Chemical and mechanical irritants

Ingredients in feminine hygiene products, for example, e.g., bubble baths, vaginal sprays and douches, can precipitate attacks of thrush by altering vaginal pH. Condoms have also been found to irritate and alter the vaginal pH.

Recurrent thrush (four or more episodes per year)

After treatment a minority of patients will present with recurrent symptoms. This may be due to poor adherence, misdiagnosis, resistant strains of *Candida*, undiagnosed diabetes or the patient having a mixed infection. Such cases are outside the remit of community pharmacy and have shown to be difficult to treat. Often specialist care is needed through genitourinary medicine clinics.

Fig. 6.2 will help in the differentiation of vaginal thrush from other conditions in which vaginal discharge is a major presenting complaint.

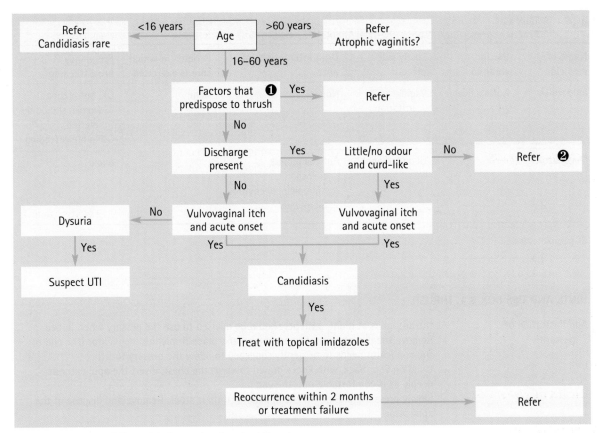

Fig. 6.2 Primer for differential diagnosis of vaginal thrush.

❶ If the person is pregnant or has diabetes then referral is the most appropriate option. If the person is suffering from medicine–induced candidiasis, the prescriber should be contacted to discuss suitable treatment options and, if appropriate, alternative therapy.

❷ Discharge that has a strong odour and is not white and curd–like should be referred, as trichomoniasis or bacterial vaginosis are more likely causes.

Evidence base for over–the–counter medication

Topical imidazoles and one systemic triazole (fluconazole) are available OTC to treat vaginal thrush. They are potent and selective inhibitors of fungal enzymes necessary for the synthesis of ergosterol, which is needed to maintain the integrity of cell membranes.

Imidazoles and triazoles have proven and comparable efficacy with clinical cure rates between 85% and 90%. Additionally, cure rates between single- or multiple-dose therapy and multiple-day therapy show no differences (Nurbhai et al., 2009). Treatment choice will, therefore, be driven by patient acceptability and cost.

Practical prescribing and product selection

Prescribing information relating to medicines for thrush reviewed in the section 'Evidence base for over-the-counter

! TRIGGER POINTS indicative of referral: Thrush

Symptoms/signs	Possible danger/reason for referral
Discharge that has a strong smell	Suggests bacterial vaginosis or trichomoniasis
Patients with diabetes	Might suggest poor diabetic control
OTC medication failure Patients predisposed to thrush Recurrent attacks	Suggests underlying problem or misdiagnosis
Women under 16 and over 60	Thrush unusual in these age groups

Table 6.6
Practical prescribing: Summary of medicines for thrush

Name of medicine	Use in children	Likely side effects	Drug interactions of note	Patients in which care is exercised	Pregnancy & breastfeeding
Imidazoles	Not applicable	Vaginal irritation	None	None	OK, but pregnant women should be referred; OK in breastfeeding
Fluconazole		GI disturbances	Anticoagulants, ciclosporin, rifampicin, phenytoin, tacrolimus		Avoid

GI, gastrointestinal.

HINTS AND TIPS BOX 6.2: THRUSH

Administration of pessaries	As the dosage is at night, patients should be advised to use the pessary when in bed • Remove the pessary from the packaging and place firmly into applicator (the end of the applicator needs to be gently squeezed to allow the pessary to fit) • Lying on your back, with knees drawn towards the chest, insert the applicator as deeply as is comfortable into the vagina • Slowly press the plunger of the applicator until it stops. Remove and dispose of the applicator • Remain in the supine position
Use of yoghurt	Some people recommended live yoghurt as a 'natural' treatment. This is based on sound rationale, as lactobacilli contained in the yoghurt produce lactic acid, which inhibits the growth of *Candida*. However, to date, there is a lack of evidence to prove or disprove this theory
General advice to help prevent infection	Avoid tight clothing, e.g., underwear, jeans, etc. Use simple, non-perfumed soaps when washing
Symptom resolution	The symptoms of thrush (burning, soreness or itching of the vagina) should disappear within 3 days of treatment. If no improvement is seen after 7 days the patient should see their GP
Vaginal douching	This should not be encouraged, has no evidence of efficacy, and is associated with serious complications such as pelvic inflammatory disease

---

medication' is discussed in the next section and summarised in Table 6.6; useful tips relating to patients presenting with thrush are given in 'Hints and Tips' in Box 6.2.

Topical imidazoles (clotrimazole, econazole, miconazole)

A number of formulations are available for local application including creams, vaginal tablets and pessaries.

Pharmacists and the public are probably most familiar with the clotrimazole range of products. All internal preparations should be administered at night. This gives the medicine time to be absorbed and eliminates the possibility of accidental loss, which is more likely to occur if the person is mobile. Slight irritation on application is infrequently reported (about 5% of users) and has been linked to the vehicle and not the active ingredient. Systemic absorption is minimal and,

6

Table 6.7
Product license restrictions – topical imidazoles

Product license restriction	Rationale
Is under 16, or over 60, years of age	Thrush less common in these age groups
Has systemic symptoms	Suggests infection from a cause other than thrush
Has symptoms that are not entirely consistent with a previous episode (e.g., discharge is coloured or malodourous; there are ulcers or blisters)	Suspect bacterial vaginitis or trichomoniasis
Has had two episodes in 6 months, and has not consulted her GP about the condition for more than a year	Good practice, as repeat infection may be due to misdiagnosis or predisposing risk factors
May be pregnant or is breastfeeding	Safe in both pregnancy and breastfeeding, although thrush is more common during pregnancy; it is also important to rule out gestational diabetes
Has had a previous sexually transmitted infection (or her partner has)	Rule out STD
Has had abnormal menstrual bleeding or lower abdominal pain	Symptoms not suggestive of thrush
Does not experience complete resolution of symptoms after 7 days of treatment	Imidazoles are highly effective, and continuing symptoms point to misdiagnosis

STD, sexually transmitted disease.

therefore, there are no interactions of note, although they may damage latex condoms and diaphragms. Consequently, the effectiveness of such contraceptives may be reduced. Topical imidazoles do have a number of product license restrictions which should be observed when recommending these products, and are listed in Table 6.7.

Fluconazole (e.g., Canesten oral)

Fluconazole is a single oral dose treatment that can be taken at any time of the day. (Note: there are also combination packs containing oral fluconazole and a tube of topical clotrimazole.) Fluconazole is generally well tolerated but can cause gastrointestinal disturbances such as nausea, abdominal discomfort, diarrhoea and flatulence in up to 10% of patients. There are a number of established, clinically important drug interactions with fluconazole. These include anticoagulants, ciclosporin, rifampicin, phenytoin and tacrolimus. However, these drug interactions relate to the use of multiple-dose fluconazole, and the relevance to single-dose fluconazole has not yet been established. It would be prudent to avoid these combinations until further evidence is available with single-dose fluconazole.

References
Ferris DG, Nyirjesy P, Sobel JD, et al. Over-the-counter antifungal drug misuse associated with patient-diagnosed vulvovaginal candidiasis. Obstet Gynecol 2002;99:419–25.
Nurbhai M, Grimshaw J, Watson M, et al. Oral versus intra-vaginal imidazole and triazole anti-fungal treatment of uncomplicated vulvovaginal candidiasis (thrush). Cochrane Database of Systematic Reviews 2007, Issue 4.

Further reading
Brown D, Binder GL, Gardner HL, et al. Comparison of econazole and clotrimazole in the treatment of vulvovaginal candidiasis. Obstet Gynecol 1980;56:121–3.
Colver H, Malu M. Vaginal discharge: recommended management in general practice. The Prescriber 2013;5 March:19–32.
Eschenbach DA, Hillier S, Critchlow C, et al. Diagnosis and clinical manifestations of bacterial vaginosis. Am J Obstet Gynecol 1988;158:819–28.
Ferris DG, Dekle C, Litaker MS. Women's use of over-the-counter antifungal medications for gynecologic symptoms. J Fam Pract 1996;42:595–600.
Fidel PL, Sobel JD. Immunopathogenesis of recurrent vulvovaginal candidiasis. Clin Microbiol Rev 1996;9:335–48.

Floyd R, Hodgson C. One-day treatment of vulvovaginal candidiasis with a 500-mg clotrimazole vaginal tablet compared with a three-day regimen of two 100-mg vaginal tablets daily. Clin Ther 1986;8:181–6.

Lebherz TB, Goldman L, Wiesmeier E, et al. A comparison of the efficacy of two vaginal creams for vulvovaginal candidiasis, and correlations with the presence of Candida species in the perianal area and oral contraceptive use. Clin Ther 1983;5:409–16.

Sobel JD, Faro S, Force RW, et al. Vulvovaginal candidiasis: epidemiologic, diagnostic and therapeutic considerations. Am J Obstet Gynecol 1998;178:203–11.

Spence D, Melville C. Vaginal discharge. Br Med J 2007;335:1147–51 (1 December), http://dx.doi.org/10.1136/bmj.39378.633287.80.

Websites

Embarrassing problems: http://www.embarrassingproblems.com/problem/vaginal-vulva-problems

NHS choices: Sex and young people: http://www.nhs.uk/Livewell/Sexandyoungpeople/Pages/Sex-and-young-people-hub.aspx

Primary dysmenorrhoea (period pain)

Background

Menstruation spans the years between menarche to menopause. Typically this will last 30 to 40 years, starting around the age of 12 and ceasing around the age of 50. The menstrual cycle usually lasts 28 days, but this can vary and last any time between 21 and 45 days. Menstruation itself lasts between 3 and 7 days. Individuals can also exhibit differences in menstrual cycle length and blood flow. Dysmenorrhoea is usually categorised as primary or secondary; primary dysmenorrhoea (PD) is defined as menstrual pain without organic pathology whereas in secondary dysmenorrhoea an identifiable pathological condition can be identified.

Prevalence and epidemiology

PD is very common but exact prevalence rates vary due to differing definitions of dysmenorrhoea used in studies, and estimates range from affecting 50–90% of menstruating women. A low percentage (7–15%) of these women report symptoms severe enough to cause school and work absence.

Aetiology

Overproduction of uterine prostaglandins E_2 and $F_{2-alpha}$ are major contributory factors in causing painful cramps. Prostaglandin production is controlled by progesterone and, before menstruation starts, progesterone levels decrease, allowing prostaglandin production to increase, and, if over produced, cramps occur. Ovulation inhibition can also improve symptoms (by using the oral contraceptive pill), as it lessens the endometrial lining of the uterus, reducing menstrual fluid volume and prostaglandin production.

Arriving at a differential diagnosis

The main consideration of the community pharmacist is to exclude conditions that have a pathological cause (secondary dysmenorrhoea). Fortunately, by far and away the most likely problem seen in primary care is PD (Table 6.8).

It is essential to take a detailed history of the patient's menstrual history as PD is a diagnosis based on exclusion. The frequency, severity and relationship of symptoms to the menstrual cycle need to be established. Asking symptom-specific questions will help the pharmacist to establish a differential diagnosis (Table 6.9).

Clinical features of PD

A typical presentation of PD is of lower abdominal cramping pains shortly before (6 hours) and for 2 or possibly 3 days after the onset of bleeding. Commonly associated symptoms include fatigue, back pain, nausea and/or vomiting and diarrhoea. It is classically associated with young women who have recently (6–12 months) started having regular periods. However, there may be a gap of months or years between menarche and onset of symptoms. This is due to as many as 50% of women being anovulatory in the first year (and still 10% of women

Table 6.8
Causes of period pain and their relative incidence in community pharmacy

Incidence	Cause
Most likely	Primary dysmenorrhoea
Likely	Secondary dysmenorrhoea
Unlikely	Pelvic inflammatory disease, dysfunctional uterine bleeding

6

	Table 6.9

Specific questions to ask the patient: Primary dysmenorrhoea

Question	Relevance
Age	PD is most common in adolescents and women in their early 20s. Secondary dysmenorrhoea usually affects women many years after the menarche, typically after the age of 30
Nature of pain	A great deal of overlap exists between PD and secondary dysmenorrhoea, but, generally, PD results in cramping, whereas secondary causes are usually described as dull, continuous diffuse pain
Severity of pain	Pain is rarely severe in PD; the severity decreases with the onset of menses. Any patient presenting with severe lower abdominal pain should be referred
Onset of pain	PD starts very shortly before or within 24 hours of the onset of menses and rarely lasts for more than 3 days. Pain associated with secondary dysmenorrhoea typically starts a few days before the onset of menses

8 years after the menarche). This is important to know, as anovulatory cycles are usually pain free.

Conditions to eliminate

Likely causes

Secondary dysmenorrhoea (e.g., endometriosis, fibroids and polyps)

Endometriosis simply means presence of endometrial tissue outside of the uterus. The exact incidence of endometriosis is unclear; however, it is the most common cause of secondary dysmenorrhoea. Reports suggest it may occur in up to 50% of menstruating women but many are asymptomatic. Any person over the age of 30, either presenting for the first time with dysmenorrhoea or who has noticed worsening symptoms, should be viewed with caution. Patients experience lower abdominal pain (aching, rather than cramping) that usually starts 5 to 7 days before menstruation begins and can be constant and severe. The pain often peaks at the onset of menstruation. Referred pain into the back and down the thighs is also possible.

Unlikely causes

Pelvic inflammatory disease

PID is an important cause of infertility and ectopic pregnancy. Many women are asymptomatic and only diagnosed during infertility investigation. It most commonly develops in sexually active women aged between 15 and 24 years old. Symptomatic cases show variable clinical presentation, but it is associated with dull bilateral lower abdominal pain and dysmenorrhoea (with pain greatest premenstrually). Other symptoms experienced include fever, malaise, vaginal discharge, irregular menses and dyspareunia.

Dysfunctional uterine bleeding

Dysfunctional uterine bleeding is a non-specific medical term defined as abnormal uterine bleeding that is not due to structural or systemic disease and includes conditions such as amenorrhoea (lack of menstruation) and menorrhagia (heavy periods), with the majority of cases attributable to menorrhagia. The pharmacist should ask the patient if their periods are different than usual.

TRIGGER POINTS indicative of referral: Primary dysmenorrhoea

Symptoms/signs	Possible danger/reason for referral
Heavy or unexplained bleeding	Possibly dysfunctional uterine bleeding
Pain experienced days before menses	Possibly secondary dysmenorrhoea
Pain that increases at the onset of menses Women over the age of 30 with new or worsening symptoms	
Accompanying systemic symptoms, such as fever and malaise	Suggests possible infection or pelvic inflammatory disease
Vaginal bleeding in postmenopausal women	Suggests potentially more sinister cause, such as carcinoma

Evidence base for over-the-counter medication

Non-steroidal anti-inflammatory drugs (NSAIDs)

The use of NSAIDs would be a logical choice because raised prostaglandin levels cause PD. In multiple clinical trials they have been shown to be effective in 80% to 85% of women. A Cochrane review (Marjoribanks et al., 2015) concluded that NSAIDs were very effective in relieving moderate to severe pain associated with PD compared with placebo. However, there was little evidence of superiority of any individual NSAID.

Hyoscine butylbromide (Buscopan)

In one study Buscopan was given to 17 patients in a double-blind placebo-crossover trial. The study failed to demonstrate a significant effect compared with placebo, or the comparator drug – aspirin, although in the authors' opinion Buscopan was a good alternative to NSAIDs.

Alverine (Spasmonal) is licensed for the treatment of dysmenorrhoea. It is an anticholinergic antispasmodic that relaxes the uterine smooth muscle; however, there is a lack of published evidence regarding its efficacy.

Low-dose combined oral contraceptives

Although not available OTC, oral contraceptives have been reported to be beneficial in treating PD. A Cochrane review (Wong et al., 2009) identified 10 trials, and found improvements in pain compared with placebo (OR = 2.01; 95% CI 1.32–3.08); therefore, if standard OTC treatment is not controlling symptoms adequately, then the patient should be best referred, as contraceptives provide an alternative treatment option.

Other treatment options

A number of alternative treatments have been tested in PD, most notably transcutaneous electrical nerve stimulation (TENS), acupuncture, exercise and dietary supplements. Of these, high frequency TENS appears to have the strongest body of evidence to support its use (Proctor et al., 2002), acupuncture appears promising (Smith et al., 2011) and

the evidence for exercise is uncertain (Brown & Brown, 2010). A wide range of dietary intervention is frequently recommended and includes vitamins B and E, fish oils and magnesium. Most trials were conducted with low patient numbers and have reported limited or no benefit except vitamin B_1 (thiamine – 100 mg), which saw a significant proportion of women with no pain compared with placebo (Proctor & Murphy, 2001). The Chinese herbal remedy *toki-shakuyaku-san*, taken for at least 6 months, may also reduce dysmenorrhoea (Proctor & Murphy, 2001).

Summary

NSAIDs (ibuprofen or naproxen) should be used as first-line therapy unless the patient is contraindicated from using an NSAID. A trial of two to three cycles should be long enough to determine whether NSAID therapy is successful. If NSAIDs are ineffective or poorly tolerated, then paracetamol should be offered.

Practical prescribing and product selection

Prescribing information relating to the medicines reviewed in the section 'Evidence base for over-the-counter medication' is discussed and summarised in Table 6.10; useful tips relating to patients presenting with PD are given in 'Hints and Tips' in Box 6.3.

Ibuprofen

There is a plethora of marketed ibuprofen products (e.g., Nurofen and Cuprofen), all of which have a standard dose for the relief of PD. Adults should take 200 to 400 mg (one or two tablets) three times a day, although most patients will need the higher dose of 400 mg three times a day. Because ibuprofen is only used for a few days each cycle,

Table 6.10
Practical prescribing: Summary of medicines for primary dysmenorrhoea

Name of medicine	Use in children	Likely side effects	Drug interactions of note	Patients in which care is exercised	Pregnancy & breastfeeding
Ibuprofen	Unlikely to be having periods. Not recommended	GI discomfort, nausea and diarrhoea	Lithium, anticoagulants, methotrexate	Elderly (increased risk of side effects)	Not applicable in pregnancy, as patients do not menstruate during pregnancy. NSAIDs OK in breastfeeding, but avoid hyoscine, if possible, due to lack of data
Naproxen					
Hyoscine		Dry mouth, sedation and constipation	Other anticholinergics, e.g., tricyclic antidepressants	Glaucoma	

HINTS AND TIPS BOX 6.3: PRIMARY DYSMENORRHOEA

Hot water bottles	The application of warmth to the lower abdomen may confer some relief of the pain

it is generally well tolerated. However, gastric irritation is possible and ibuprofen can cause peptic ulcers or bronchospasm in asthmatics who have a history of hypersensitivity to aspirin or NSAIDs. Ibuprofen can interact with many medicines, although most are not clinically significant (see Table 6.10).

Naproxen (Feminax Ultra)

Naproxen is indicated for primary dysmenorrhoea for women aged between 15 and 50 years old. The dose is two tablets (500 mg) initially, followed 6 to 8 hours later by a second tablet (250 mg), if needed. No more than three tablets should be taken in a 24-hour period. The same side effects, cautions and contraindications with ibuprofen apply to naproxen.

Hyoscine hydrobromide (Buscopan Cramps)

The dosage frequency for adults is two tablets four times a day. It is contraindicated in patients with narrow-angle glaucoma and myasthenia gravis, and care should be exercised in patients whose conditions are characterised by tachycardia (e.g., hyperthyroidism and cardiac problems). Anticholinergic side effects such as dry mouth, visual disturbances and constipation can be experienced but are generally mild and self-limiting. Side effects are potentiated if it is given with tricyclic antidepressants, antihistamines, butyrophenones, phenothiazines and disopyramide.

References

Brown J, Brown S. Exercise for dysmenorrhoea. Cochrane Database of Systematic Reviews 2010, Issue 2. Art.No.: CD004142. http://dx.doi.org/10.1002/14651858.CD004142.pub2.

Marjoribanks J, Ayeleke RO, Farquhar C, et al. Nonsteroidal anti-inflammatory drugs for dysmenorrhoea. Cochrane Database of Systematic Reviews 2015, Issue 7. Art. No.: CD001751. http://dx.doi.org/10.1002/14651858.CD001751.pub3.

Proctor M, Murphy PA. Herbal and dietary therapies for primary and secondary dysmenorrhoea. Cochrane Database of Systematic Reviews 2001, Issue 2. Art. No.: CD002124. http://dx.doi.org/10.1002/14651858.CD002124.

Proctor M, Farquhar C, Stones W, et al. Transcutaneous electrical nerve stimulation for primary dysmenorrhoea. Cochrane Database of Systematic Reviews 2002, Issue 1. Art. No.: CD002123. http://dx.doi.org/10.1002/14651858.CD002123.

Smith CA, Zhu X, He L, et al. Acupuncture for primary dysmenorrhoea. Cochrane Database of Systematic Reviews 2011, Issue 1. Art. No.: CD007854. http://dx.doi.org/10.1002/14651858.CD007854.pub2.

Wong CL, Farquhar C, Roberts H, et al. Oral contraceptive pill for primary dysmenorrhoea. Cochrane Database of Systematic Reviews 2009, Issue 4. Art. No.: CD002120. http://dx.doi.org/10.1002/14651858.CD002120.pub3.

Further reading

Auld B, Sinha P. Dysmenorrhoea: diagnosis and current management. The Prescriber 2006:33–40.

Harlow SD, Ephross SA. Epidemiology of menstruation and its relevance to women's health. Epidemiol Rev 1995;17:265–86.

Kemp JH. 'Buscopan' in spasmodic dysmenorrhoea. Curr Med Res Opin 1972;1:19–25.

Websites

Endometriosis UK: http://www.endo.org.uk/
Endometriosis SHE Trust: http://www.shetrust.org.uk/
Royal College of Obstetricians and Gynaecologists: http://www.rcog.org.uk

Premenstrual syndrome

Background

Premenstrual syndrome (PMS) is a broad term that encompasses a wide range of symptoms – both physical and psychological. Symptoms range from mild to very severe; severe symptoms, especially mood symptoms, affect approximately 5% of patients and can interfere with day-to-day functioning and relationships. In these women a diagnosis of premenstrual dysphoric disorder is given.

Prevalence and epidemiology

The exact prevalence of PMS is hard to determine because of varying definitions attributed to PMS, and the number of people that do not seek medical help. Surveys have shown that over 90% of women have experienced PMS symptoms, but only a fifth seek medical help, yet 13–25% have taken time off work because of PMS symptoms. There appears to be no marked racial or ethnic differences in the prevalence, but age appears to be a risk factor – most women tend to be over 30 years old.

Aetiology

The precise pathophysiology of PMS is still unclear. A number of theories have been put forward, for example, excess oestrogen, a lack of progesterone or ovarian function. Most researchers now believe PMS is a complex interaction between ovarian steroids and the neurotransmitters serotonin and γ-aminobutyric acid (GABA).

Arriving at a differential diagnosis

Owing to the varying and wide-ranging symptoms associated with PMS, the pharmacist must endeavour to differentiate PMS from other gynaecological and mental health disorders. Careful questioning of when the symptoms occur and what symptoms are experienced will hopefully give rise to a differential diagnosis of PMS, although this might not be easy. It is important not to focus on one cycle's symptoms, but ask the patient to describe their symptoms over previous cycles. A diary over three cycles should be maintained to allow a fuller picture of symptoms to be elucidated (symptom diaries are available such as the Daily Record of Severity of Problems – see www.rcog.org.uk). Asking symptom-specific questions will help the pharmacist establish a differential diagnosis (Table 6.11).

Clinical features of PMS

Many symptoms have been attributed to PMS, although the most common symptoms are listed in Table 6.12.

Conditions to eliminate

Primary dysmenorrhoea

Abdominal cramps and suprapubic pain might be experienced by PMS sufferers, although these symptoms are uncommon. Key distinguishing features between PMS and primary dysmenorrhoea are the lack of behavioural and mood symptoms in primary dysmenorrhoea and the difference in the timing of symptoms in relation to the menstrual cycle.

Mental health disorders

Depression and anxiety are common mental health disorders, which often go undiagnosed and can be encountered by community pharmacists. Patients with PMS might experience symptoms similar to such conditions, namely low or sad mood, loss of interest or pleasure and prominent anxiety or worry. Other symptoms may include disturbed sleep and appetite, dry mouth and poor concentration. However, the symptoms are not cyclical and are not associated with other symptoms of PMS such as breast tenderness and bloating.

Table 6.12
Common symptoms of PMS

Physical	Behavioural	Mood
Swelling	Sleep disturbances	Irritability
Breast tenderness	Appetite changes	Mood swings
Aches	Poor concentration	Anxiety/tension
Headache	Decreased interest	Depression
Bloating/weight	Social withdrawal	Feeling out of control

Table 6.11
Specific questions to ask the patient: Premenstrual syndrome

Question	Relevance
Onset of symptoms	Symptoms that are experienced 7–14 days before, and that disappear a few hours after the onset of menses, are suggestive of PMS
Age of patient	PMS is most common in women aged in their 30s and 40s
Presenting symptoms	Patients with PMS will normally have symptoms suggestive of mental health disorders, such as low mood, insomnia and irritability. This can make excluding mental health disorders, such as depression, difficult. However, the cyclical nature of the symptoms in conjunction with symptoms such as breast tenderness, bloatedness and fluid retention point to PMS

<table>
<tr><td colspan="2">TRIGGER POINTS indicative of referral: Premenstrual syndrome</td></tr>
<tr><td>Symptoms/signs</td><td>Possible danger/reason for referral</td></tr>
<tr><td>Psychological symptoms alone</td><td>If not occurring in sync with usual menstrual cycle, these could indicate potential anxiety or depressive disorders</td></tr>
<tr><td>Severe or disabling symptoms</td><td>May indicate a more severe form, such as premenstrual dysphoric disorder</td></tr>
<tr><td>Symptoms that either worsen or stay the same after the onset of menses</td><td>Does not suggest PMS, as symptoms should abate once menstruation starts</td></tr>
</table>

depression (Wyatt et al., 1999). Caution is needed in the review findings, as most included trials were of poor quality.

Vitex agnus-castus (VAC), from the fruit of the chaste tree, is also promoted for various menstrual issues, including PMS. A recent, well-conducted systematic review found four studies using VAC at doses of 20 to 40 mg daily and, in all studies, it was found to reduce physical and psychological symptoms by more than 50% compared with control (Jang et al., 2014). The same review located one study that compared VAC to fluoxetine 20 to 40 mg daily and found no significant difference in efficacy between the two. However, it must be noted that although the quality of the studies was assessed in the systematic review, most studies involving VAC lacked information on randomisation and concealment of allocation.

Summary

The evidence is limited for dietary and herbal supplements in the treatment of PMS. However, calcium supplements, vitamin B_6 and Vitex agnus-castus have the best evidence of effectiveness, and could be considered in mild to moderate PMS.

Practical prescribing and product selection

Prescribing information relating to medicines for PMS reviewed in the section 'Evidence base for over-the-counter medication' is discussed and summarised in Table 6.13.

Calcium

Calcium supplementation should provide at least 1200 mg of elemental calcium per day. It is important to ensure that a product taken by the patient provides the required amount of elemental calcium. For example, a calcium lactate 300 mg tablet provides only 39 mg of elemental

Evidence base for over-the-counter medication

There are many drug and non-drug treatments advocated for the treatment of PMS, yet most lack evidence from well-conducted RCTs. A lack of evidence or no evidence exists to support the use of reflexology, exercise, chiropractic manipulation, bright light therapy and relaxation. With regard to herbal, vitamin or mineral supplementation, only calcium supplements have good evidence of effectiveness (Whelan et al., 2009). Calcium supplementation at doses of 1200 mg per day for 3 months has shown that overall PMS symptoms are significantly reduced in the luteal phase compared with placebo (Ward & Holimon, 1999).

Trials involving vitamin B_6 have shown that overall symptoms of PMS improve over a period of 2 to 6 months and also help with behavioural/mood symptoms such as

Table 6.13
Practical prescribing: Summary of medicines used in premenstrual syndrome

Name of medicine	Use in children	Likely side effects	Drug interactions of note	Patients in which care is exercised	Pregnancy & breastfeeding
Pyridoxine	Not applicable	Very high doses can cause toxicity (>500 mg daily)	Levodopa when administered alone	None	Not applicable in pregnancy, as patients do not menstruate during pregnancy; OK in breastfeeding
Calcium		Nausea and flatulence	None	Renally impaired patients	
VAC		Skin reactions	None known	None	

calcium; calcium carbonate 1.25 g tablets (e.g., Calcichew) provide 500 mg of elemental calcium per tablet. Calcium supplements can cause mild gastrointestinal disturbances, such as nausea and flatulence. If the patient is taking tetracycline antibiotics or iron, then a 2-hour gap should elapse between doses to avoid decreased absorption of the antibiotic or iron.

Vitamin B₆ (pyridoxine)

There is no definitive dose of vitamin B_6 required to alleviate symptoms of PMS. However, doses of up to 100 mg daily have been shown to help reduce symptoms. Side effects are extremely rare with doses at this level, although, at higher doses, it can cause numbness and peripheral neuropathy. A number of drug interactions have been observed in patients taking vitamin B_6, most notably phenytoin, phenobarbital and levodopa. Only the vitamin B_6/levodopa interaction is significant and should be avoided. Although doses as low as 5 mg vitamin B_6 will reduce the effects of levodopa, the problem of this interaction in clinical practice is almost always negated, as combinations of levodopa/carbidopa (Sinemet) or levodopa/benserazide (Madopar) are unaffected by vitamin B_6.

Vitex agnus-castus

The key clinical trials using VAC used a dose of 20 to 40 mg of VAC extract, equating to approximately 180 to 360 mg of crude dried fruit per day. There are a number of preparations available in the UK; however there is little standardisation of dosing. VAC is generally well tolerated with no known interactions but limited adverse effects, mainly skin reactions, can occur.

References
Jang SH, Kim DI, Choi MS. Effects and treatment methods of acupuncture and herbal medicine for premenstrual syndrome/premenstrual dysphoric disorder: systematic review. BMC Complement Altern Med 2014;14(1):11.
Ward MW, Holimon TD. Calcium treatment for premenstrual syndrome. Ann Pharmacother 1999;33:1356–8.
Whelan AM, Jurgens TM, Naylor H. Herbs, vitamins and minerals in the treatment of premenstrual syndrome: a systematic review. Can J Clin Pharmacol 2009;16(3):e407–e429.
Wyatt KM, Dimmock PW, Jones PW, et al. Efficacy of vitamin B-6 in the treatment of premenstrual syndrome: systematic review. Br Med J 1999;318:1375–81.

Further reading
RCOG. Management of premenstrual syndrome. Royal College of Obstetricians and Gynaecologists. 2007. Available at: https://www.rcog.org.uk/en/guidelines-research-services/guidelines/gtg48/ (accessed 13 August, 2015).
Gianetto-Berruti A, Feyles V. Premenstrual syndrome. Minerva Ginecol 2002;54:85–95.
Thys-Jacobs S, Starkey P, Bernstein D, et al. Calcium carbonate and the premenstrual syndrome: effects on premenstrual and menstrual symptoms. Am J Gynecol 1998;179:444–52.

Website
National Association for Premenstrual Syndrome: http://www.pms.org.uk/

Heavy menstrual bleeding (menorrhagia)

Background

Heavy menstrual bleeding (HMB) has been quantified (in research settings) as between 60 mL to 80 mL of blood loss per cycle – but this is impractical in a clinical setting. A more useful and practical definition is excessive menstrual blood loss over several consecutive cycles, which interferes with a woman's physical, social, emotional and/or material quality of life.

Prevalence and epidemiology

The prevalence of HMB is difficult to establish due to varying definitions. However, 5% of women aged between 30 and 49 years old consult their GP each year (Vessey et al., 1992) and a third of women describe their periods as being heavy.

Aetiology

In approximately half of cases no identifiable cause can be found. Identifiable causes can result from uterine and pelvic pathology (e.g., fibroids, polyps and carcinoma), systemic disorders (e.g., hypothyroidism) and iatrogenic factors (e.g., medication and intrauterine devices).

Arriving at a differential diagnosis

The main consideration of the community pharmacist is to exclude sinister pathology. A detailed history of the patient's menstrual cycle is essential. Asking symptom-specific questions will help the pharmacist establish a differential diagnosis (Table 6.14).

? Table 6.14
Specific questions to ask the patient: Heavy menstrual bleeding

Question	Relevance
Timing of bleeding	Symptoms that might suggest structural or pathological abnormality include bleeding at times other than at menses
Effect on quality of life	An assessment should be made to determine what effect menstrual bleeding is having on the patient
Symptoms in relation to normal cycles	Patients will show cycle-to-cycle variation in the amount of blood loss. It is important to discuss with the patient this normal variation and to determine from the patient whether the patient feels blood loss is within the normal range

Clinical features of HMB

The key symptom will be blood loss that is perceived to be greater than normal. The patient's bleeding pattern should be the same as during normal menses but heavier.

Conditions to eliminate

Medicine-induced menstrual bleeding

Occasionally, medicines can change menstrual bleeding patterns (Table 6.15). If an adverse drug reaction is suspected then the pharmacist should contact the prescriber and discuss other treatment options. Additionally, the incidence of menstrual pain is higher in patients who have had an intrauterine device fitted.

Endometrial and cervical carcinoma

These are characterised by inappropriate uterine bleeding and usually occur in postmenopausal women. Bleeding starts as slight and intermittent but, over time, becomes heavy and continuous. Irregular bleeding between periods, especially if associated with postcoital bleeding, is extremely significant and suggests a precancerous state or cancer of the cervix.

Table 6.15
Medication that can alter menstrual bleeding

Anticoagulants
Cimetidine
Monoamine oxidase inhibitors
Phenothiazines
Steroids
Thyroid hormones

! TRIGGER POINTS indicative of referral: Menorrhagia

Symptoms/signs	Possible danger/reason for referral
Intermenstrual bleeding Postcoital bleeding Pelvic pain	Possibly a sign of cervical/ endometrial cancer
Treatment failure	May indicate alternative diagnosis or more serious pathology

Evidence base for over-the-counter medication

Tranexamic acid has been in clinical use in the UK for approximately 30 years and has established itself as a clinically effective medicine in decreasing menstrual blood loss. It reduces blood loss by up to 50%. It provides symptomatic relief and does not resolve underlying causes.

Practical prescribing and product selection

Tranexamic acid is an antifibrinolytic that stops the conversion of plasminogen to plasmin – an enzyme that digests fibrin and thus brings about clot dissolution. NICE guidelines (2007) state that if the patient history suggests no abnormalities, then drug treatment can be given (see 'Hints and Tips' in Box 6.4). This is either hormonal (currently still POM) or non-hormonal (NSAIDs or tranexamic acid). As an OTC product, it is restricted to women with a history of heavy bleeding who have regular (21–35 day) cycles that show no more than 3 days of individual variability in cycle duration.

HINTS AND TIPS BOX 6.4: HEAVY MENSTRUAL BLEEDING (HMB)

Which treatment?	If menorrhagia/HMB coexists with dysmenorrhoea, the use of NSAIDs should be preferred to tranexamic acid
Treatment failure (NICE guidance)	If there is no improvement in symptoms within 3 menstrual cycles, then use of NSAIDs and/or tranexamic acid should be stopped

Tranexamic acid

Tranexamic acid should be taken once bleeding starts. The dosage is two tablets three times a day for a maximum of 4 days. The dosage can be increased to two tablets four times a day in very heavy menstrual bleeding. The maximum dose is eight tablets (4 g) daily. Side effects are unusual. Those reported include mild nausea, vomiting and diarrhoea (affecting between 1% and 10% of patients).

Visual disturbances and thromboembolic events have been reported but are very rare. The causal relationship of thromboembolic events and tranexamic acid is unclear, and NICE guidelines state that no increase in the overall rate of thrombosis has been identified with those taking tranexamic acid. Nevertheless, women at high risk of thrombosis have been excluded from pharmacy supply.

Tranexamic acid should not be taken in patients on anticoagulants, taking the combined oral contraceptive, unopposed oestrogen or tamoxifen. In breastfeeding women one small, unpublished study suggests that only low levels of tranexamic acid pass into breast milk and that waiting 3 to 4 hours before breastfeeding will minimise any risk.

References

NICE guidelines. Heavy menstrual bleeding (Jan 2007). Available from https://www.nice.org.uk/guidance/cg44 (accessed 13 August 2015).

Vessey MP, Villard-Mackintosh L, McPherson K, et al. The epidemiology of hysterectomy: findings in a large cohort study. Br J Obstet Gynaecol 1992;99(5):402–7.

Self-assessment questions

The following questions are intended to supplement the text. Two levels of questions are provided; multiple-choice questions and case studies. The multiple-choice questions are designed to test factual recall, and the case studies allow knowledge to be applied to a practice setting.

Multiple-choice questions

6.1 Which of the following is NOT a product license restriction on the OTC sale of tranexamic acid?

    a. A woman with polycystic ovary syndrome
    b. A woman over the age of 45
    c. A woman with a 2-day variation in a menstrual cycle lasting 30 days
    d. A woman taking unopposed tamoxifen
    e. A woman taking an oral contraceptive

6.2 Which of the following would you NOT recommend as suitable OTC treatment for vulvovaginal candidiasis?

    a. Clotrimazole 10% vaginal cream
    b. Fluconazole 150 mg oral capsule
    c. Clotrimazole 500 mg pessary
    d. Ketoconazole 2% cream
    e. Clotrimazole 1% topical cream

6.3 A 39-year-old woman presents with what she describes as 'period pain'. On further questioning you ascertain that the aching pain, which can be quite severe, seems to be worse about a week before her period and is also worse during intercourse. Which condition is she most likely to be suffering from?

    a. Pelvic inflammatory disease
    b. Primary dysmenorrhoea
    c. Endometrial carcinoma
    d. Endometriosis
    e. Cervical carcinoma

6.4 Which of the following symptoms are NOT commonly associated with premenstrual syndrome?

    a. Sleep disturbances
    b. Breast tenderness
    c. Vaginal discharge
    d. Headache
    e. Fluid retention

6.5 Which set of symptoms most closely match that of vaginal thrush?

    a. Itch and discharge described as having an offensive odour
    b. Itch and burning sensation and curd-like discharge
    c. Little itching but frothy yellow discharge
    d. Little or no itch but increased urgency and pain on passing urine
    e. Little itching but associated with blood stained discharge

6.6 Which of the following symptoms is commonly associated with trichomoniasis?

    a. Frothy, green-yellow vaginal discharge
    b. Clear, watery vaginal discharge
    c. Cottage-cheese like vaginal discharge
    d. White, fishy-smelling vaginal discharge
    e. Small ulcers on the external genitalia

6.7 A woman presents with what she thinks is cystitis. Which of the following symptoms would cause you to refer her to the doctor?

    a. Pain when passing urine
    b. Increased frequency of urination
    c. Increased urgency of urination
    d. Pain in the loin area
    e. Voiding small amounts of urine

6.8 Which patient group is NOT considered to be at risk of developing an upper UTI?

    a. A woman whose symptoms have been present for 9 days
    b. Diabetic patients
    c. Pregnant women
    d. Immunocompromised patients
    e. Symptoms that are abrupt in onset

Questions 6.9 to 6.14 concern the following conditions:

A. Primary dysmenorrhoea
B. Pelvic inflammatory disease
C. Endometriosis
D. Menorrhagia
E. Endometrial carcinoma
F. Bacterial vaginosis
G. Thrush

Select from A to G, which:

6.9 Most common in sexually active women aged between 15 and 24 years old

6.10 Is caused by the overproduction of uterine prostaglandins

6.11 The key symptom is blood loss perceived to be greater than normal

6.12 Pain typically presents shortly before and for 2 to 3 days after commencement of menses

6.13 Usually occurs in postmenopausal women

6.14 Is associated with strong odour

Questions 6.15 to 6.17: For each of these questions *one or more* of the responses is (are) correct. Decide which of the responses is (are) correct. Then choose:

A. If a, b and c are correct
B. If a and b only are correct
C. If b and c only are correct
D. If a only is correct
E. If c only is correct

Directions summarised

A	B	C	D	E
a, b and c	a and b only	b and c only	a only	c only

6.15 A pharmacist should refer patients with premenstrual syndrome when:

a. They have cyclical mood swings
b. They complain of breast tenderness
c. They are under the age of 30 when first presenting with symptoms

6.16 Which of the following drugs can predispose women to thrush?

a. Non-steroidal anti-inflammatory drugs (NSAIDs)
b. Broad-spectrum antibiotics
c. Hormone replacement therapy

6.17 Which of the symptoms listed are indicative of referral?

a. Intermenstrual bleeding
b. Postcoital bleeding
c. Dyspareunia

Questions 6.18 to 6.20: These questions consist of a statement in the left-hand column, followed by a statement in the right-hand column. You need to:

● decide whether the first statement is true or false
● decide whether the second statement is true or false

Then choose:

A. If both statements are true, and the second statement is a correct explanation of the first statement
B. If both statements are true, but the second statement is NOT a correct explanation of the first statement
C. If the first statement is true, but the second statement is false
D. If the first statement is false, but the second statement is true
E. If both statements are false

Directions summarised

	1st statement	2nd statement	
A	True	True	2nd explanation is a correct explanation of the first
B	True	True	2nd statement is not a correct explanation of the first
C	True	False	
D	False	True	
E	False	False	

First statement *Second statement*

6.18 Poorly controlled diabetics are more likely to suffer from thrush

Hyperglycaemia encourages the proliferation of *C. albicans*

6.19 Cystitis symptoms lasting longer than 5–7 days should be referred

NSAIDs have been shown to cause cystitis

6.20 Tranexamic acid stops the conversion of plasminogen to plasmin

Patients should start taking tranexamic acid 1 day before their period starts

6

Case study

A woman aged about 30 comes into your pharmacy and asks to speak to you. She tells you that she thinks she has thrush again. When she had similar symptoms before, she saw the doctor, who prescribed her a cream to use. Although it was effective, it was messy to use, so she asks whether there is anything else she could use instead.

a. **What questions do you need to ask?**

It is best to confirm her self-diagnosis. Although she has had similar symptoms, it is always best to double check; therefore ask questions on the nature of the symptoms, e.g., itch and discharge. It is also worth finding out how long ago she saw the doctor to check for frequency of recurrence.

b. **What other factors should be considered?**

Questions should be aimed at deciding whether the patient is suitable for an OTC product, either internal or oral. Questions of this nature are generally linked to ensuring that the patient does not fall outside the product license restrictions of an imidazole vaginal pessary or oral fluconazole.

c. **In addition to supplying a product, is there anything else you could recommend?**

- *Avoid local irritants – perfumed products such as vaginal deodorants, soaps, bubble bath*
- *Avoid wearing tight-fitting trousers or tights. Loose-fitting cotton underwear allows the skin to breathe more*
- *Spermicides such as nonoxynol-9 may disturb the vaginal flora and precipitate infection*
- *Probiotics (e.g., live yoghurt) may be used orally or topically. Although there is no evidence they are effective, they will not cause any harm, and can be cooling to the affected area when used topically. However, these are messy to use, which is something the patient wants to avoid.*

CASE STUDY 6.2

Mrs PR, a 26-year-old woman, presents to the pharmacy Saturday afternoon asking for something for cystitis. The counter assistant finds out that the patient has had the symptoms for about 3 days and has tried no medication to relieve the symptoms. At this point the patient is referred to the pharmacist.

a. What are your initial thoughts about possible diagnoses?

Based on her age and presenting symptoms a self-diagnosis of cystitis is likely. Kidney infections are common and the major other condition to consider; her age also means that STIs are possible.

b. What questions do you need to ask?

Obviously finding out more about the presenting symptoms is important, as this allows you to gain a picture of the problem. However, once a general symptom profile has been established, you should use targeted questions to aid the diagnosis. These questions should be discriminatory between the likely causes of her symptoms to allow you to arrive at a diagnosis. Three questions that would help are:

- *Location of the pain*
- *Kidney infections have loin pain; cystitis does not*
- *Associated symptoms*
- *Kidney infections often have systemic symptoms*
- *Any factors that might have precipitated the attack*

Sexual activity can predispose to greater risk of STIs, although this could be a difficult question to ask in a pharmacy setting

You find out that Mrs PR is suffering from pain on urination, discomfort and she is going to the toilet frequently but has no other symptoms. She has had these symptoms previously, about 2 years ago, but they went away on their own after a day or two. She takes no medicine from her doctor.

c. What course of action are you going to take?

Symptoms suggest an uncomplicated, acute urinary tract infection and empirical treatment could be instigated, but the patient should be told that, if treatment fails, then she should visit the doctor. Advice about adequate fluid intake should also be given.

Mrs PR returns to the pharmacy on Monday evening with a prescription for erythromycin 250 mg qds × 20.

d. Is this an appropriate antibiotic for a urinary tract infection?

Trimethoprim (or nitrofurantoin) is first-line treatment, unless local health poilicies advocate against its use due to resistance. Enquiry should be made with the patient about previous treatments, as she may not be able to tolerate trimethoprim. Additionally, the course is for 5 days and normally a 3-day course is sufficient (good evidence exists for 3-day treatment courses).

CASE STUDY 6.3

A girl in her late teens/early 20s asks for some painkillers for period pain. The following questions are asked, and responses received.

Information gathering	Data generated
What symptoms experiencing	General aching pain in tummy
How long had the symptoms	2 days
Severity of pain	4/10 (Using a scale 1–10, where 1 is no or little pain, and 10 is excruciating pain)
Any other symptoms	Felt a little sick
When is your period due	Any time now
Additional questions asked	No systemic symptoms No discharge or unusual bleeding
Previous history of presenting complaint	Had period pain before but this seems worse than previous times

Information gathering	Data generated
Past medical history	None
Drugs (OTC, Rx and compliance)	Paracetamol for pain. Helps a little but wants something a bit stronger
Allergies	Not asked (not applicable)
Social history	Not asked (not applicable)
Family history	Not asked (not applicable)

Epidemiology dictates that the most likely cause of period pain seen in primary care is primary dysmenorrhoea.

Diagnostic pointers with regard to symptom presentation

The next table summarises the expected findings for questions when related to the different conditions that can be seen by community pharmacists.

CASE STUDY 6.3 (Continued)

	Age	Pain timing to period	Nature & severity of pain	Bleeding pattern	Discharge
Primary dysmenorrhoea	Under 30	Just prior	Aching, mild to moderate	Normal	Unusual
Secondary dysmenorrhoea	Over 30	Days before	Cramping, moderate to severe	Possible	Unusual
PID	Young sexually active	Not associated with menstruation	Dull and can vary in severity	Irregular	Yes
Medicines	Any	N/A	None	Irregular	N/A
Dysfunctional uterine bleeding	Any	N/A	None	Irregular	No
Carcinoma	Postmenopausal	N/A	No (only in late stage of disease)	Irregular	Rare

When this information is applied to that gained from our patient we see that her symptoms strongly suggest primary dysmenorrhoea. A degree of caution needs to be exercised because her symptoms seem worse than previous episodes and simple analgesia seems to be ineffective.

	Age	Pain timing to period	Nature & severity of pain	Bleeding pattern	Discharge
Primary dysmenorrhoea	✓	✓	✓	✓	✓
Secondary dysmenorrhoea	✗	✗	✗?	✓?	✓
PID	✓	✗	✗	✗	✗
Medicines	Not applicable (no medicines taken)				
Dysfunctional uterine bleeding	✓	N/A	✗	✗	✗
Carcinoma	✗	N/A	✗	✗	✗

Course of action:

Treat her symptoms this time but review over the next few cycles.

CASE STUDY 6.4

A female patient in her early 40s presents complaining of thrush. The following questions are asked, and responses received.

Information gathering	Data generated
What symptoms experiencing	Moderate itching
How long had the symptoms	Last 1 or 2 days
Any other symptoms	No other symptoms
Additional questions asked	Slight non-odourous discharge No changes to feminine hygiene products
Previous history of presenting complaint	Similar to last symptoms which cleared with Canesten but finds cost OTC too much so wants a prescription
Past medical history	Diabetic

Information gathering	Data generated
Drugs (OTC, Rx)	Insulin
Allergies	None known
Social history	Not asked
Family history	Mum diabetic. Dad died about 5 years ago from a fatal myocardial infarction.

Epidemiology dictates that bacterial vaginosis is most prevalent in primary care.

Diagnostic pointers with regard to symptom presentation

The next table summarises the expected findings for questions when related to the three commonest conditions in which discharge is present.

CASE STUDY 6.4 (Continued)

	Timing	Discharge	Odour	Itch
Thrush	Acute and onset quick	White curd- or cottage-cheese-like (1 in 5 patients)	Little or none	Prominent
Bacterial vaginosis	Acute but onset slower	White and thin (1 in 2 patients)	Strong and fishy, which might be worse during menses and after sex	Slight
Trichomoniasis	Acute but onset slower	Green-yellow and can be frothy	Malodorous	Slight

When this information is applied to that gained from our patient we see that her symptoms support a differential diagnosis of thrush.

	Timing	Discharge	Odour	Itch
Thrush	✓	?	✓	✓
Bacterial vaginosis	?	✓	✗	✗
Trichomoniasis	✗?	✓	✗	✗

It is worth remembering that certain disease states and actions can precipitate thrush and should be excluded. Symptoms do not appear to be brought on by any changes in toiletries but the patient is diabetic. The patient has had symptoms previously (although questioning did not reveal when the last episode was) and it is possible that the symptoms are as a consequence of her diabetes.

Course of action:

Treatment could be given but the patient should be advised to see her doctor to check her diabetic control.

Answers

1 = c	2 = d	3 = d	4 = c	5 = c	6 = a	7 = d	8 = e	9 = F	10 = A
11 = D	12 = A	13 = E	14 = F	15 = E	16 = C	17 = A	18 = A	19 = B	20 = C

Gastroenterology

In this chapter

Background

The main function of the gastrointestinal (GI) tract is to break down food into a suitable energy source to allow normal physiological function of cells. Needless to say, the process is complex and involves many different organs. Consequently, there are many conditions that affect the GI tract, some of which are acute and self-limiting and respond well to over-the-counter (OTC) medication, and others that are serious and require referral.

General overview of the anatomy of the GI tract

It is vital that pharmacists have a sound understanding of GI tract anatomy. Many conditions will present with similar symptoms and from similar locations, for example abdominal pain, and the pharmacist will need a basic knowledge of GI tract anatomy – and in particular of where each organ of the GI tract is located – to facilitate a correct differential diagnosis (see Fig. 7.15).

Oral cavity

The oral cavity comprises the cheeks, hard and soft palates and tongue.

Stomach

The stomach is roughly 'J' shaped and receives food and fluid from the oesophagus. It empties into the duodenum. It is located slightly left of the midline and anterior (below) to the rib cage. The lesser curvature of the stomach sits adjacent to the liver.

Liver

The liver is located below the diaphragm and mostly right of the midline in the upper right quadrant of the abdomen. The liver performs many functions, including carbohydrate, lipid and protein metabolism and the processing of many medicines.

Gall bladder

The gall bladder is a pear-shaped sac that lies deep to the liver and hangs from the lower front margin of the liver. Its function is to store and concentrate bile made by the liver.

Pancreas

The pancreas lies behind the stomach. It is essential for producing digestive enzymes transported to the duodenum via the pancreatic duct and secretion of hormones such as insulin.

Small intestine

The small intestine is where most of the absorption of nutrients and medicines occur. It comprises three sections: the duodenum, the jejunum and the ileum. The duodenum starts at the exit of the stomach and its main roles are to neutralise stomach acid and start the chemical digestion of chyme (the partly digested food from the stomach). The jejunum is a small section that joins the duodenum and ileum. In the ileum the mucosa becomes highly folded to form villi that increase the surface area and facilitate the absorption of soluble molecules.

Large intestine

The large intestine starts with the caecum, which is where the appendix connects to the gut. This is followed by the colon, and ends with the rectum. The role of the large intestine is largely to absorb water, and to expel waste.

History taking and physical examination

A thorough patient history is essential, as physical examination of the GI tract in a community pharmacy is limited to inspection of the mouth. This should allow confirmation of the diagnoses for conditions such as mouth ulcers and oral thrush. A description of how to examine the oral cavity appears in the following section.

Conditions affecting the oral cavity

Background

The process of digestion starts in the oral cavity. The tongue and cheeks position large pieces of food so that the teeth can tear and crush food into smaller particles. Saliva moistens, lubricates and begins the process of digesting carbohydrates (by secreting amylase enzymes) before swallowing.

The physical examination

The oral cavity (Fig. 7.1) can be easily observed in the pharmacy, provided the mouth can be viewed with a good light source, preferably a pen torch. Before performing the examination it is important to explain to the patient fully what you are about to do and gain their consent.

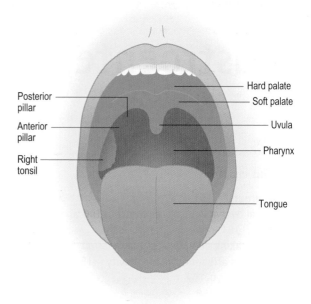

Posterior pillar — Anterior pillar — Right tonsil — Hard palate — Soft palate — Uvula — Pharynx — Tongue

Fig. 7.1 The oral cavity.

Steps involved in performing an oral examination are detailed as follows:

1. Examine the area where the lesion(s)/pain originates from. Look at the size/shape/colour of the lesion(s). Note any redness or swelling local to the area.

2. Once the presenting problem has been inspected check the rest of the oral cavity for any further signs or symptoms. It is possible that other parts of the mouth are affected but have not been noticed by the patient.

3. While inspecting the mouth also check for signs of a healthy mouth – i.e., no signs of tooth decay or periodontal disease (bleeding gums).

Mouth ulcers

Background

Aphthous ulcers, more commonly known as mouth ulcers, is a collective term used to describe various different clinical presentations of superficial, painful oral lesions that occur in recurrent bouts at intervals between a few days to a few months. The majority of patients (80%) who present in a community pharmacy will have minor aphthous ulcers (MAU). It is the community pharmacists' role to exclude more serious pathology, for example, systemic causes and carcinoma.

Prevalence and epidemiology

The prevalence and epidemiology of MAU is poorly understood but has been reported to affect 20% of the UK population. They occur in all ages, but it has been reported that they are more common in patients aged between 10 and 40, and up to 66% of young adults give a history consistent with MAU.

Aetiology

The cause of MAU is unknown, although about 40% of people have a family history of oral ulceration. A number of theories have been put forward to explain why people get MAU, including a genetic link, stress, trauma, food sensitivities, nutritional deficiencies (iron, zinc and vitamin B_{12}) and infection, but none have so far been proven.

Arriving at a differential diagnosis

There are three main clinical presentations of ulcers: minor, major or herpetiform. Although it is most likely the patient will be suffering from MAU (Table 7.1), it is essential that these are differentiated from other causes and referred to the GP for further evaluation.

A number of ulcer-specific questions should always be asked of the patient (Table 7.2) and an inspection of the oral cavity should also be performed to help aid the diagnosis.

Table 7.1
Causes of ulcers and their relative incidence in community pharmacy

Incidence	Cause
Most likely	Minor aphthous ulcers (MAUs)
Likely	Major aphthous ulcers, trauma
Unlikely	Herpetiform ulcers, herpes simplex, oral thrush, medicine-induced
Very unlikely	Oral carcinoma, erythema multiforme (Stevens–Johnson syndrome), Behçet's syndrome, hand, foot and mouth disease

Clinical features of minor aphthous ulcers

The ulcers of MAU are roundish, grey-white in colour and painful. They are small – usually less than 1 cm in diameter – and shallow with a raised red rim. Pain is the key presenting symptom and can make eating and drinking difficult, although pain subsides after 3 or 4 days. They rarely occur on the gingival mucosa and occur singly or in small crops of up to five ulcers. It normally takes 7 to 14 days for the ulcers to heal but recurrence typically occurs after an interval of 1 to 4 months (Fig. 7.2).

Table 7.2
Specific questions to ask the patient: Mouth ulcers

Question	Relevance
Number of ulcers	MAUs occur singly or in small crops. A single large ulcerated area is more indicative of pathology outside the remit of the community pharmacist Patients with numerous ulcers are more likely to be suffering from major or herpetiform ulcers rather than MAU
Location of ulcers	Ulcers on the side of the cheeks, tongue and inside of the lips are likely to be MAUs Ulcers located towards the back of the mouth are more consistent with major or herpetiform ulcers
Size and shape	Irregular-shaped ulcers tend to be caused by trauma. If trauma is not the cause, then referral is necessary to exclude sinister pathology If ulcers are large or very small, they are unlikely to be caused by MAUs
Painless ulcers	Any patient presenting with a painless ulcer in the oral cavity must be referred. This can indicate sinister pathology such as leukoplakia or carcinoma
Age	MAUs in young children (<10 years old) are not common and other causes such as primary infection with herpes simplex should be considered If ulcers appear for the first time after adolescence, then the diagnostic probability is increased for them to be caused by things other than MAUs

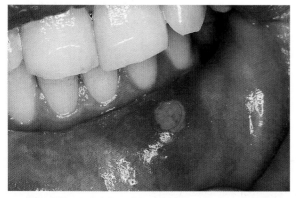

Fig. 7.2 Minor aphthous ulcer. Reproduced from R Cawson et al., 2002, Essentials of oral pathology and oral medicine, 7th edition, Churchill Livingstone, with permission.

Conditions to eliminate

Likely causes

Major aphthous ulcers

These are characterised by large (>1 cm in diameter), numerous ulcers, occurring in crops of 10 or more. The ulcers often coalesce to form one large ulcer. The ulcers are slower to heal than MAU, typically taking 3 to 4 weeks to heal (Fig. 7.3).

Trauma

Trauma to the oral mucosa will result in damage and ulceration. Trauma may be mechanical (e.g., tongue biting)

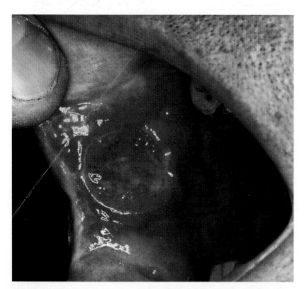

Fig. 7.3 Major aphthous ulcer. Reproduced from R Cawson et al., 2002, Essentials of oral pathology and oral medicine, 7th edition, Churchill Livingstone, with permission.

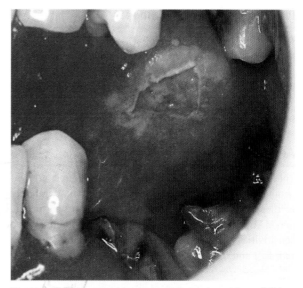

Fig. 7.4 Ulcer caused by trauma. Reproduced from D Wray et al., 1999, Textbook of general and oral medicine, by Churchill Livingstone, with permission.

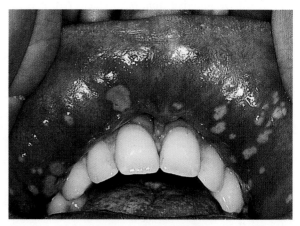

Fig. 7.5 Herpetiform ulcer. Reproduced from R Cawson et al., 2002, Essentials of oral pathology and oral medicine, 7th edition, Churchill Livingstone, with permission.

or thermal, resulting in ulcers with an irregular border. Patients should be able to recall the traumatic event and have no history of similar ulceration or signs of systemic infection (Fig. 7.4).

Unlikely causes

Herpetiform ulcers

Herpetiform ulcers are pinpoint and often occur in large crops of up to 100 at a time. They are located in the posterior part of the mouth, an unusual location for MAU (Fig. 7.5). They usually heal within 14 days.

Oral thrush

Oral thrush usually presents as creamy-white, soft elevated patches. It is covered in more detail in the next section and the reader is referred to page 158 for differential diagnosis of thrush from other oral lesions.

Herpes simplex

Herpes simplex virus is a common cause of oral ulceration in children. Primary infection results in ulceration of any part of the oral mucosa, especially the gums, tongue and cheeks. The ulcers tend to be small and discrete and many in number. Before the eruption of ulcers the person might show signs of systemic infection, such as fever and pharyngitis.

Medicine-induced ulcers

A number of case reports have been received of medication causing ulcers. These include cytotoxic agents, nicorandil, alendronate, non-steroidal anti-inflammatory drugs (NSAIDs) and beta-blockers. Ulcers are often seen at the start of therapy or when the dose is increased.

Very unlikely causes

Oral carcinoma

Globally the incidence of oral cancers is increasing. In the UK it accounts for 3% of all new cancer cases, and in 2011, over 6000 cases of oral cancer were confirmed; in 2012 more than 2000 people died from oral cancers. It is twice as common in men than in women. Incidence rates increase sharply beyond 45 years of age and three-quarters of cases were diagnosed in 50-74 year olds. Smoking has been linked to 65% of oral cancer cases in the UK. Excess alcohol consumption is also a known risk factor.

The majority of cancers are noted on the side of the tongue, mouth and lower lip. Initial presentation ranges from painless spots, lumps or ulcers in the mouth or lip area that fail to resolve. Over time these become painful, change colour, crust over or bleed. The painless nature of early symptoms leads people to seek help only when other symptoms become apparent. Symptoms therefore can be present for a number of weeks before the patient presents to a health care practitioner. Urgent referral is needed as survival rates increase dramatically if the disease is diagnosed in its early stages.

Erythema multiforme

Infection or drug therapy can cause erythema multiforme, although in about 50% of cases no cause can be found.

Symptoms are sudden in onset, causing widespread ulceration of the oral cavity. In addition the patient can have annular and symmetric erythematous skin lesions located towards the extremities. Conjunctivitis and eye pain is also common.

Behcet's syndrome

Most patients will suffer from recurrent, painful major aphthous ulcers that are slow to heal. Lesions are also observed in the genital region and eye involvement (iridocyclitis) is common.

Hand, foot and mouth disease

Hand, foot and mouth disease (HFMD) is generally a mild disease that is usually caused by the Coxsackie virus A16. Although mainly seen in children under 10 years of age, it can appear in older children and adults. As the name suggests, in addition to mouth lesions patients also present with blisters on their hands and feet. The person may also have cold-like symptoms and fever. It is important to identify the disease as it is very contagious, and good hygiene is required to prevent it from spreading to others.

Fig. 7.6 will aid the differentiation between serious and non-serious conditions that cause mouth ulcers.

! TRIGGER POINTS indicative of referral: Mouth ulcers

Symptoms/signs	Possible danger/reason for referral
Children under age 10	MAU rare & Hand, foot and mouth disease possible in this age group
Ulcers greater than 1 cm in diameter Ulcers in crops of five to ten, or more Duration longer than 14 days	Suggests other causes of ulceration outside scope of community pharmacist
Painless ulcer Eye involvement	Possible sinister pathology

Evidence base for over-the-counter medication

A wide range of products are used for the temporary relief and treatment of mouth ulcers. These products contain corticosteroids, local anaesthetics, antibacterials, astringents and antiseptics.

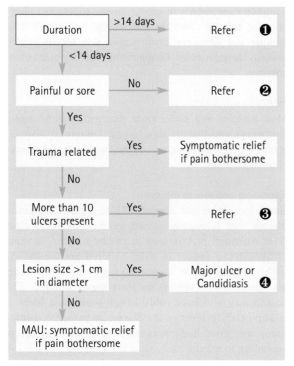

Fig. 7.6 Primer for differential diagnosis of mouth ulcers.

❶ Duration
MAUs normally resolve in 7 to 14 days. Ulcers that fail to heal within this time need referral to exclude other causes.

❷ Painless ulcers
These can indicate sinister pathology, especially if the patient is over 50 years old. In addition, it is likely that the ulcer will have been present for some time before the patient presented to the pharmacy.

❸ Numerous ulcers
Crops of 5 to 10 or more ulcers are rare in MAU. Referral is necessary to determine the cause.

❹ Major ulcer or candidiasis
See Fig. 7.9 for primer for differential diagnosis of oral thrush.

Corticosteroids

Very few randomised controlled trials have been conducted using topical corticosteroids. Those conducted involved small patient numbers or products that are not commercially available OTC. A review in BMJ Best Practice recommended topical corticosteroids as one of the mainstays of treatment for patients with MAU (Scully, 2014). However, this conclusion is based on low quality evidence.

Hydrocortisone sodium succinate pellets

Only one trial conducted by Truelove & Morris-Owen (1958) could be found that investigated the efficacy of hydrocortisone sodium succinate pellets. The authors recruited 52 patients suffering from various forms of oral ulceration. Twenty-three patients were suffering from minor aphthous ulceration. They stated that 22 of the 23 patients obtained rapid relief of pain, and the healing rate of the ulcers was accelerated.

Antibacterial agents (e.g., chlorhexidine)

A number of randomised controlled trials have investigated antibacterial mouthwashes containing chlorhexidine gluconate. Data from some, but not all, studies have found that they reduced the pain and severity of each episode of ulceration (Scully, 2014).

Products containing anaesthetic or analgesics

There is very little trial data to support the pain-relieving effect of anaesthetics or analgesics in MAU, apart from choline salicylate. However, these preparations are clinically effective in other painful oral conditions. It is therefore not unreasonable to expect some relief of symptoms to be shown when using these products to treat MAU.

Choline salicylate

Choline salicylate has been shown to exert an analgesic effect in a number of small studies. However, only one study by Reedy (1970) involving 27 patients evaluated choline salicylate in the treatment of oral aphthous ulceration. No significant differences were found between choline salicylate and placebo in ulcer resolution but choline salicylate was found to be significantly superior to placebo in relieving pain.

Benzydamine

Benzydamine mouthwash has been studied in a small, low-quality trial for its effect in managing recurrent aphthous stomatitis (Scully, 2014). The study found that benzydamine was not significantly different from placebo in terms of ulcer severity or ulcer pain. However, nearly half the patients preferred benzydamine because of its transient topical analgesic effect.

Protectorants

Pastes that contain gelatin, pectin and carmellose sodium stick when in contact with wet mucosal surfaces are advocated, yet there is a paucity of data to support their efficacy.

Practical prescribing and product selection

Prescribing information relating to the medicines used for ulcers reviewed in the section 'Evidence base for over-the-counter medication' is discussed and summarised in Table 7.3; useful tips relating to patients presenting with ulcers are given in 'Hints and Tips' in Box 7.1.

Hydrocortisone sodium succinate pellets

Each pellet contains 2.5 mg hydrocortisone in the form of the ester hydrocortisone sodium succinate. The dose for adults and children over 12 is one pellet to be dissolved in close proximity to the ulcers four times a day for up to 5 days. It does not interact with any medicines, can be taken by all patient groups, has no side effects and appears to be safe in pregnancy.

Antibacterial agents (e.g., chlorhexidine)

Chlorhexidine (e.g., Corsodyl) mouthwash is indicated as an aid in the treatment and prevention of gingivitis and in the maintenance of oral hygiene, which includes the management of aphthous ulceration. Ten mL of the mouthwash should be rinsed around the mouth for about 1 minute twice a day. It can be used by all patient groups, including those who are pregnant and breastfeeding. Side effects associated with its use include reversible tongue and tooth discolouration, burning of the tongue and taste disturbance.

HINTS AND TIPS BOX 7.1: ULCERS

Protectorant products	Apply after food, as food is likely to rub off these products

Choline salicylate (Bonjela Cool, Bonjela Adult)

Adults and children over 16 years old should apply the gel, using a clean finger, over the ulcer when needed, but limit this to every 3 hours. It is a safe medicine and can be given to all patient groups. It is not known to interact with any medicines or cause any side effects.

Local anaesthetics (lidocaine e.g., Anbesol range, Iglu gel, Medijel) and benzocaine (e.g., Oralgel range)

All local anaesthetics have a short duration of action; frequent dosing is therefore required to maintain the anaesthetic effect. They are thus best used on a when-needed basis, although the upper limit on the number of applications allowed does vary, depending on the concentration of anaesthetic included in each product. They appear to be free from any drug interactions, have minimal side effects and can be given to most patients. A small percentage of patients might experience a hypersensitivity reaction with lidocaine or benzocaine; this appears to be more common with benzocaine.

Table 7.3
Practical prescribing: Summary of medicines for ulcers

Name of medicine	Use in children	Likely side effects	Drug interactions of note	Patients in which care is exercised	Pregnancy & breastfeeding
Corticosteroid	>12 years	None	None	None	OK
Choline salicylate	>16 years	None	None	None	OK
Lidocaine	>7 years (Iglu)*	Can cause sensitisation reactions	None	None	OK
Benzocaine	>12 years				
Chlorhexidine	>12 years	None	None	None	OK
Benzydamine	>12 years	May cause stinging	None	None	OK
Carmellose	No age limit stated*	None	None	None	OK

*Children should not be routinely given products, as ulcers are rare in this age group.

Benzydamine

For dosing and administration of the oral rinse see page 33.

Protectorants

This can be applied as frequently as required. There are no apparent interactions, and can be used in all patient groups.

References

Reedy BL. A topical salicylate gel in the treatment of oral aphthous ulceration. Practitioner 1970;204:846–50.

Scully C. 2014. Aphthous ulcers. BMJ Best Practice. April 2014. Available at: http://bestpractice.bmj.com.ezproxy.newcastle.edu.au/best-practice/monograph/564.html [Accessed 5 September 2014].

Truelove SC, Morris-Owen RM. Treatment of aphthous ulceration of the mouth. BMJ 1958;1:603–7.

Further reading

Brocklehurst P, Tickle M, Glenny AM, et al. Systemic interventions for recurrent aphthous stomatitis (mouth ulcers). Cochrane Database of Systematic Reviews 2012, Issue 9. Art. No.: CD005411. http://dx.doi.org/10.1002/14651858.CD005411.pub2

Browne RM, Fox EC, Anderson RJ. Topical triamcinolone acetonide in recurrent aphthous stomatitis. A clinical trial. Lancet 1968;1:565–7.

MacPhee IT, Sircus W, Farmer ED, et al. Use of steroids in treatment of aphthous ulceration. Br Med J 1968;2(598):147–9.

Scully C, Gorsky M, Lozada-Nur F. The diagnosis and management of recurrent aphthous stomatitis: a consensus approach. J Am Dent Assoc 2003;134:200–7.

Zakrzewska JM. Fortnightly review: oral cancer. Br Med J 1999;318:1051–4.

Websites

The Behçet's Syndrome Society: http://behcets.org.uk
The British Dental Health Foundation: https://www.dentalhealth.org

Oral thrush

Background

Oropharyngeal candidiasis (oral thrush) is an opportunistic mucosal infection and is unusual in healthy adults. If oral thrush is suspected in this population community pharmacists should determine whether any identifiable risk factors are present. A healthy adult with no risk factors generally requires referral to the doctor.

Prevalence and epidemiology

The very young (neonates) and the very old are most likely to suffer from oral thrush. It has been reported that 5% of newborn infants and 10% of debilitated elderly patients suffer from oral thrush. Most other cases will be associated with underlying pathology such as diabetes, xerostomia (dry mouth) and patients who are immunocompromised or would be attributable to identifiable risk factors such as recent antibiotic therapy, inhaled corticosteroids and ill-fitting dentures.

Aetiology

It is reported that *Candida albicans* is found in the oral cavity of 30–60% of healthy people in developed countries (Gonsalves et al., 2007). Prevalence in denture wearers is even higher. It is transmitted directly between infected people or via objects that can hold the organism. Changes to the normal environment in the oral cavity will allow *C. albicans* to proliferate.

Arriving at a differential diagnosis

Oral thrush is not difficult to diagnose, provided a careful history is taken and an oral examination performed. It is the role of the pharmacist to eliminate underlying pathology and exclude risk factors. A number of other conditions need to be considered (Table 7.4) and specific questions asked of the patient to aid in differential diagnosis (Table 7.5). After questioning the pharmacist should inspect the oral cavity to confirm the diagnosis.

Clinical features of oral thrush

The classic presentation of oral thrush is mouth pain and soreness associated with creamy-white, soft elevated

Table 7.4 Causes of oral lesions and their relative incidence in community pharmacy	
Incidence	**Cause**
Most likely	Thrush
Likely	Minor aphthous ulcers, medicine-induced thrush, ill-fitting dentures
Unlikely	Lichen planus, underlying medical disorders, e.g., diabetes, xerostomia (dry mouth) and immunosuppression, major and herpetiform ulcers, herpes simplex
Very unlikely	Leukoplakia, squamous cell carcinoma

Table 7.5 Specific questions to ask the patient: Oral thrush	
Question	**Relevance**
Size and shape of lesion	Typically patients with oral thrush present with 'patches'. They tend to be irregularly shaped and vary in size from small to large
Associated pain	Thrush almost always causes some degree of discomfort or pain. Painless patches, especially in people over 50 years of age, should be referred to exclude sinister pathology, such as leukoplakia
Location of lesions	Oral thrush often affects the tongue and cheeks, although if precipitated by inhaled steroids, the lesions appear on the pharynx

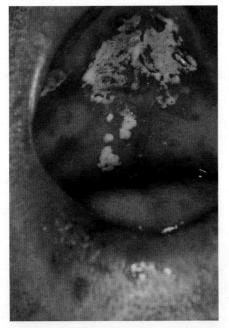

Fig. 7.7 Oral candidiasis. Reproduced from CD Forbes and WF Jackson, 2004, Illustrated pocket guide to clinical medicine, 2nd edition, Mosby, with permission.

patches that can be wiped off, revealing underlying erythematous mucosa (Fig. 7.7). Altered taste and a burning tongue can also be present. Lesions can occur anywhere in the oral cavity but usually affect the tongue, palate, lips and cheeks. Patients sometimes complain of malaise and loss of appetite. In neonates, spontaneous resolution usually occurs but can take a few weeks.

Conditions to eliminate

Likely causes

Minor aphthous ulcers
Mouth ulcers are covered in more detail on page 153 and the reader is referred to this section for differential diagnosis of these from oral thrush.

Medicine-induced thrush
Inhaled corticosteroids and antibiotics are often associated with causing thrush. In addition, medicines that cause dryness of the mouth can also predispose people to thrush. Always take a medicine history to determine whether medicines could be a cause of the symptoms.

Denture wearers
Wearing dentures, especially if they are not taken out at night, not kept clean, or do not fit well can predispose people to thrush.

Unlikely causes

Lichen planus
Lichen planus is a dermatological condition with lesions similar in appearance to plaque psoriasis. In about 50% of people the oral mucous membranes are affected. The cheeks, gums or tongue develop white, slightly raised painless lesions that look a little like a spider's web. Other symptoms can include soreness of the mouth and a burning sensation. Occasionally, lichen planus of the mouth occurs without any skin rash.

Underlying medical disorders
As stated previously, oral thrush is unusual in the adult population. Patients are at greater risk of developing thrush if they suffer from medical conditions such as diabetes, xerostomia (dry mouth) or are immunocompromised.

Other forms of ulceration (e.g., major and herpetiform ulcers, herpes simplex)
These are covered in more detail on page 154, and the reader is referred to this section for differential diagnosis of these from oral thrush.

Very unlikely causes

Leukoplakia
Leukoplakia is a predominantly white lesion of the oral mucosa that cannot be characterised as any other definable lesion and is therefore a diagnosis based on exclusion (Fig. 7.8). It is often associated with smoking and is a precancerous lesion, although epidemiological data suggest that annual transformation rate to squamous cell carcinoma is approximately 1%. Patients present with a symptomless white patch on the tongue or cheek that develops over a

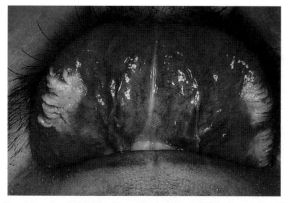

Fig. 7.8 Leukoplakia. Reproduced from CD Forbes and WF Jackson, 2004, Illustrated pocket guide to clinical medicine, 2nd edition, Mosby, with permission.

period of weeks. The lesion cannot be wiped off, unlike oral thrush. Most cases are seen in people over the age of 40; it is more common in men. Suspected cases require referral.

Squamous cell carcinoma

Squamous cell carcinoma is covered in more detail on page 155, and the reader is referred to this section for differential diagnosis of these from oral thrush.

Fig. 7.9 will aid the differentiation of thrush from other oral lesions.

> ❗ **TRIGGER POINTS indicative of referral: Oral thrush**

Symptoms/signs	Possible danger/reason for referral
Diabetic patients	May indicate poor diabetic control
Duration greater than 3 weeks	Unlikely to be thrush and needs further investigation by a doctor
Immuno-compromised patients	Likely to have severe and extensive involvement. Outside community pharmacist's remit
Painless lesions	Sinister pathology

Evidence base for over-the-counter medication

Only Daktarin oral gel (miconazole) is available OTC to treat oral thrush. It has proven efficacy and appears to have clinical cure rates between 80% and 90%. In comparative trials, Daktarin appears to have superior cure rates than the POM Nystatin.

Practical prescribing and product selection

Prescribing information relating to Daktarin Oral gel reviewed in the section 'Evidence base for over-the-counter medication' is discussed and summarised in Table 7.6; useful tips relating to the application of Daktarin are given in 'Hints and Tips' in Box 7.2.

The dose of gel is four times a day in all age groups, although the volume administered varies dependent on the age of the patient. For those aged between 4 and 24 months, 1.25 mL (one-quarter measuring spoon) of gel should be applied, and for adults and children over 2 years of age, 2.5 mL (one-half measuring spoon) of gel is applied.

It can occasionally cause nausea and vomiting. The manufacturers state that it can interact with a number of medicines, namely mizolastine, cisapride, triazolam, midazolam, quinidine, pimozide, HMG-CoA reductase inhibitors and anticoagulants. However, there is a lack of published data to determine how clinically significant these interactions are except with warfarin. Co-administration of warfarin with miconazole increases warfarin levels markedly, and the patient's INR (internationalised normalised ratio) should be monitored closely. The manufacturers advise that Daktarin should be avoided in pregnancy but published data do not support an association between miconazole and congenital defects. It appears to be safe to use while breastfeeding.

References
Gonsalves WC, Chi A, Neville BW. Common oral lesions: Part I. Superficial mucosal lesions. Am Fam Physician 2007;75:501–7.

Further reading
Hoppe JE, Hahn H. Randomized comparison of two nystatin oral gels with miconazole oral gel for treatment of oral thrush in infants. Antimycotics Study Group. Infection 1996;24:136–9.
Hoppe JE. Treatment of oropharyngeal candidiasis in immunocompetent infants: a randomized multicenter study of miconazole gel vs. nystatin suspension. The Antifungals Study Group. Pediatr Infect Dis J 1997;16:288–93.
Parvinen T, Kokko J, Yli-Urpo A. Miconazole lacquer compared with gel in treatment of denture stomatitis. Scand J Dent Res 1994;102:361–6.

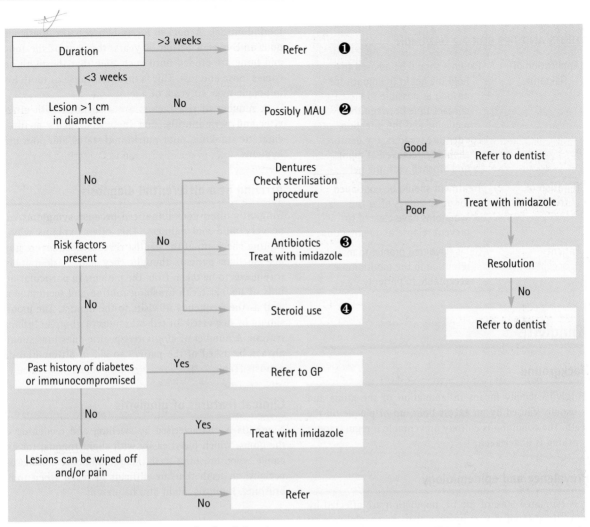

Fig. 7.9 Primer for differential diagnosis of oral thrush.

❶ **Duration**
Any lesion lasting more than 3 weeks must be referred to exclude sinister pathology.

❷ **MAU**
See Fig. 7.6 for primer for differential diagnosis of mouth ulcers.

❸ **Antibiotics**
Broad-spectrum antibiotics, e.g., amoxicillin and macrolides, can precipitate oral thrush by altering normal flora of the oral cavity.

❹ **Inhaled corticosteroids**
High-dose inhaled corticosteroids can cause oral thrush. Patients should be encouraged to use a spacer and wash their mouth out after inhaler use to minimise this problem.

Table 7.6
Practical prescribing: Summary of medicines for oral thrush

Name of medicine	Use in children	Likely side effects	Drug interactions of note	Patients in which care is exercised	Pregnancy & breastfeeding
Daktarin	>4 months	Nausea and vomiting (approx. 5% of patients)	Warfarin	None	OK

HINTS AND TIPS BOX 7.2 DAKTARIN

Application of Daktarin	Patients should be advised to hold the gel in the mouth for as long as possible to increase contact time between the medicine and the infection. For denture wearers, the dentures should be removed at night and brushed with the gel
Duration of treatment	Treatment should be continued for up to 2 days after the symptoms have cleared to prevent relapse and reinfection
Patient acceptability	Gel is flavoured orange to make retention in the mouth more acceptable to patients

Gingivitis

Background

Gingivitis simply means inflammation of the gums and is usually caused by an excess build-up of plaque on the teeth. The condition is entirely preventable if regular tooth brushing is undertaken.

Prevalence and epidemiology

It is estimated 50% of the UK population are affected by gum disease and that more than 85% of people over 40 will experience gingival disease. Men more than women tend to suffer from severe gingivitis.

Aetiology

After tooth brushing, the teeth soon become coated in a mixture of saliva and gingival fluid, known as pellicle. Oral bacteria and food particles adhere to this coating and begin to proliferate, forming plaque; subsequent brushing of the teeth removes this plaque build-up. However, if plaque is allowed to build up for 3 or 4 days, bacteria begin to undergo internal calcification, producing calcium phosphate, better known as tartar (or calculus). This adheres tightly to the surface of the tooth and retains bacteria in situ. The bacteria release enzymes and toxins that invade the gingival mucosa, causing inflammation of the gingiva (gingivitis). If the plaque is not removed, the inflammation travels downwards, involving the periodontal ligament and associated tooth structures

(periodontitis). A pocket forms between the tooth and gum and, over a period of years, the root of the tooth and bone are eroded until such time that the tooth becomes loose and lost. This is the main cause of tooth loss in people over 40 years of age.

A number of risk factors are associated with gingivitis and periodontitis, and include diabetes mellitus, cigarette smoking, poor nutritional status and poor oral hygiene.

Arriving at a differential diagnosis

Gingivitis often goes unnoticed because symptoms can be very mild and painless. This often explains why a routine check-up at the dentist reveals more severe gum disease than patients thought they had. A dental history needs to be taken from the patient, in particular details of his/her tooth brushing routine and technique as well as the frequency of visits to the dentist. The mouth should be inspected for tell-tale signs of gingival inflammation. A number of gingivitis-specific questions should always be asked of the patient to aid in differential diagnosis (Table 7.7).

Clinical features of gingivitis

Gingivitis is characterised by swelling and reddening of the gums, which bleed easily with slight trauma, for example when brushing teeth. Plaque might be visible; especially on teeth that are difficult to reach when tooth brushing. Halitosis might also be present.

Table 7.7
Specific questions to ask the patient: Gingivitis

Question	Relevance
Tooth-brushing technique	Overzealous tooth brushing can lead to bleeding gums and gum recession. Make sure the patient is not 'over-cleaning' his or her teeth. An electric toothbrush might be helpful for people who apply too much force when brushing teeth
Bleeding gums	Gums that bleed without exposure to trauma and is unexplained or unprovoked need referral to exclude underlying pathology

Conditions to eliminate

Periodontitis   tooth structure → lose tooth.

If gingivitis is left untreated, it will progress into periodontitis. Symptoms are similar to gingivitis but the patient will experience spontaneous bleeding, taste disturbances, halitosis and difficulty while eating. Periodontal pockets might be visible, and the patient might complain of loose teeth. Referral to a dentist is needed for evaluation and removal of tartar.

Medicine-induced gum bleeding

Medicines such as warfarin, heparin and NSAIDs might produce gum bleeding. It is also worth noting that a number of medicines can cause gum hypertrophy, notably phenytoin and ciclosporin. It has also been seen in patients taking nifedipine.

Spontaneous bleeding

A number of conditions can produce spontaneous gum bleeding, for example agranulocytosis and leukaemia. Other symptoms should be present, for example, progressive fatigue, weakness and signs of systemic illness such as fever. Immediate referral to the doctor is needed.

! TRIGGER POINTS indicative of referral: Gingivitis

Symptoms/signs	Possible danger/reason for referral
Foul taste associated with gum bleeding Loose teeth	Suspect periodontitis
Spontaneous gum bleeding	Suspect periodontitis or more sinister pathology
Signs of systemic illness	Indicator of more serious underlying pathology

Evidence base for over-the-counter medication

Put simply, there is no substitute for good oral hygiene. Prevention of plaque build-up is the key to healthy gums and teeth. Twice-daily brushing is recommended to maintain oral hygiene at adequate levels. Brushing teeth with a fluoride toothpaste to prevent tooth decay should preferably take place after eating. Flossing is recommended three times a week to access areas that a toothbrush might miss and is associated with less gum bleeding compared with toothbrushing alone (Sambunjak et al., 2011).

A Cochrane review concluded that powered toothbrushes (with rotation oscillation action – where brush heads rotate in one direction, and then in the opposite direction) are more effective than manual brushing at plaque removal (Yaacob et al., 2014).

There is a plethora of oral hygiene products marketed to the public. These products should be reserved for established gingivitis or in those patients who have a poor tooth-brushing technique.

Mouthwashes contain chlorhexidine, hexetidine and hydrogen peroxide. Of these, chlorhexidine in concentrations of either 0.1% or 0.2% has been proven the most effective antibacterial in reducing plaque formation and gingivitis (Ernst et al., 1998). In clinical trials it has been shown to be consistently more effective than placebo and comparator medicines; and there appears to be no difference in effect between concentrations. It has even been used as a positive control.

Practical prescribing and product selection

Prescribing information relating to the medicines used for gingivitis reviewed in the section 'Evidence base for over-the-counter medication' is discussed and summarised in Table 7.8; useful tips relating to products for oral care are given in 'Hints and Tips' in Box 7.3.

All mouthwashes have minimal side effects and can be used by all patient groups. They are rinsed around the mouth between 30 seconds and 1 minute, then spat out.

Chlorhexidine gluconate (e.g., Corsodyl 0.2%, Eludril 0.1%) الفم

Corsodyl is suitable for adults and children over 12 years old with a standard dose of 10 mL twice a day. Eludril can be given from 6 years upwards and the dose is 10–15 mL two or three times a day. Although chlorhexidine is free from side effects, patients should be warned that prolonged use may stain the tongue and brown the teeth. This can be reduced or removed by brushing teeth before use. If this fails to remove the staining, then it can be removed by a dentist. Corsodyl and Eludril are also available as a spray as well as a gel (1%) formulation of Corsodyl. All products are only licensed for adults and children over 12 years of age.

Hexetidine (Oraldene)

Adults and children over 6 years of age should use a 15 mL dose two or three times a day.

Hydrogen peroxide (e.g., Peroxyl)

Adults and children over 6 years of age should use 10 mL rinsed around the mouth up to four times a day.

Table 7.8
Practical prescribing: Summary of medicines for gingivitis

Name of medicine	Use in children	Likely side effects	Drug interactions of note	Patients in which care is exercised	Pregnancy & breastfeeding
Chlorhexidine	>6 years (Eludril mouthwash)	Staining of teeth and tongue. Mild irritation	None	None	OK
Hexetidine	>6 years	Mild irritation or numbness of tongue		None	OK
Hydrogen peroxide		Mucosal irritation, but rare			

HINTS AND TIPS BOX 7.3 TOOTH PROTECTION

Dental flossing	Correct technique is important otherwise gums can be traumatised. A piece of floss about 8 inches long should be wrapped around the ends of the middle fingers of each hand, leaving 2 to 3 inches between the first finger and thumb. The floss should be placed between two teeth and curved in to a 'C' shape around one tooth and slid up between the gum and tooth until resistance is felt, then moved vertically up and down several times to remove plaque
Using fluoride	Fluoride does reduce dental caries. Drinking water in some parts of the UK contains measurable concentrations of fluoride. Therefore fluoride toothpastes or fluoride supplementation is not needed However, most people in Britain require fluoride supplementation which is normally through toothpaste. Most packs of toothpaste state how many parts per million of fluoride the toothpaste contains; 500 ppm is a low level, 1000–1500 ppm is a high level. A low-dose toothpaste should be used for children under 7 to avoid dental fluorosis which causes tooth discolouration Oral fluoride supplements can also be given where fluoride in water is less than 0.7 parts per million. (see BNF for dosing)

References

Ernst CP, Prockl K, Willershausen B. The effectiveness and side effects of 0.1% and 0.2% chlorhexidine mouthrinses: a clinical study. Quintessence Int 1998;29:443–8.

Sambunjak D, Nickerson JW, Poklepovic T, et al. Flossing for the management of periodontal diseases and dental caries in adults. Cochrane Database of Systematic Reviews 2011, Issue 12. Art. No.: CD008829. http://dx.doi.org/10.1002/14651858.CD008829.pub2.

Yaacob M, Worthington HV, Deacon SA, et al. Powered versus manual toothbrushing for oral health. Cochrane Database of Systematic Reviews 2014, Issue 6. Art. No.: CD002281. http://dx.doi.org/10.1002/14651858.CD002281.pub3.

Further reading

Brecx M, Brownstone E, MacDonald L, et al. Efficacy of Listerine, Meridol and chlorhexidine mouthrinses as supplements to regular tooth cleaning measures. J Clin Periodontol 1992;19:202–7.

Hase JC, Ainamo J, Etemadzadeh H, et al. Plaque formation and gingivitis after mouthrinsing with 0.2% delmopinol hydrochloride, 0.2% chlorhexidine digluconate and placebo for 4 weeks, following an initial professional tooth cleaning. J Clin Periodontol 1995;22:533–9.

Jones CM, Blinkhorn AS, White E. Hydrogen peroxide, the effect on plaque and gingivitis when used in an oral irrigator. Clin Prev Dent 1990;12:15–8.

Kelly M. Adult Dental Health Survey: Oral Health in the United Kingdom 1998. London: TSO; 2000.

Lang NP, Hase JC, Grassi M, et al. Plaque formation and gingivitis after supervised mouthrinsing with 0.2% delmopinol hydrochloride, 0.2% chlorhexidine digluconate and placebo for 6 months. Oral Dis1998;4:105–13.

Maruniak J, Clark WB, Walker CB, et al. The effect of 3 mouthrinses on plaque and gingivitis development. J Clin Periodontol1992;19:19–23.

Websites

The British Dental Association: http://www.bda.org/
The British Fluoridation Society: http://www.bfsweb.org/
The British Dental Health Foundation: https://www.dentalhealth.org/
The American Academy of Periodontology: http://www.perio.org/

Dyspepsia

Background

Confusion surrounds the terminology associated with upper abdominal symptoms, and the term *dyspepsia* is used by different authors to mean different things. It is therefore an umbrella term generally used by healthcare professionals to refer to a group of upper abdominal symptoms that arise from five main conditions:

- non-ulcer dyspepsia/functional dyspepsia (indigestion)
- gastro-oesophageal reflux disease (GORD, heartburn)
- gastritis
- duodenal ulcers
- gastric ulcers

These five conditions represent 90% of dyspepsia cases presented to the GP.

The National Institute for Health and Care Excellence (nice.org.uk/cg184) issued guidance on the management of dyspepsia and GORD in adults in primary care (2014). This guidance has specific information on pharmacist management of dyspepsia and specific reference is made to this guidance.

Prevalence and epidemiology

The exact prevalence of dyspepsia is unknown. This is largely because of the number of people who self-medicate or do not report mild symptoms to their doctor. However, it is clear that dyspepsia is extremely common. Between 25% and 40% of the general population in Western society are reported to suffer from dyspepsia, and virtually everyone at some point in their lives will experience an episode. Estimates also suggest that 10% of people suffer on a weekly basis and that 2% to 5% of all doctor consultations are for dyspepsia. The prevalence of dyspepsia is modestly higher in women than in men.

Aetiology

The aetiology of dyspepsia differs depending on its cause. Decreased muscle tone leads to lower oesophageal sphincter incompetence (often as a result of medicines or overeating) and is the principal cause of GORD. Increased acid production results in inflammation of the stomach (gastritis) and is usually attributable to *Helicobacter pylori* infection, or acute alcohol indigestion. The presence of *H. pylori* is central to duodenal and gastric ulceration – *H. pylori* is present in 95% of duodenal ulcers and 80% of gastric ulcers. The exact mechanism by which it causes ulceration is still unclear but the bacteria do produce toxins that stimulate the inflammatory cascade. Increasingly common are medicine-induced ulcers, most notably NSAIDs and low-dose aspirin.

Finally, when no specific cause can be found for a patient's symptoms, the complaint is said to be non-ulcer dyspepsia. (Some authorities do not advocate the use of this term, preferring the term 'functional dyspepsia'.)

Arriving at a differential diagnosis

Overwhelmingly, patients who present in a community pharmacy with dyspepsia are likely to be suffering from GORD, gastritis or non-ulcer dyspepsia (Table 7.9). Research has shown that even those patients who meet NICE guidelines for endoscopical investigation are found to have either gastritis/hiatus hernia (30%), oesophagitis (10–17%) or no abnormal findings (30%). It has also been reported that a medical practitioner with an average list size will only see one new case of oesophageal cancer and one new case of stomach cancer every 4 years. Despite these statistics, a thorough medical and drug history should be taken to enable the community pharmacist to rule out serious pathology. ALARM symptoms (see 'Trigger points for referral'), which would warrant further investigation, are surprisingly common, and it is important that patients exhibiting these symptoms are referred. A number of dyspepsia-specific questions should always be asked of the patient to aid in differential diagnosis (Table 7.10).

Clinical features of dyspepsia

Patients with dyspepsia present with a range of symptoms commonly involving:

- vague abdominal discomfort (aching) above the umbilicus associated with belching
- bloating
- flatulence
- a feeling of fullness
- nausea and/or vomiting
- heartburn

Table 7.9
Causes of upper GI symptoms and their relative incidence in community pharmacy

Incidence	Cause
Most likely	Non-ulcer dyspepsia
Unlikely	Medicine induced, peptic ulcers, irritable bowel syndrome, biliary disease
Very unlikely	Gastric and oesophageal cancers, atypical angina

Table 7.10
Specific questions to ask the patient: Dyspepsia

Question	Relevance
Age	Young adults are likely to suffer from dyspepsia with no specific pathological condition, unlike patients over 50 years of age, in which a specific pathological condition becomes more common
Location	Dyspepsia is experienced as pain above the umbilicus and centrally located (epigastric area). Pain below the umbilicus will not be due to dyspepsia Pain experienced behind the sternum (breastbone) is likely to be heartburn If the patient can point to a specific area of the abdomen, then it is unlikely to be dyspepsia
Nature of pain	Pain associated with dyspepsia is described as aching or discomfort. Pain described as gnawing, sharp or stabbing is unlikely to be dyspepsia
Radiation	Pain that radiates to other areas of the body is indicative of more serious pathology and the patient must be referred. The pain might be cardiovascular in origin, especially if the pain is felt down the inside aspect of the left arm
Severity	Pain described as debilitating or severe must be referred to exclude more serious conditions
Associated symptoms	Persistent vomiting with or without blood is suggestive of ulceration or even cancer and must be referred Black and tarry stools indicate a bleed in the GI tract and must be referred
Aggravating or relieving factors	Pain shortly after eating (1–3 hours) and relieved by food or antacids are classic symptoms of ulcers Symptoms of dyspepsia are often brought on by certain types of food, for example, caffeine-containing products and spicy food
Social history	Bouts of excessive drinking are commonly implicated in dyspepsia. Likewise, eating food on the move or too quickly is often the cause of the symptoms. A person's lifestyle is often a good clue to whether these are contributing to his or her symptoms

Although dyspeptic symptoms are a poor predictor of disease severity or underlying pathology, retrosternal heartburn is the classic symptom of GORD.

Conditions to eliminate

Unlikely causes

Peptic ulceration
Ruling out peptic ulceration is probably the main consideration for community pharmacists when assessing patients with symptoms of dyspepsia. Ulcers are classed as either gastric or duodenal. They occur most commonly in patients aged between 30 and 50. Typically the patient will have well-localised, mid-epigastric pain described as 'constant', 'annoying' or 'gnawing/boring'. In gastric ulcers the pain comes on whenever the stomach is empty, usually 30 minutes after eating and is generally relieved by antacids or food, and aggravated by alcohol and caffeine. Gastric ulcers are also more commonly associated with weight loss and GI bleeds than duodenal ulcers. Patients can experience weight loss of 5 to 10 kg and, although this could indicate carcinoma, especially in people aged over 40, on investigation a benign gastric ulcer is found most of the time. NSAID use is associated with a three- to four-fold increase in gastric ulcers.

Duodenal ulcers tend to be more consistent in symptom presentation. Pain occurs 2 to 3 hours after eating, and pain that awakens a person at night is highly suggestive of duodenal ulcer.

If ulcers are suspected, referral to the GP is necessary, as peptic ulcers can only be conclusively diagnosed by endoscopy.

Medicine-induced dyspepsia
A number of medicines can cause gastric irritation, leading to or provoking GI discomfort, or they can decrease oesophageal sphincter tone, resulting in reflux. Aspirin and NSAIDs are very often associated with dyspepsia and can affect up to 25% of patients. Table 7.11 lists other medicines commonly implicated in causing dyspepsia.

Irritable bowel syndrome
Patients younger than age 45 who have uncomplicated dyspepsia, lower abdominal pain and altered bowel habits

Table 7.11
Medicines that commonly cause dyspepsia/ abdominal discomfort

Acarbose (1%–10%)
Antibiotics, e.g., macrolides and tetracyclines
Anticoagulants
Angiotensin-converting enzyme (ACE) inhibitors
Alcohol (in excess)
Bisphosphonates
Calcium antagonists
Iron
Metformin
Metronidazole
Nitrates
Oestrogens
Orlistat (>10%)
Potassium supplements
SSRIs
Sildenafil (1% to 10%)
Steroids
Theophylline

SSRI, selective serotonin reuptake inhibitor.

are likely to have irritable bowel syndrome (IBS). For further details on IBS see page 187.

Biliary disease

Acute cholecystitis (inflammation of the gall bladder) and cholelithiasis (presence of gall stones in the bile ducts, also called biliary colic) are characterised by persistent and steady severe pain. Pain can vary from sharp, cramping or dull in nature. Classically, the onset is sudden and starts a few hours after a meal, frequently awakening the patient in the early hours of the morning. The pain can also be felt in the epigastric area and radiate to the tip of the right scapula in cholelithiasis (see Fig. 7.18). Fatty foods often aggravate the pain. The incidence increases with increasing age and is most common in people over 50 years of age. It is also more prevalent in women than in men.

Very unlikely causes

Gastric carcinoma
Gastric carcinoma is the third most common GI malignancy after colorectal and pancreatic cancer. However, only 2% of patients who are referred by their GP for an endoscopy have malignancy. It is therefore a rare condition and community pharmacists are extremely unlikely to encounter a patient with carcinoma. One or more ALARM symptoms should be present, plus symptoms such as nausea and vomiting.

Oesophageal carcinoma
In its early stages, oesophageal carcinoma might go unnoticed. Over time, however, as the oesophagus becomes constricted, patients will complain of difficulty in swallowing and experience a sensation of food sticking in the oesophagus. As the disease progresses, weight loss becomes prominent despite the patient maintaining a good appetite.

Atypical angina
Not all cases of angina have classic textbook presentation of pain in the retrosternal area with radiation to the neck, back or left shoulder that is precipitated by temperature changes or exercise. Patients can complain of dyspepsia-like symptoms and feel generally unwell. These symptoms might be brought on by a heavy meal. In such cases antacids will fail to relieve symptoms and referral is needed.

Fig. 7.10 will aid differentiation of the causes of dyspepsia.

! TRIGGER POINTS indicative of referral: Dyspepsia

Symptoms/signs	Possible danger/ reason for referral
ALARM signs and symptoms Anaemia (signs include tiredness, pale complexion, shortness of breath) Loss of weight Anorexia Recent onset of progressive symptoms Melaena, dysphagia and haematemesis	Symptoms requiring further investigation
Pain described as severe, debilitating or that awakens the patient at night Persistent vomiting	Suggests ulceration
Referred pain	Possible cardiovascular or biliary cause

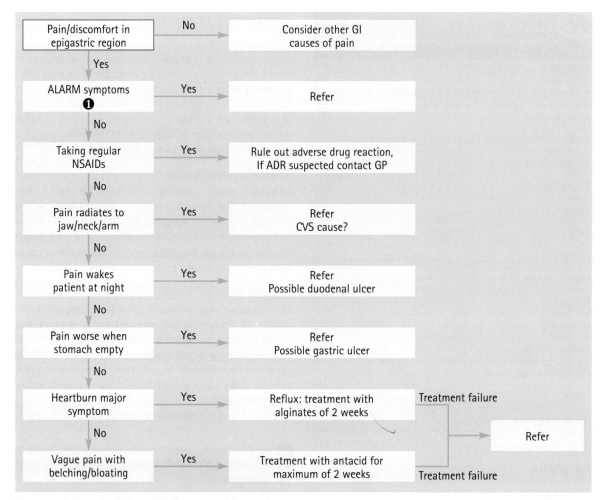

Fig. 7.10   Primer for differential diagnosis of dyspepsia.

❶ ALARM symptoms
These include anaemia (signs can include tiredness and pale complexion), loss of weight, anorexia, dark stools, difficulty in swallowing and vomiting blood.

Evidence base for over-the-counter medication

In accordance with NICE guidelines, the group of patients that should be treated by pharmacists are classed as having 'uninvestigated dyspepsia' (i.e., those who have not had endoscopical investigation). OTC treatment options consist of antacids, H_2 antagonists, alginates and proton pump inhibitors (PPIs). Before treatment is instigated lifestyle advice should be given where appropriate. Although there is no strong evidence that dietary changes will lessen dyspepsia symptoms, a general healthier lifestyle will have wider health benefits. Recommendations should include:

1. Move to a lower fat diet
2. Alcohol intake kept to recommended levels
3. Stop smoking
4. Decrease weight
5. Reduce caffeine intake

It might also be possible to identify factors that precipitate or worsen symptoms. Commonly implicated foods that precipitate dyspepsia are spicy or fatty foods, caffeine, chocolate and alcohol. Bending is also said to worsen symptoms.

Antacids

Antacids have been used for many decades to treat dyspepsia and have proven efficacy in neutralising stomach acid. However, the neutralising capacity of each antacid varies, dependent on the metal salt used. In addition, the solubility of each metal salt differs, which affects their onset and duration of action. Sodium and potassium salts are the most highly soluble, which makes them have a quicker onset, but are shorter acting. Magnesium and aluminium salts are less soluble, so have a slower onset, but greater duration of action. Calcium salts have the advantage of being quick acting yet have a prolonged action.

It is therefore commonplace for manufacturers to combine two or more antacid ingredients together to ensure a quick onset (generally sodium salts, e.g., sodium bicarbonate) and prolonged action (aluminium, magnesium or calcium salts).

Alginates

Alginate products are promoted as **first-line treatment for patients suffering from GORD**. When in contact with gastric acid the alginate precipitates out, forming a sponge-like matrix that floats on top of the stomach contents. Alginate preparations are also commonly combined with antacids to help neutralise stomach acid. In clinical trials alginate-containing products have demonstrated superior symptom control compared with placebo and antacids. However, PPIs and H_2 antagonists do have superior efficacy to alginates.

H_2 antagonists

Just one H_2 antagonist is currently available OTC in the UK; ranitidine. Cimetidine and famotidine were also available OTC but withdrawn by the manufacturer, and nizatidine has exemption from POM control but currently there is no marketed product.

There is a paucity of publicly available trial data supporting their use at non-prescription doses.

However, the inhibitory effects of OTC doses of ranitidine on gastric acid have been investigated in healthy volunteers. Trials showed conclusively that ranitidine, and its comparator drug, famotidine, did significantly raise intragastric pH compared with placebo, although antacids (calcium carbonates) had a significantly quicker onset of action but with shorter duration.

Proton pump inhibitors

A number of trials have compared PPIs with H_2 antagonists for non-ulcer dyspepsia and GORD-like symptoms

(Moayyedi et al., 2006; Talley et al., 2002; van Pinxteren, 2006). Results indicate that PPIs, even at half the standard POM dose, are generally superior to H_2 antagonists in treating dyspeptic symptoms.

Summary

Antacids will work for the majority of people presenting at the pharmacy with mild dyspeptic symptoms. They can be used as first-line therapy unless heartburn predominates, then an alginate or alginate/antacid combination can be used. H_2 antagonists appear to be equally as effective as antacids but are considerably more expensive. Proton pump inhibitors are the most effective and could be considered first-line, especially for those patients who suffer from moderate to severe or recurrent symptoms. Like H_2 antagonists they are expensive in comparison to simple antacids and might influence patient choice or pharmacist recommendation.

Practical prescribing and product selection

Prescribing information relating to the medicines used for dyspepsia reviewed in the section 'Evidence base for over-the-counter medication' is discussed and summarised in Table 7.12.

Antacids

The majority of marketed antacids are combination products containing two, three or even four constituents. The rationale for combining different salts together appears to be twofold. First, to ensure the product has quick onset (containing sodium or calcium) and a long duration of action (containing magnesium, aluminium or calcium). Second, to minimise any side effects that might be experienced from the product. For example, magnesium salts tend to cause diarrhoea and aluminium salts constipation; however, if both are combined in the same product, then neither side effect is noticed. Useful tips relating to antacids are given in 'Hints and Tips' in Box 7.4.

Antacids can affect the absorption of a number of medications via chelation and adsorption. Commonly affected medicines include tetracyclines, quinolones, imidazoles, phenytoin, penicillamine and bisphosphonates. In addition, the absorption of enteric-coated preparations can be affected due to antacids increasing the stomach pH. The majority of these interactions are easily overcome by leaving a minimum gap of 1 hour between the respective doses of each medicine.

Most patient groups can take antacids, although patients on salt-restricted diets (e.g., patients with coronary

Table 7.12
Practical prescribing: Summary of medicines for dyspepsia

Name of medicine	Use in children	Likely side effects	Drug interactions of note	Patients in which care is exercised	Pregnancy & breastfeeding
Antacids Sodium only	>12 years	None	None	Patients with heart disease	OK
Calcium only		Constipation	Tetracyclines, quinolones, imidazoles, phenytoin, penicillamine and bisphosphonates	None	OK
Magnesium only		Diarrhoea			
Aluminium only		Constipation			
Alginates	>12 years*	None	None	Patients with heart disease	OK
H_2 antagonists	>16 years	Abdominal pain, diarrhoea, constipation and headache reported but uncommon	None	None	Experience has shown them to be OK. Reported diarrhoea with famotidine during breastfeeding
PPIs Omeprazole, Esomeprazole	>18 years	Headache, diarrhoea, constipation, nausea and vomiting, abdominal pain, flatulence	Azole antifungals, clopidogrel, diazepam, fluvoxamine, cilostazol	None	Manufacturers advise avoidance but limited information indicates that maternal PPI doses produce low levels in milk and would not be expected to cause any adverse effects in breastfed infants
Pantoprazole		As above plus	Azole antifungals, atazanavir		

*Certain products can be given to children but dyspepsia is unusual in children and it might be prudent to refer such patients to their GP.

heart disease) should ideally avoid sodium-containing antacids. In addition, antacids should not be recommended in children because dyspepsia is unusual in children under 12 years of age, and, indeed, all products are licensed for use only for children aged 12 and over.

Alginates (e.g., the Gaviscon range)

Products containing alginates are combination preparations that contain an alginate with antacids. They are best given after each main meal and before bedtime, although they can be taken on a when-needed basis. They can be given during pregnancy and breastfeeding and to most patient groups, but, as with antacids, patients on salt-restricted diets should ideally avoid sodium-containing alginate preparations. They are reported not to have any side effects or interactions with other medicines. Like antacids, most alginate-based products are licensed for use in children over 12 years of age, but some products can be used in children aged 6 years and older (e.g., Gaviscon Cool liquid).

H_2 antagonists

Sales of H_2 antagonists are restricted to adults and children over the age of 16. They possess no clinically important drug

HINTS AND TIPS BOX 7.4 ANTACIDS

Type of formulation?	Ideally, antacids should be given in the liquid form because the acid-neutralising capacity and speed of onset is greater than that of tablet formulations
Overuse of antacids	Misuse and chronic use of antacids will result in significant systemic absorption, leading to various unwanted medical conditions. Milk-alkali syndrome has been reported with chronic abuse of calcium-containing antacids, as has osteomalacia with aluminium-containing products Antacid therapy should ideally not be longer than 2 weeks. If symptoms have not resolved in this time, then other treatments and/or evaluation from the GP should be recommended
When is the best time to take antacids?	Antacids should be taken after food because gastric emptying is delayed in the presence of food. This allows antacids to exert their effect for up to 3 hours
Salt (sodium) content	Be aware that some antacid preparations do contain significant amounts of sodium – for example Gaviscon Advance contains 4.6 mmol of sodium per 10 mL. UKMi have produced a document detailing medicines with high sodium content which is located on the NICE evidence webpages (http://www.evidence.nhs.uk)
The elderly	Avoid constipating products, as the elderly are prone to constipation
Possible solutions to minimise symptoms	Simple suggestions such as eating less but more often or eating smaller meals might help control symptoms. Avoid eating late at night and lying flat at night – use a pillow to prop up the person

interactions, and side effects are rare. They have been used in pregnancy and breastfeeding, with ranitidine having been used most. Data suggests that they can be used in pregnancy and breastfeeding, although manufacturers advise patients to speak to the doctor or pharmacist before taking.

Ranitidine (e.g., Zantac and Gavilast range, Ranicalm)
Dosing for ranitidine (Zantac 75) is similar to famotidine in that one tablet should be taken straight away but, if symptoms persist, then a further tablet should be taken 1 hour later. The maximum dose is 300 mg (four tablets) in 24 hours. The General Sales List version of ranitidine cannot be used for prevention of heartburn, and the maximum dose (for Zantac 75 Relief and Ranicalm) is only two tablets in 24 hours.

Proton pump inhibitors
All are only available to adults and people aged 18 years and over. If symptoms have not been controlled within 2 weeks, the patient should be referred to his/her doctor.

Omeprazole (Dexcel Heartburn Relief Tablets, Boots Acid Reflux Tablets)
This is marketed for the relief of reflux-like symptoms (e.g., heartburn) associated with acid-related dyspepsia.

Omeprazole can cause a number of common side effects (>1 in 100), which include headache, diarrhoea, constipation, abdominal pain, nausea, vomiting and flatulence. Drug interactions with omeprazole are possible because it is metabolised in the liver by cytochrome P450 isoenzymes. These include 'azole' antifungals (decrease in azole bioavailability), diazepam (enhanced diazepam side effects), fluvoxamine (increased omeprazole levels), cilostazol (increased cilostazol levels) and clopidogrel (reduced clopidogrel levels). Other interactions listed in the manufacturer's literature include phenytoin and warfarin, but their clinical significance appears low.

It appears to be safe in pregnancy and excreted in only small amounts of breast milk and is not contraindicated when used as a POM medicine; however, for pharmacy use it is not recommended.

Esomeprazole (Nexium Control)
Nexium Control is indicated for the short-term treatment of reflux symptoms (e.g., heartburn and acid regurgitation) in adults. The recommended dose is 20 mg (one tablet) once daily with its side-effects and cautions in use being the same as omeprazole.

Pantoprazole (Pantoloc Control)
Pantoprazole has a license for the short-term symptomatic treatment of GORD-like symptoms (e.g., heartburn). The

dosage is one 10mg tablet each day. Manufacturers advise avoidance in pregnancy and breastfeeding women. However, limited data in breastfeeding indicates that maternal pantoprazole doses of 40mg daily produce low levels in milk and would not be expected to cause any adverse effects in breastfed infants.

References

Moayyedi P, Soo S, Deeks J, et al. Pharmacological interventions for non-ulcer dyspepsia. Cochrane Database of Systematic Reviews, 2006, Issue 4. Art. No.: CD001960. http://dx.doi.org/10.1002/14651858.CD001960.pub3.

Talley NJ, Moore MG, Sprogis A, et al. Randomised controlled trial of pantoprazole versus ranitidine for the treatment of uninvestigated heartburn in primary care. Med J Aust 2002;177(8):423–7.

van Pinxteren B, Sigterman KE, Bonis P, et al. Short-term treatment with proton pump inhibitors, H2-receptor antagonists and prokinetics for gastro-oesophageal reflux disease-like symptoms and endoscopy negative reflux disease. Cochrane Database of Systematic Reviews, 2006, Issue 3. Art. No.: CD002095. http://dx.doi.org/10.1002/14651858.CD002095.pub3.

Further reading

Castell DO, Dalton CB, Becker D, et al. Alginic acid decreases postprandial upright gastroesophageal reflux. Comparison with equal-strength antacid. Dig Dis Sci 1992;37:589–93.

Dowswell T, Neilson JP. Interventions for heartburn in pregnancy. Cochrane Database of Systematic Reviews, 2008, Issue 4. Art. No.: CD007065. http://dx.doi.org/10.1002/14651858.CD007065.pub2.

Drake D, Hollander D. Neutralizing capacity and cost effectiveness of antacids. Ann Intern Med 1981;94:215–7.

Feldman M. Comparison of the effects of over-the-counter famotidine and calcium carbonate antacid on postprandial gastric acid. A randomized controlled trial. JAMA1996;275:1428–31.

Halter F. Determination of neutralization capacity of antacids in gastric juice. Z Gastroenterol 1983;21:S33–40.

Netzer P, Brabetz-Hofliger A, Brundler R, et al. Comparison of the effect of the antacid Rennie versus low dose H2 receptor antagonists (ranitidine, famotidine) on intragastric acidity. Ailment Pharmacol Ther 1998;12:337–42.

Reilly TG, Singh S, Cottrell J, et al. Low dose famotidine and ranitidine as single post-prandial doses: a three-period placebo-controlled comparative trial. Ailment Pharmacol Ther 1996;10:749–55.

Smart HL, Atkinson M. Comparison of a dimethicone/antacid (Asilone gel) with an alginate/antacid (Gaviscon liquid) in the management of reflux oesophagitis. J R Soc Med 1990;83:554–6.

Websites

British Society of Gastroenterology: http://www.bsg.org.uk/

CORE–research charity into gut and liver disease: http://www.corecharity.org.uk/

American Gastroenterological Association: http://www.gastro.org/

Gastroenterological Society of Australia: www.gesa.org.au

New Zealand Society of Gastroenterology: www.nzsg.org.nz/cms2/guidelines

Diarrhoea

Background

Diarrhoea can be defined as an increase in frequency of the passage of soft or watery stools relative to the usual bowel habit for that individual. It is not a disease but a sign of an underlying problem such as an infection or gastrointestinal disorder. It can be classed as acute (less than 7 days), persistent (more than 14 days) or chronic (lasting longer than a month). Most patients will present to the pharmacy with a self-diagnosis of acute diarrhoea. It is necessary to confirm this self-diagnosis because patients' interpretations of their symptoms might not match closely with the medical definition of diarrhoea.

Prevalence and epidemiology

The exact prevalence and epidemiology of diarrhoea is not well known. This is probably due to the number of patients who do not seek care or who self-medicate. However, acute diarrhoea does generate high medical consultation rates. It has been reported that children under the age of 5 years have between one and three bouts of diarrhoea per year and adults, on average, just under one episode of diarrhoea per year. Many of these cases are thought to be food related.

Aetiology

The aetiology of diarrhoea depends on its cause. Acute gastroenteritis, the most common cause of diarrhoea in all age groups, is usually viral in origin. Commonly implicated viruses are the rotavirus (now vaccine preventable – see page 177), Norovirus and small, round structured virus. Viruses tend to cause diarrhoea by blunting the villi of the upper small intestine, decreasing the absorptive surface. Bacterial causes of diarrhoea are normally as a result of eating contaminated food or drink and cause diarrhoea by a number of mechanisms.

For example, enterotoxigenic *E. coli* produce enterotoxins that affect gut function with secretion and loss of fluids; enteropathogenic *E. coli* interferes with normal mucosal function; and enteroinvasive *E. coli*, *Shigella* and *Salmonella* species cause injury to the mucosa of the small intestine and deeper tissues.

Other organisms, for example *Staphylococcus aureus* and *Bacillus cereus,* produce preformed enterotoxins which on ingestion stimulate the active secretion of electrolytes into the intestinal lumen.

Arriving at a differential diagnosis

The most common causes of diarrhoea are viral or bacterial infection (Table 7.13) and the community pharmacist can appropriately manage the vast majority of cases. The main priority is identifying those patients that need referral and how quickly they need to be referred. Dehydration is the main complicating factor, especially in the very young and very old. A number of diarrhoea-specific questions should always be asked of the patient to aid in differential diagnosis (Table 7.14).

Table 7.13
Causes of diarrhoea and their relative incidence in community pharmacy

Incidence	Cause
Most likely	Viral and bacterial infection
Likely	Medicine induced
Unlikely	Irritable bowel syndrome, giardiasis, faecal impaction
Very unlikely	Ulcerative colitis and Crohn's disease, colorectal cancer, malabsorption syndromes

Clinical features of acute diarrhoea

Symptoms are normally rapid in onset, with the patient having a history of prior good health. Nausea and vomiting might be present before or during the bout of

Table 7.14
Specific questions to ask the patient: Diarrhoea

Question	Relevance
Frequency and nature of the stools	Patients with acute self-limiting diarrhoea will be passing watery stools more frequently than normal Diarrhoea associated with blood and mucous (dysentery) requires referral to eliminate invasive infection such as *Shigella, Campylobacter, Salmonella* or *E. coli* O157 Bloody stools is also associated with conditions such as inflammatory bowel disease
Periodicity	A history of recurrent diarrhoea of no known cause should be referred for further investigation
Duration	A person who presents with a history of chronic diarrhoea should be referred. The most frequent causes of chronic diarrhoea are IBS, inflammatory disease and colon cancer
Onset of symptoms	Ingestion of bacterial pathogens can give rise to symptoms in a matter of a few hours (toxin-producing bacteria) after eating contaminated food or up to 3 days later. It is therefore important to ask about food consumption over the last few days, establish if anyone else ate the same food and to check the status of his or her health
Timing of diarrhoea	Patients who experience diarrhoea first thing in the morning might well have underlying pathology such as IBS Nocturnal diarrhoea is often associated with inflammatory bowel disease
Recent change of diet	Changes in diet can cause changes to bowel function, for example, when away on holiday. If the person has recently been to a non-Western country, then giardiasis is a possibility
Signs of dehydration	Mild (<5%) dehydration can be vague but include tiredness, anorexia, nausea and light-headedness Moderate (5% to10%) dehydration is characterised by dry mouth, sunken eyes, decreased urine output, moderate thirst and decreased skin turgor (pinch test of 1–2 seconds or longer)

acute diarrhoea. Abdominal cramping, flatulence and tenderness are also often present. If rotavirus is the cause the patient might also experience viral prodromal symptoms such as cough and cold. Acute infective diarrhoea is usually watery in nature with no blood present. Complete resolution of symptoms should be observed in 2 to 4 days. However, diarrhoea caused by the rotavirus can persist for longer.

Conditions to eliminate

Likely causes

Medicine-induced diarrhoea
Many medicines can induce diarrhoea (Table 7.15). If medication is suspected as the cause of the diarrhoea the patient's doctor should be contacted and an alternative suggested.

Table 7.15
Examples of medicines known to cause diarrhoea (frequently defined as very common [>10%] or common [1% to 10%])

α-blocker	Prazosin
ACE inhibitor	Lisinopril, perindopril
Angiotensin receptor blocker	Telmisartan
Acetylcholinesterase inhibitor	Donepezil, galantamine, rivastigmine
Antacid	Magnesium salts
Antibacterial	All
Antidiabetic	Metformin, acarbose
Antidepressant	SSRIs, clomipramine, venlafaxine
Anti-emetic	Aprepitant, dolasetron
Anti-epileptic	Carbamazepine, oxcarbamazepine, tiagabine, zonisamide, pregabalin, levetiracetam
Antifungal	Caspofungin, fluconazole, flucytosine, nystatin (in large doses), terbinafine, voriconazole
Antimalarial	Mefloquine
Antiprotozoal	Metronidazole, sodium stibogluconate
Antipsychotic	Aripiprazole
Antiviral	Abacavir, emtricitabine, stavudine, tenofovir, zalcitabine, zidovudine, amprenavir, atazanavir, indinavir, lopinavir, nelfinavir, saquinavir, efavirenz, ganciclovir, valganciclovir, adefovir, oseltamivir, ribavirin, fosamprenavir
Beta-blocker	Bisoprolol, carvedilol, nebivolol
Bisphosphonate	Alendronic acid, disodium etidronate, ibandronic acid, risedronate, sodium clodronate, disodium pamidronate, tiludronic acid
Cytokine inhibitor	Adalimumab, infliximab
Cytotoxic	All classes of cytotoxics
Dopaminergic	Levodopa, entacapone

Table 7.15 Examples of medicines known to cause diarrhoea (defined as very common [>10%] or common [1% to 10%]) (Continued)	
Growth hormone antagonist	Pegvisomant
Immunosuppressant	Ciclosporin, mycophenolate, leflunomide
NSAID	All
Ulcer healing	Proton pump inhibitors
Vaccines	Pediacel, haemophilus, meningococcal
Miscellaneous	Calcitonin, strontium ranelate, colchicine, dantrolene, olsalazine, anagrelide, nicotinic acid, pancreatin, eplerenone, acamprosate

Reproduced with permission from R Walker and C Whittlesea, Clinical pharmacy and therapeutics, 5th edition, 2011, Churchill Livingstone.

Unlikely causes

Irritable bowel syndrome
Patients younger than 45 years of age with lower abdominal pain and a history of alternating diarrhoea and constipation are likely to have IBS. For further details on IBS see page 187.

Giardiasis
Giardiasis, a protozoan infection of the small intestine, is contracted through drinking contaminated drinking water. It is an uncommon cause of diarrhoea in Western society. However, with more people taking foreign holidays to non-Western countries, enquiry about recent travel should be made. The patient will present with watery and foul-smelling diarrhoea, accompanied with symptoms of bloating, flatulence and epigastric pain. If giardiasis is suspected, the patient must be referred to a GP for confirmation and appropriate antibiotic treatment.

Faecal impaction
Faecal impaction is most commonly seen in the elderly and those with poor mobility. Patients might present with continuous soiling as a result of liquid passing around hard stools and mistakenly believe they have diarrhoea. On questioning, the patient might describe the passage of regular, poorly formed hard stools that are difficult to pass. Referral is needed, as manual removal of the faeces is often needed.

Very unlikely causes

Ulcerative colitis and Crohn's disease
Both conditions are characterised by chronic inflammation at various sites in the GI tract and follow periods of remission and relapse. They can affect any age group, although peak incidence is between 20 and 30 years of age. In mild cases of both conditions, diarrhoea is one of the major presenting symptoms, although blood in the stool is usually present. Patients often have lower abdominal pain and suffer from urgency, nocturnal diarrhoea and early morning rushes. In the acute phase, patients will appear unwell and have malaise.

Malabsorption syndromes
Lactose intolerance is often diagnosed in infants under 1 year old. In addition to more frequent loose bowel movements, symptoms such as fever, vomiting, perianal excoriation and a failure to gain weight might occur.

Coeliac disease has a bimodal incidence: first, in early infancy when cereals become a major constituent of the diet, and second, during the fourth and fifth decades. Steatorrhoea (fatty stools) is common and might be observed by the patient as frothy or floating stools in the toilet pan. Bloating and recurrent abdominal pain are usually present. Weight loss in the presence of a normal appetite is also observed.

Colorectal cancer
Any middle-aged patient presenting with a longstanding change of bowel habit must be viewed with suspicion. Persistent diarrhoea accompanied by a feeling that the bowel has not really been emptied is suggestive of neoplasm. This is especially true if weight loss is also present.

Fig. 7.11 will aid differentiation of diarrhoeal cases that require referral.

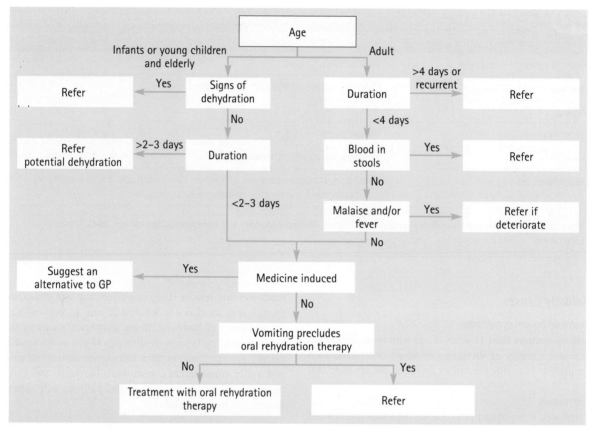

Fig. 7.11   Primer for differential diagnosis of diarrhoea.

TRIGGER POINTS indicative of referral: Diarrhoea

Symptoms/signs	Possible danger/ reason for referral
Change in bowel (long-term) habit in patients over 50 years	Sinister pathology?
Diarrhoea following recent travel to tropical or subtropical climate	Giardiasis?
Duration longer than 2–3 days in children and elderly	At risk of dehydration and associated complications
Patients unable to drink fluids	
Presence of blood or mucous in the stool	Outside scope of community pharmacist
Suspected faecal impaction in the elderly	
Severe abdominal pain	
Steatorrhoea	Malabsorption syndrome?

Evidence base for over-the-counter medication

Acute infectious diarrhoea still remains one of the leading causes of death in developing countries, despite advances in its treatment. In developed and Western countries diarrhoeal disease is primarily of economic and socially disruptive significance. Goals of OTC treatment are therefore concentrated on relief of symptoms. Given most causes of diarrhoea only last 24 to 48 hours, the main aim of treatment should be to reduce any potential dehydration caused by fluid loss. Agents that change the motility of the gut to reduce diarrhoea (e.g., loperamide) should be reserved for situations where staying at home and resting would be impractical or inconvenient.

Before considering treatment it is important to stress to patients the importance of hand washing. Interventions that promote hand washing can reduce diarrhoea episodes by about one-third (Ejemot et al., 2008).

Oral rehydration solution (ORS)

ORS represents one of the major advances in medicine. It has proved to be a simple, highly effective treatment, which has decreased mortality and morbidity associated with acute diarrhoea in developing countries. The formula recommended by the World Health Organisation (WHO) contains glucose (75 mmol/L), sodium (75 mmol/L), potassium (20 mmol/L), chloride (65 mmol/L) and citrate (10 mmol/L) in an almost isotonic fluid. Until recently, the WHO oral rehydration solution contained 90 mmol/L sodium but a systematic review (Hahn et al., 2002) concluded that ORS, with a reduced osmolarity compared with the standard WHO formula, was associated with fewer complications in children with mild to moderate diarrhoea. Based on this and other findings, the WHO oral rehydration solution now has a reduced osmolarity of 245 mm/L, which contains 75 mmol/L of sodium. A number of similar preparations are available commercially in the form of sachets that require reconstitution in clean water before use; however, commercially available solutions in the UK contain lower sodium concentrations (50–60 mmol/L of sodium), as diarrhoea tends to be isotonic, and therefore replacement of large quantities of sodium is less important.

Rice-based ORS

In many developing countries a glucose substitute was added to electrolytes because of glucose unavailability. These products were found to be quite successful. Clinical trials have subsequently shown rice-based ORS to be highly efficacious, well tolerated and potentially more effective than conventional ORS.

Loperamide

Loperamide is a synthetic opioid analogue and is thought to exert its action via opiate receptors slowing intestinal tract time and increasing the capacity of the gut. It has been extensively researched, with many published trials investigating its effectiveness in acute infectious diarrhoea. The majority of well-designed, double-blind, placebo-controlled trials have consistently shown it to be significantly better than placebo and comparable to diphenoxylate. Loperamide is also available compounded with simethicone. However, there is little evidence of better efficacy in terms of diarrhoeal symptoms with the combination.

Bismuth subsalicylate

Bismuth-containing products have been used for many decades. Its use has declined over time as other products have become more popular. However, bismuth subsalicylate has been shown to be effective in treating traveller's diarrhoea. A review paper by Steffen (1990) concluded that bismuth subsalicylate was clinically superior to placebo, decreasing the number of unformed stools and increasing

the number of patients who were symptom free. However, two of the trials reviewed showed bismuth subsalicylate to be significantly slower in symptom resolution than its comparator drug loperamide.

Kaolin and morphine

The constipating side effect of opioid analgesics can be used to treat diarrhoea. However, kaolin and morphine products have no evidence of efficacy and should not be recommended. It remains a popular home remedy, especially with the elderly.

Rotavirus vaccine

In 2006, two new oral vaccines were licensed by the European Medicines Agency and the US Food and Drug Administration. Clinical trials have shown them to be effective (Soares-Weiser et al., 2012).

From 2013, the rotavirus vaccine (Rotarix) was added to the routine UK childhood vaccination schedule. The oral vaccine is given as two doses, the first at 2 months and the second at 3 months, alongside their other routine childhood vaccinations. Due to its introduction, the rotavirus vaccine has prevented more than 70% of cases.

Summary

Since diarrhoea results in fluid and electrolyte loss, it is important to re-establish normal fluid balance and so ORS is first-line treatment for all age groups, especially children and the frail elderly. Loperamide is a useful adjunct in reducing the number of bowel movements but should be reserved for those patients who will find it inconvenient to use a restroom.

Practical prescribing and product selection

Prescribing information relating to the medicines used for diarrhoea reviewed in the section 'Evidence base for over-the-counter medication' is discussed and summarised in Table 7.16; useful tips relating to patients presenting with diarrhoea are given in 'Hints and Tips' in Box 7.5.

ORS (Dioralyte, Dioralyte Relief (rice-based), Electrolade, Oralyte)

ORS can be given to all patient groups, has no side effects or drug interactions. The volume of solution given is dependent on how much fluid is lost. As infants and the elderly are more at risk of developing dehydration, they should be encouraged to drink as much ORS as possible. In adults, 2 L of ORS should be given in the first 24 hours, followed by unrestricted normal fluids with 200 mL of

Table 7.16
Practical prescribing: Summary of medicines for diarrhoea

Name of medicine	Use in children	Likely side effects	Drug interactions of note	Patients in which care is exercised	Pregnancy & breastfeeding
ORS	Infant upwards	None	None	None	OK
Loperamide	>12 years	Abdominal cramps, nausea, vomiting, tiredness	None	None	OK
Bismuth	>16 years	Black stools or tongue	Quinolone antibiotics	None	Avoid in breastfeeding if possible as It has a n theory avoid in bf because it has a salicylate content and risk of association with Reye's syndrome.
Morphine salts	>12 years	None	None	None	OK

HINTS AND TIPS BOX 7.5 DIARRHOEA

Reconstitution of ORS	All proprietary sachets require 200 mL of water per sachet to reconstitute Different brands come in different flavours: • Dioralyte – blackcurrant and citrus • Dioralyte Relief – apricot, raspberry or blackcurrant • Electrolade – banana, blackcurrant, lemon and lime and orange Once reconstituted, ORS must be stored in the fridge and drunk within 24 hours Note: Oralyte is sold as a ready-to-drink product and requires no reconstitution.
Rough guidelines for referral for children	<1 year old: refer if duration >1 day <3 years old: refer if duration >2 days >3 years old: refer if duration >3 days
Kaolin and morphine	Subject to abuse. Store out of sight
Alternative to ORS	Patients can be advised to increase their intake of fluids, particularly fruit juices with their glucose and potassium content, and soups because of their sodium chloride content

rehydration solution per loose stool or vomit. The solution is best sipped every 5 to 10 minutes rather than drunk in large quantities less frequently. In infants, 1 to 1¹/₂ times the usual feed volume should be given.

Loperamide (e.g., Diah-Limit, Imodium range)

The dose is two capsules immediately, followed by one capsule after each further bout of diarrhoea. It has minimal CNS side effects, although CNS depressant effects and respiratory depression have been reported at high doses. OTC doses are therefore limited to 16 mg a day and cannot be used in children under 12. Loperamide has an excellent safety record, although abdominal cramps, nausea, vomiting, tiredness, drowsiness, dizziness and dry mouth have been reported. Loperamide is available in a range of formulations, such as dispersible tablets, melt-tabs and liquid.

Bismuth (Pepto-Bismol Liquid 87.6 mg/5 mL bismuth subsalicylate and Chewable tablet 262.5 mg)

Pepto-Bismol should only be given to people over the age of 16. The dose is 30 mL or two tablets taken every 30 min to 1 hour when needed, with a maximum of eight doses in 24 hours. Bismuth subsalicylate is well tolerated and has a favourable side effect profile, although black stools are commonly observed (caused by unabsorbed bismuth compound). Occasional use is not known to cause problems during pregnancy and breastfeeding, but the manufacturers state it should not be used. Bismuth can decrease the bioavailability of quinolone antibiotics therefore a minimum 2-hour gap should be left between doses of each medicine.

Morphine (e.g., Kaolin and morphine, J Collis Browne's mixture)

Morphine is generally well tolerated at OTC doses, with no side effects reported. The products can be given to all patient groups, including pregnant and breastfeeding women. There are no drug interactions of note. The standard dose for adults and children over 12 years of age is 10 mL every 6 hours.

References

Ejemot-Nwadiaro RI, Ehiri JE, Meremikwu MM, et al. Hand washing for preventing diarrhoea. Cochrane Database of Systematic Reviews 2008, Issue 1. Art. No.: CD004265. http://dx.doi.org/10.1002/14651858.CD004265.pub2.

Hahn S, Kim Y, Garner P. Reduced osmolarity oral rehydration solution for treating dehydration caused by acute diarrhoea in children. Cochrane Database of Systematic Reviews 2002, Issue 1. Art. No.: CD002847. http://dx.doi.org/10.1002/14651858.CD002847.

Soares-Weiser K, MacLehose H, Bergman H, et al. Vaccines for preventing rotavirus diarrhoea: vaccines in use. Cochrane Database of Systematic Reviews 2012, Issue 2. Art. No.: CD008521. http://dx.doi.org/10.1002/14651858. CD008521.pub2.

Steffen R. Worldwide efficacy of bismuth subsalicylate in the treatment of travelers' diarrhea. Rev Infect Dis 1990;12:S80-86.

Further reading

Amery W, Duyck F, Polak J, et al. A multicentre double-blind study in acute diarrhoea comparing loperamide (R 18553) with two common antidiarrhoeal agents and a placebo. Curr Ther Res Clin Exp 1975;17:263-70.

Chassany O, Michaux A, Bergman JF. Drug-induced diarrhoea. Drug Safe 2000;22:53-72.

Cornett JWD, Aspeling RL, Mallegol D. A double blind comparative evaluation of loperamide versus diphenoxylate with atropine in acute diarrhea. Curr Ther Res 1977;21:629-37.

Gavin N, Merrick N, Davidson B. Efficacy of glucose-based oral rehydration therapy. Pediatrics 1996;98:45-51.

Islam A, Molla AM, Ahmed MA, et al. Is rice based oral rehydration therapy effective in young infants? Arch Dis Child 1994;71:19-23.

Molla AM, Sarker SA, Hossain M, et al. Rice-powder electrolyte solution as oral-therapy in diarrhoea due to Vibrio cholerae and Escherichia coli. Lancet 1982;1(8285):1317-9.

Nelemans FA, Zelvelder WG. A double-blind placebo controlled trial of loperamide (Imodium) in acute diarrhea. J Drug Res 1976;2:54-9.

Patra FC, Mahalanabis D, Jalan KN, et al. Is oral rice electrolyte solution superior to glucose electrolyte solution in infantile diarrhoea? Arch Dis Child 1982;57:910-2.

Selby W. Diarrhoea – differential diagnosis. Aust Fam Physician 1990;19:1683-6.

Websites

Crohn's and colitis UK: https://www.crohnsandcolitis.org.uk/

Constipation

Background

Constipation, like diarrhoea, means different things to different people. Constipation arises when the patient experiences a reduction in his/her normal bowel habit accompanied with more difficult defecation and/or hard stools. In Western populations 90% of people defecate between three times a day and once every 3 days. However, many people still believe that anything other than one bowel movement a day is abnormal.

Prevalence and epidemiology

Constipation is very common. It occurs in all age groups but is especially common in the elderly. It has been estimated that 25% to 40% of all people over the age of 65 have constipation. The majority of the elderly have normal frequency of bowel movements but strain at stool. This is probably a result of a sedentary lifestyle, a decreased fluid intake, poor nutrition, avoidance of fibrous foods and chronic illness. Women are two to three times more likely to suffer from constipation than men and 40% of women in late pregnancy experience constipation.

Aetiology

The normal function of the large intestine is to remove water and various salts from the colon, drying and expulsion of the faeces. Any process that facilitates water resorption will generally lead to constipation. The most common cause of constipation is an increase in intestinal tract transit time of food, which allows greater water resorption from the large bowel, leading to harder stools that are more difficult to pass. This is most frequently caused by a deficiency in dietary fibre, a change in lifestyle and/or environment and medication. Occasionally, patients ignore the defecation reflex as it may be inconvenient for them to defecate.

Arriving at a differential diagnosis

The first thing a pharmacist should do is to establish the patient's current bowel habit compared with normal. This should establish whether the patient is suffering from constipation. Questioning should then concentrate on determining the cause because constipation is a symptom and not a disease and can be caused by many different conditions. Constipation does not usually have sinister pathology, and the most common cause in the vast majority of non-elderly adults will be a lack of dietary fibre (Table 7.17). However, constipation can be caused by medication and many disease states including neurological disorders (e.g., multiple sclerosis, Parkinson's disease), metabolic and endocrine conditions (diabetes, hypothyroidism) and neoplasm. A number of constipation-specific questions should always be asked of the patient to aid in differential diagnosis (Table 7.18).

Table 7.17
Causes of constipation and their relative incidence in community pharmacy

Incidence	Cause
Most likely	Eating habits/lifestyle
Likely	Medication
Unlikely	Irritable bowel syndrome, pregnancy, depression, functional disorders (children)
Very unlikely	Colorectal cancer, hypothyroidism

Clinical features of constipation

Besides the inability to defecate, patients might also have abdominal discomfort and bloating. In children, parents might also notice the child is more irritable and have a decreased appetite. Specks of blood in the toilet pan might be present and are usually due to straining at stool. In the vast majority of cases blood in the stool does not indicate sinister pathology. Those patients presenting with acute constipation with no other symptoms apart from very small amounts of bright red blood can be managed in the pharmacy; however, if blood loss is substantial (stools appear tarry, red or black) or the patient has other associated symptoms such as malaise and/or abdominal distension and is over 40 years old, then referral is needed.

Table 7.18
Specific questions to ask the patient: Constipation

Question	Relevance
Change of diet or routine	Constipation usually has a social or behavioural cause. There will usually be some event that has precipitated the onset of symptoms
Pain on defecation	Associated pain when going to the toilet is usually due to a local anorectal problem. Constipation is often secondary to the suppression of defecation because it induces pain. These cases are best referred for physical examination
Presence of blood	Bright red specks in the toilet or smears on toilet tissue suggest haemorrhoids or a tear in the anal canal (fissure). However, if blood is mixed in the stool (melaena), then referral to the GP is necessary. A stool that appears black and tarry is suggestive of an upper GI bleed
Duration (chronic or recent?)	If a patient suffers from longstanding constipation and has been previously seen by the GP then treatment could be given. However, cases of more than 14 days with no identifiable cause or previous investigation by the GP should be referred
Lifestyle changes	Changes in job or marital status can precipitate depressive illness that can manifest with physiological symptoms, such as constipation

Conditions to eliminate

Likely causes

Medicine-induced constipation

Many medicines are known to cause constipation. Most exert their action by decreasing gut motility, although opioids tend to raise sphincter tone and reduce sensitivity to rectal distension. A detailed medication history should always be sought from the patient and Table 7.19 lists the commonly implicated medicines that cause constipation.

Unlikely causes

Irritable bowel syndrome

Patients younger than 45 years of age with lower abdominal pain and a history of alternating diarrhoea and constipation are likely to have IBS. For further details on IBS see page 187.

Pregnancy

Constipation is common in pregnancy, especially in the third trimester. A combination of increased circulating progestogen, displacement of the uterus against the colon by the foetus, decreased mobility and iron supplementation all contribute to an increased incidence of constipation while pregnant. Most patients complain of hard stools rather than a decrease in bowel movements. If a laxative is used, a bulk-forming laxative should be recommended.

Depression

Upwards of 20% of the population will suffer from depression at some time. Many will present with physical as well as emotional symptoms. It has been reported that a third of all patients suffering from depression present with gastrointestinal complaints in a primary care setting. Core

Table 7.19
Examples of medicines known to cause constipation (frequently defined as very common [>10%] or common [1%–10%])

α-blocker	Prazosin
Antacid	Aluminium and calcium salts
Anticholinergic	Trihexyphenidyl, hyoscine, oxybutynin, procyclidine, tolterodine
Antidepressant	Tricyclics, SSRIs, reboxetine, venlafaxine, duloxetine, mirtazapine
Anti-emetic	Palonosetron, dolasetron, aprepitant
Anti-epileptic	Carbamazepine, oxcarbazepine
Antipsychotic	Phenothiazines, haloperidol, pimozide and atypical antipsychotics such as amisulpride, aripiprazole, olanzapine, quetiapine, risperidone, zotepine, clozapine
Antiviral	Foscarnet
Beta-blocker	Oxprenolol, bisoprolol, nebivolol; other beta-blockers tend to cause constipation more rarely
Bisphosphonate	Alendronic acid
CNS stimulant	Atomoxetine
Calcium channel blocker	Diltiazem, verapamil
Cytotoxic	Bortezomib, buserelin, cladribine, docetaxel, doxorubicin, exemestane, gemcitabine, irinotecan, mitoxantrone, pentostatin, temozolomide, topotecan, vinblastine, vincristine, vindesine, vinorelbine
Dopaminergic	Amantadine, bromocriptine, cabergoline, entacapone, tolcapone, levodopa, pergolide, pramipexole, quinagolide
Growth hormone antagonist	Pegvisomant

(Continued)

Table 7.19
Examples of medicines known to cause constipation (frequently defined as very common [>10%] or common [1%–10%]) (Continued)

Immunosuppressant	Basiliximab, mycophenolate, tacrolimus
Lipid-lowering agent	Cholestyramine, colestipol, rosuvastatin, atorvastatin (other statins uncommon), gemfibrozil
Iron	Ferrous sulphate
Metabolic disorders	Miglustat
Muscle relaxant	Baclofen
NSAID	Meloxicam; other NSAIDs, e.g., aceclofenac and COX-2 inhibitors reported as uncommon
Smoking cessation	Bupropion
Opioid analgesic	All opioid analgesics and derivatives
Ulcer healing	All proton pump inhibitors, sucralfate

Reproduced with permission from R Walker and C Whittlesea, Clinical pharmacy and therapeutics, 5th edition, 2011, Churchill Livingstone.

symptoms of persistent low mood and loss of interest in most activities should trigger referral.

Functional causes in children
Constipation in children is common and the cause can be varied. Constipation is not normally a result of organic disease but stems from poor diet or a traumatic experience associated with defecation, for example, unwillingness to defecate due to association of prior pain on defecation.

Very unlikely causes

Colorectal cancer
Colorectal carcinomas are rare in patients under the age of 40. However, the incidence of carcinoma increases with increasing age and any patient over the age of 40 presenting for the first time with a marked change in bowel habit should be referred. Sexes appear to be equally affected. The patient might complain of abdominal pain, rectal bleeding and tenesmus. Weight loss – a classic textbook sign of colon cancer – is common but observed only in the latter stages of the disease. Therefore a patient is unlikely to have noticed a marked weight loss when visiting a pharmacy early in the disease progression.

Hypothyroidism
The signs and symptoms of hypothyroidism are often subtle and insidious in onset. Patients might experience weight gain, lethargy, cold intolerance, coarse hair and dry skin as well as constipation. Hypothyroidism affects ten times more women than men and peak incidence is in the fifth or sixth decade. Constipation is often less pronounced than lethargy and cold intolerance.

Fig. 7.12 will aid differentiation between common causes of constipation and more serious causes.

! TRIGGER POINTS indicative of referral:

Symptoms/signs	Possible danger/reason for referral
Pain on defecation, causing patient to suppress defecation reflex	Check for anal fissure
Patients over 40 years of age with sudden change in bowel habits with no obvious cause	Danger symptom for rectal carcinoma
Greater than 14 days' duration with no identifiable cause	Suspect underlying cause that requires fuller investigation by GP
Tiredness	Check for anaemia or thyroid dysfunction

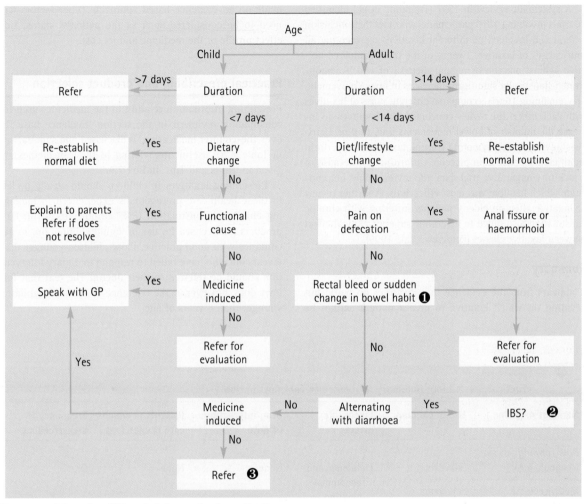

Fig. 7.12 Primer for differential diagnosis of constipation.

❶ Patients with unexplained constipation of recent onset accompanied with rectal bleeding should be referred for further investigation; most likely a colonoscopy or sigmoidoscopy and stool culture to eliminate carcinoma.

❷ See Fig. 7.13 for primer for differential diagnosis of IBS.

❸ If no obvious cause of constipation can be found, referral to the GP is needed for further evaluation.

Evidence base for over-the-counter medication

For uncomplicated constipation, non-drug treatment is advocated as first-line treatment for all patient groups, as simple dietary and lifestyle modifications (increasing exercise) will relieve the majority of acute cases of constipation. Advice includes increasing fluid and fibre intake. Dietary fibre increases stool bulk, stool water content and colonic bacterial load. Fibre intake should be increased to approximately 30 g day in the form of fruit, vegetables, cereals, grain foods and wholemeal bread. It is important to remind patients that adequate fluid intake (2 L per day) is needed when following a high-fibre diet, and patients might experience excessive gas production, colicky abdominal pain and bloating. Effects of a high-fibre diet are usually seen in 3 to 5 days.

If medication is required, four classes of OTC laxatives are available: bulk-forming agents, stimulants, osmotics and stool softeners. Despite their widespread use, surprisingly few well-designed trials have substantiated clinical efficacy.

A systematic review in 1997 (Tramonte et al.) identified 36 trials involving 1815 participants who met their inclusion criteria and involved 25 different laxatives representing all four classes of laxative. Twenty of the trials compared laxative against placebo or regular diet, 13 of which demonstrated statistically significant increases in bowel movement. The remaining 16 trials compared different types of laxatives with each other. The review concluded that laxatives do increase the number of bowel movements and, in 9 of 11 trials studying overall symptom control, laxatives did perform significantly better than placebo. Unfortunately, because of a lack of comparative trial data, the review could not conclude which laxative was most efficacious. A further review of laxative effect in elderly patients suffering with chronic constipation also failed to determine superior clinical effect between laxative classes (Petticrew et al., 1999).

Summary

It appears from the evidence that laxatives do work, but deciding on which laxative to give a patient cannot be made on an evidence-based approach. Other factors will need to be considered such as the patients' status, side effect profile of the medicine and its cost.

Practical prescribing and product selection

Prescribing information relating to the medicines used for constipation reviewed in the section 'Evidence base for over-the-counter medication' is discussed and summarised in Table 7.20; useful tips relating to these medicines are given in 'Hints and Tips' in Box 7.6.

Prescribing laxatives in children should ideally be left to those healthcare professionals experienced in managing childhood constipation (BNF edition 70, 2016). OTC products are licensed for use in young children but in accordance with good practice, those children younger than 6 years old who have failed to respond to dietary intervention should be referred to their doctor. The text that follows does, however, make reference to dosing in children younger than 6 years of age.

Table 7.20
Practical prescribing: Summary of medicines for constipation

Name of medicine	Use in children	Likely side effects	Drug interactions of note	Patients in which care is exercised	Pregnancy & breastfeeding
Bulk forming					
Ispaghula husk	>6 years	Flatulence and abdominal bloating	None	None	OK
Methylcellulose	>12 years				
Sterculia	>6 years				
Stimulant					
Senna	>6 years	Abdominal pain	None	None	OK, but use other laxatives in preference to stimulants in pregnancy and breastfeeding
Glycerol	Infant upwards*				
Sodium picosulfate	>10 years				
Bisacodyl	>4 years				
Osmotic					
Lactulose	Infant upwards*	Flatulence, abdominal pain and colic	None	None	OK
Magnesium hydroxide	Not recommended				
Stool softeners					
Docusate	>6 months*	None reported	None	None	OK

*If prescribing to children less than 6 years of age, then the pharmacist must be competent in prescribing laxatives for children.

HINTS AND TIPS BOX 7.6: CONSTIPATION

Administration of suppositories	1. Wash your hands 2. Lie on one side with your knees pulled up towards your chest 3. Gently push the suppository, pointed end first, into your back passage with your finger 4. Push the suppository in as far as possible 5. Lower your legs, roll over onto your stomach and remain still for a few minutes. 6. If you feel your body trying to expel the suppository, try to resist this. Lie still and press your buttocks together 7. Wash your hands
Sachets containing Ispaghula husk	Once the granules have been mixed with water, the drink should be taken as soon as the effervescence subsides because the drink 'sets' and becomes undrinkable
Prolonged use of lactulose	In children this can contribute to the development of dental caries. Patients should be instructed to pay careful attention to dental hygiene
Lactulose taste	The sweet taste is unpalatable to many patients, especially if high doses need to be taken
Bisacodyl	Bisacodyl tablets are enteric coated and therefore patients should be told to avoid taking antacids and milk at the same time because the coating can be broken down, leading to dyspepsia and gastric irritation
Laxative abuse	Some people, especially young women, use laxatives as a slimming aid. Any very slim person who is regularly purchasing laxatives should be politely asked about why they are taking the laxatives. An opening question could be phrased, 'We've noticed that you have been buying quite a lot of these, and we are concerned that you should be better by now. Is there anything we can do for you to help?'
Onset of action	Stimulants are the quickest-acting laxative, usually within 6–12 hours. Lactulose and bulk-forming laxatives may take 48–72 hours before an effect is seen. Stool softeners are the slowest in onset, taking up to 3 days or more to work.
Which laxative to use in pregnancy?	Fibre supplementation and bulk-forming agents are considered to be safe and should therefore be first-line treatments wherever possible. Stimulant laxatives and macrogols also appear to be safe in pregnancy. Stimulant laxatives are more effective than bulk-forming laxatives but are more likely to cause diarrhoea and abdominal pain
Avoid drinks with caffeine	These can act as a diuretic and serve to make constipation worse
Combining laxatives	There is little evidence on the beneficial effect of combining different classes of laxatives. However, in refractory cases this approach might be justifiable

Bulk-forming laxatives (e.g., ispaghula husk, methylcellulose and sterculia)

Bulk-forming laxatives exert their effect by mimicking increased fibre consumption, swelling in the bowel and increasing faecal mass. In addition they also encourage the proliferation of colonic bacteria, and this helps further increase faecal bulk and stool softness. Patients should be advised to increase their fluid intake while taking bulk-forming medicines. Their effect is usually seen in 12 to 36 hours but can take as long as 72 hours. Side effects commonly experienced include flatulence and abdominal distension. They are well tolerated in pregnancy and breastfeeding and have no teratogenic effects. They appear to have no drug interactions of any note.

Ispaghula husk

Ispaghula husk is widely available as either granules (Fybogel, Ispagel) or powder (Regulan). All have to be reconstituted with water before taking. The dose for adults and children over 12 years old can range from one to six sachets a day, depending on the brand used and the severity of the condition. Fybogel is probably the most familiar branded product used

OTC in the UK – adults should take one sachet or two level, 5 mL spoonfuls twice a day and for children aged between 6 and 12, ½ to one 5 mL spoonful twice daily.

Methylcellulose (Celevac)

Methylcellulose is only available as Celevac tablets. The adult dose is three to six tablets twice daily, and each dose should be taken with at least 300 mL of liquid.

Sterculia (Normacol and Normacol Plus granules or sachets)

Both products contain 62% sterculia, but Normacol Plus also contains 8% frangula. The dose for both products is the same. Adults and children over 12 years of age should take either one or two sachets or heaped 5 mL spoonfuls, once or twice daily after meals. For children aged between 6 and 12, the dose is half that of the adult dose.

The granules should be placed dry on the tongue and swallowed immediately with plenty of water or a cool drink. They can also be sprinkled onto, and taken with, soft food, such as yoghurt.

Stimulant laxatives (e.g., bisacodyl, glycerol, senna, sodium picosulfate)

Stimulant laxatives increase GI motility by directly stimulating colonic nerves. It is this action that, presumably, causes abdominal pain and is the main side effect associated with stimulant laxatives. Additionally, stimulant laxatives are associated with the possibility of nerve damage in long-term use and are the most commonly abused laxatives. Their onset in action is quicker than other laxative classes, with patients experiencing a bowel movement in 6 to 12 hours when taken orally. They can be taken by all patient groups, have no drug interactions and are safe in pregnancy and breastfeeding. However, because of their stimulant effect on uterine contractions, they are best avoided in pregnancy if possible.

Bisacodyl (Dulcolax)

Bisacodyl is available as either tablets or suppositories and can be given to patients over 4 years of age, although OTC products restrict use to those over the age of 10. The dose for children is 5 mg (one paediatric suppository) and for adults and children over 10 years, the dose is 5 to 10 mg (one to two tablets or one Dulcolax 10 mg suppository).

Glycerol suppositories

Glycerol suppositories are normally used when a bowel movement is needed quickly. The patient should experience a bowel movement in 15 to 30 minutes. Varying sizes are made to accommodate use in different ages. The 1-g suppositories are designed for infants, the 2-g for children and the 4-g for adults.

Senna (e.g., Senokot, Ex-Lax Senna)

Senna is available as syrup, tablets or granules. Dosing of proprietary products differs from those recommended in the BNF and BNF-C. Proprietary products tend to have lower dosing schedules than those advocated in the BNF/BNF-C. These are: adults and children over 12 years of age should take 15 mg each day (two tablets or 10 mL), preferably at bedtime; children over 6 years of age should take half the adult dose (7.5 mg, one tablet or 5 mL).

Sodium picosulfate (e.g., Dulcolax Pico)

Adults and children over 10 years of age should take 5 to 10 mg (5–10 mL) at night.

Osmotic laxatives (e.g., lactulose, macrogols and magnesium salts)

These act by retaining fluid in the bowel by osmosis or by changing the pattern of water distribution in the faeces. Flatulence, abdominal pain and colic are frequently reported. They can be taken by all patient groups, have no drug interactions and are safely used in pregnancy and breastfeeding.

Lactulose

Lactulose is given twice daily for all ages. The dose for adults is initially 15 mL (adjusted upward depending on response), for children between 5 and 18 years of age, the dose is 5 to 20 mL, for those between 1 and 5 years of age, the dose is 2.5 to 10 mL and for children under 1 year of age, the dose is 2.5 mL. It has been reported that up to 20% of patients experience troublesome flatulence and cramps, although these often settle after a few days. It may take 48 hours or longer for it to work.

Macrogols (e.g., Movicol, Dulcobalance)

Macrogols are available as powders that are reconstituted with water. They are licensed for chronic constipation and should therefore not be routinely recommended by pharmacists because treatment should be only instigated in those presenting with acute constipation.

Magnesium salts

Magnesium, when used as a laxative, is usually given as magnesium hydroxide. The adult dose ranges between 30 to 45 mL when needed. It is generally not recommended for use in children but is commonly prescribed in the elderly.

Stool softeners (liquid paraffin and docusate sodium)

Liquid paraffin has been traditionally used to treat constipation. However, the adverse side effect profile of liquid paraffin now means it should never be recommended because other, safer and more effective medications are available.

Docusate sodium

Docusate sodium is a non-ionic surfactant that has stool-softening properties that allows penetration of intestinal fluids into the faecal mass. It also has weak stimulant properties. Docusate is available as either capsules (DulcoEase, Dioctyl) or solution (Docusal). It can be given in children aged 6 months and over. Children between the age of 6 months and 2 years should take 12.5 mg (5 mL of Docusal paediatric solution) three times a day. For children aged between 2 and 12, the dose is 12.5 to 25 mg (5–10 mL) three times a day. Adults and children over 12 years old should take up to 500 mg daily in divided doses. In contrast to liquid paraffin, docusate sodium seems to be almost free of any side effects. Docusate sodium can be given to all patient groups.

References
Petticrew M, Watt I, Brand M. What's the 'best buy' for treatment of constipation? Results of a systematic review of the efficacy and comparative efficacy of laxatives in the elderly. Br J Gen Pract 1999;49:387–93.
Tramonte SM, Brand MB, Mulrow CD, et al. The treatment of chronic constipation in adults. A systematic review. J Gen Intern Med 1997;12:15–24.

Further reading
Borum ML. Constipation: evaluation and management. Primary Care 2001;28:577–90.
Gattuso JM, Kamm MA. Adverse effects of drugs used in the management of constipation and diarrhoea. Drug Saf 1994;10:47–65.
Gerber PD, Barrett JE, Barrett JA, et al. The relationship of presenting physical complaints to depressive symptoms in primary care patients. J Gen Intern Med 1992;7:170–3.
Herz MJ, Kahan E, Zalevski S, et al. Constipation: a different entity for patients and doctors. Fam Pract 1996;13:156–9.
Higgins PDR, Johnson JF. Epidemiology of constipation in North America: a systemic review. Am J Gast 2004;99:750–9.
Jewell D, Young G. Interventions for treating constipation in pregnancy. Cochrane Database of Systematic Reviews 2001, Issue 2. Art. No.: CD001142. http://dx.doi.org/10.1002/14651858.CD001142.
Leng-Peschlow E. Senna and its rational use. Pharmacology 1992;44:S1–52.

Paraskevaides EC. Fatal lipid pneumonia and liquid paraffin. Br J Clin Pract 1990;44:509–10.
Talley NJ, Fleming KC, Evans JM, et al. Constipation in an elderly community: a study of prevalence and potential risk factors. Am J Gastroenterol 1996;9:19–25.

7

Irritable bowel syndrome (IBS)

Background

IBS is one of the most common GI tract conditions seen in primary care. It can be defined as a functional bowel disorder (i.e., absence of abnormality) in which abdominal pain and bloating is associated with a change in bowel habit. The diagnosis is suggested by the presence of longstanding colonic symptoms without any deterioration in the patient's general condition.

Prevalence and epidemiology

IBS is common and is often managed through self-care. Adult prevalence rates in Western countries are reported to be between 10% and 20%, with approximately twice as many women than men affected. It most commonly affects people between 20 and 30 years old, but recent trends indicate that there is a significant prevalence of IBS in older people.

Aetiology

No anatomic cause can be found to explain the aetiology of IBS, but it is now clearly understood to be multifactorial. Many factors can contribute to disease expression and include motility dysfunction, diet and genetics. In a small proportion of cases symptoms appear after bacterial gastroenteritis. Psychological factors also influence symptom reporting and consultation, and some studies have shown patients who suffer from higher levels of stress or depression experience worse symptoms compared with other patients. Flare-up of symptoms has also been associated with periods of increased stress. Symptoms of diarrhoea and constipation appear to be linked with hyperactivity of the small intestine and colon in response to food ingestion and parasympathomimetic drugs. Excessive parasympathomimetic activity might account for mucous associated with the stool.

Arriving at a differential diagnosis

IBS is essentially a diagnosis of exclusion, and a careful and thorough history of the patient is essential. A number of IBS-specific questions should always be asked of the patient to aid in differential diagnosis (Table 7.21).

Table 7.21
Specific questions to ask the patient: Irritable bowel syndrome

Question	Relevance
Age	IBS usually affects people under the age of 45 Particular care is required in labelling middle-aged (i.e., over 45 years old) and elderly patients with IBS when presenting with bowel symptoms for the first time. Such patients are best referred for further evaluation to eliminate organic bowel disease
Periodicity	IBS tends to be episodic. The patient might have a history of being well for a number of weeks or months in between bouts of symptoms. Often patients can trace their symptoms back many years, even to childhood
Presence of abdominal pain	The nature of pain experienced by patients with IBS is very varied, ranging from localised and sharp to diffuse and aching. It is therefore not very discriminatory; however, the patient will probably have experienced similar abdominal pain in the past. Any change in the nature and severity of the pain is best referred for further evaluation
Location of pain	Pain from IBS is normally located in the left lower quadrant. For further information on other conditions that cause pain in the lower abdomen see page 198
Diarrhoea and constipation	Patients with IBS do not have textbook definitions of constipation or diarrhoea but bowel function will be different than normal Constipation-predominant IBS is more common in women

Clinical features of IBS

IBS is characterised by abdominal pain or discomfort, located especially in the left lower quadrant of the abdomen, which is often relieved by defecation or the passage of wind. Altered defecation, either constipation or diarrhoea, with associated bloating is also normally present. People with IBS can present with 'diarrhoea predominant', 'constipation predominant' or alternating symptom profiles. During bouts of diarrhoea, mucous tends to be visible on the stools. Patients might also complain of increased stool frequency but pass normal or pellet-like stools. Diarrhoea on awakening and shortly after meals is also observed in many patients. IBS is likely if the patient has had any of the following symptoms for 6 months:

- Abdominal pain or discomfort
- Bloating
- Change in bowel habit

Conditions to eliminate

Constipation and diarrhoea

Because the major presenting symptom of IBS is an alteration in defecation, it is necessary to differentiate IBS from acute and chronic causes of constipation and diarrhoea. For further information on differentiating these conditions from IBS, please refer to page 180 (for constipation) and page 174 (for diarrhoea).

Fig. 7.13 will aid differentiation of IBS from other abdominal conditions.

TRIGGER POINTS indicative of referral: IBS

Symptoms/signs	Possible danger/reason for referral
Blood in the stool	The presence of blood in the stool is unusual in IBS and can suggest inflammatory bowel disease
Fever Nausea and/or vomiting Severe abdominal pain	Not usually associated with IBS. Suggests origin of symptoms from other abdominal causes
Children under age 16 Patients over age 45 with recent change to bowel habit	IBS is unusual in these age groups. Refer for further investigation.
Steatorrhoea	Associated with malabsorption syndromes

Evidence base for over-the-counter medication

Before medicines are recommended, it might be useful to discuss if stress is a factor and if this can be avoided. In

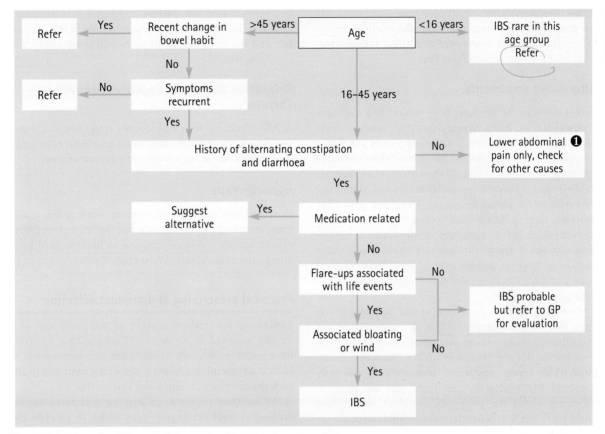

Fig. 7.13 Primer for differential diagnosis of irritable bowel syndrome.

❶ **Lower abdominal pain**
See Fig. 7.29 for primer for differential diagnosis of abdominal pain.

addition, dietary modification has shown to be effective for some patients. (see 'Hints and Tips' in Box 7.7) If diet is deemed a major contributor towards symptoms, then food avoidance can be tried. Suspected food products must be excluded from the diet for a minimum of 2 weeks and then gradually reintroduced to determine whether the food item triggers symptoms.

Antispasmodics are considered first-line pharmacological intervention for IBS, although the evidence base for them is weak; these include mebeverine, alverine, hyoscine and peppermint oil. In addition, bulk-forming and stimulant laxatives can be used to treat constipation-predominant IBS and loperamide for diarrhoea-predominant IBS. Both laxatives and diarrhoeals can be taken on a regular basis using the lowest effective dose. The following text only concentrates on the evidence for those products specifically marketed for the treatment of IBS.

Antispasmodics

The Cochrane review by Ruepert et al. (2011) concluded that antispasmodics as a class of medicines compared with placebo provided a statistically significant benefit for abdominal pain, global assessment and IBS symptom scores. However, as the authors acknowledge, antispasmodics are pharmacologically diverse and in their review it was not possible to include all compounds (due to limited number of studies) at subgroup analysis. Therefore in this review, it was not possible to determine the individual effectiveness of certain OTC antispasmodics. No data was reviewed for alverine and only one trial was included that considered mebeverine. In that trial (Kruis et al., 1986) no statistically significant effect for improvement of global assessment was found for mebeverine. Similarly, for hyoscine, no statistically significant effect for improvement of global assessment was found. The only OTC product which the review found evidence of efficacy was peppermint oil. For peppermint oil a statistically significant effect for improvement of global assessment and effect for improvement of IBS symptom score was found.

Alternative treatments

Herbal remedies for IBS have been subject to a Cochrane review (Liu et al., 2006). Seventy-five trials were reviewed, involving 71 different herbal medicines versus placebo or conventional pharmacological treatment. When compared against placebo, STW 5 and STW5-II, Padma Lax, Tongxie Yaofang and Ayurvedic preparation showed significant improvement of global symptoms. Compared with conventional therapy (in 65 trials testing 51 different herbal medicines), 22 herbal medicines demonstrated a statistically significant benefit for symptom improvement. Most trials were, however, deemed to be of poor methodological quality and authors concluded that findings should be interpreted with caution.

Probiotics, such as *Lactobacillus* and *Bifidobacterium* have also been promoted for IBS. A systematic review identified 18 studies using probiotics either alone or in combination for the treatment of IBS (Moayyedi et al., 2010). The results suggested probiotics significantly improved IBS symptoms and there was no apparent difference across the probiotics. However, the authors noted that there was potential publication bias in the review, with an over-representation of small, positive studies, and therefore these estimates of efficacy are likely to be overestimates. The authors concluded that probiotics appear to be effective in IBS, however, the size of the effect and the effectiveness of individual probiotics is still to be established.

Relaxation therapy & Cognitive Behavioural Therapy

A 2009 Cochrane review (Zijdenbos et al.) concluded that cognitive behavioural therapy might be effective, although studies included in the review were of poor quality.

Hypnotherapy

Hypnotherapy might be effective in treating IBS symptoms, including abdominal pain, but studies reviewed were of poor quality and small size, and so findings need to be interpreted with caution (Webb et al., 2007).

Practical prescribing and product selection

Prescribing information relating to the medicines used for IBS reviewed in the section 'Evidence base for over-the-counter medication' is discussed and summarised in Table 7.22; useful tips relating to the treatment of patients with IBS are given in 'Hints and Tips' in Box 7.7.

All marketed products can be given to children (see individual entries) but anyone aged under 16 suspected of having IBS should be referred to a doctor as IBS in this age group is unusual.

Table 7.22
Practical prescribing: Summary of IBS medicines

Name of medicine	Use in children*	Likely side effects	Drug interactions of note	Patients in which care is exercised	Pregnancy & breastfeeding
Hyoscine	>6 years	Constipation and dry mouth	Tricyclic antidepressants, neuroleptics, antihistamines and disopyramide	Glaucoma, myasthenia gravis and prostate enlargement	Avoid if possible, although single doses in breastfeeding are acceptable
Mebeverine	>10 years	None	None	None	OK
Peppermint oil	>15 years	Heartburn	None	None	OK in pregnancy; try to avoid in breastfeeding, as it may reduce milk supply
Alverine	>12 years	Rash	None	None	OK

*IBS is unusual in children. Any person under 16 years of age presenting with IBS-like symptoms should be referred for further evaluation

HINTS AND TIPS BOX 7.7 IRRITABLE BOWEL SYNDROME

Dietary advice (taken from NICE CG61)

Have regular meals and avoid missing meals

Drink at least eight cups of fluid per day, especially non-caffeinated drinks

Reduce intake of alcohol and fizzy drinks

Consider limiting intake of high-fibre food

Reduce intake of 'resistant starch' often found in processed or re-cooked foods

Limit fresh fruit to 3 portions per day

Hyoscine butylbromide (Buscopan IBS Relief, Buscopan Cramps)

The recommended starting dose for adults is one tablet three times a day, although this can be increased to two tablets four times a day if necessary. Buscopan Cramps can be given to children over the age of 6 (one tablet three times a day). It is a quaternary derivative of hyoscine, so it does not readily cross the blood-brain barrier and therefore sedation is not normally encountered, although it might cause dry mouth and constipation. Because of its anticholinergic effects, it is best avoided with other medicines that also have anticholinergic effects, for example, antihistamines, tricyclic antidepressants, neuroleptics and disopyramide. It can be given during pregnancy and breastfeeding but avoided if possible. It should also be avoided in patients with glaucoma, myasthenia gravis and prostate enlargement.

Mebeverine (Colofac IBS)

Adults and children over 10 should take one tablet three times a day, preferably 20 minutes before meals. Mebeverine is not known to interact with other medicines, has no cautions in its use and can be given in pregnancy and breastfeeding although there is a lack of detailed studies. It is associated with very few side effects although allergic reactions have been reported.

Alverine (Spasmonal)

Adults and children over 12 years of age should take one or two capsules three times a day before food. Like mebeverine, it is not known to interact with other medicines, has no cautions in its use and can be given in pregnancy and whilst breastfeeding. It has no interactions with other medicines and can be used by all patient groups. Rash is the most common side effect, although nausea, headache, dizziness, itching and allergic reactions have been reported.

Peppermint oil (e.g., Colpermin IBS Relief)

Adults and children over 15 years of age can take peppermint oil. The dosage is one capsule three times a day before food, which can be increased to two capsules three times a day in severe symptoms. It often causes heartburn and rarely allergic rashes have been reported. It is safe to use in pregnancy but in theory can decrease breast milk production. It has no drug interactions and can be used by all patient groups.

References

Kruis W, Weinzierl M, Schussler P, et al. Comparison of the therapeutic effect of wheat bran, mebeverine and placebo in patients with the irritable bowel syndrome. Digestion 1986;34:196–201.

Liu JP, Yang M, Liu Y, et al. Herbal medicines for treatment of irritable bowel syndrome. Cochrane Database of Systematic Reviews 2006, Issue 1. Art. No.: CD004116. http://dx.doi.org/10.1002/14651858.CD004116.pub2.

Moayyedi P, Ford AC, Talley NJ, et al. The efficacy of probiotics in the treatment of irritable bowel syndrome: a systematic review. BMJ 2010;59(3):325.

Ruepert L, Quartero AO, de Wit NJ, et al. Bulking agents, antispasmodics and antidepressants for the treatment of irritable bowel syndrome. Cochrane Database of Systematic Reviews 2011, Issue 8. Art. No.: CD003460. http://dx.doi.org/10.1002/14651858.CD003460.pub3.

Webb AN, Kukuruzovic R, Catto-Smith AG, et al. Hypnotherapy for treatment of irritable bowel syndrome. Cochrane Database of Systematic Reviews 2007, Issue 4. Art. No.: CD005110. http://dx.doi.org/10.1002/14651858.CD005110.pub2.

Zijdenbos IL, de Wit NJ, van der Heijden GJ, et al. Psychological treatments for the management of irritable bowel syndrome. Cochrane Database of Systematic Reviews 2009, Issue 1. Art. No.: CD006442. http://dx.doi.org/10.1002/14651858.CD006442.pub2.

Further reading

Agrawal A, Whorwell PJ. Irritable bowel syndrome: diagnosis and management. Br Med J 2006;332:280–3.

Jamieson DJ, Steege JF. The prevalence of dysmenorrhea, dyspareunia, pelvic pain and irritable bowel syndrome in primary care practices. Obstet Gynecol 1996;87:55–8.

Nunan D, Boughtflower J, Roberts NW, et al. Physical activity for treatment of irritable bowel syndrome. Cochrane Database of Systematic Reviews 2015, Issue 1. Art. No.: CD011497. http://dx.doi.org/10.1002/14651858.CD011497.

Poynard T, Regimbeau C, Benhamou Y. Meta-analysis of smooth muscle relaxants in the treatment of irritable bowel syndrome. Aliment Pharmacol Ther 2001;15:355–61.

Ritchie JA, Truelove SC. Treatment of irritable bowel syndrome with lorazepam, hyoscine butylbromide and ispaghula husk. BMJ 1979;1(6160):376–8.

Tudor GJ. A general practice study to compare alverine citrate with mebeverine hydrochloride in the treatment of irritable bowel syndrome. Br J Clin Pract 1986;40:276–8.

Whitehead WE, Crowell MD, Robinson JC, et al. Effects of stressful life events on bowel symptoms: subjects with irritable bowel syndrome compared with subjects without bowel dysfunction. Gut 1992;33:825–30.

Websites

Irritable Bowel Syndrome Self Help and Support Group: http://www.ibsgroup.org

A register of IBS therapists specialising in hypnotherapy can be found at http://www.ibs-register.co.uk

Haemorrhoids

Background

Haemorrhoids (piles) are the most common problem affecting the anorectal region. Patients might feel embarrassed talking about symptoms and it is therefore important that any requests for advice are treated sympathetically and away from others to avoid embarrassment.

Prevalence and epidemiology

The exact prevalence of haemorrhoids is unknown but it is estimated that one in two people will experience at least one episode at some point during their lives. Haemorrhoids can occur at any age but are rare in children and adults under the age of 20. It affects both sexes equally and is more common with increasing age; especially in people between 45 to 65 years of age. There is a high incidence of haemorrhoids in pregnant women.

Aetiology

The cause of haemorrhoids is probably multifactorial with anatomical (degeneration of elastic), physiological (increased anal canal pressure) and mechanical (straining at stool) processes implicated. Haemorrhoids have been traditionally described as engorged veins of the haemorrhoidal plexus. The analogy of varicose veins of the anal canal is often used but is misleading. Current thinking favours the theory of prolapsed anal cushions. Anal cushions maintain fine continence and are submucosal vascular structures suspended in the canal by a connective tissue framework derived from the internal anal sphincter and longitudinal muscle. Within each of the three cushions is a venous plexus that is fed by arteriovenous blood supply. Veins in these cushions fill with blood when sphincters inside them relax and empty when the sphincters contract. Fragmentation of the connective tissue supporting the cushions leads to their descent. The prolapsed anal cushion has impaired venous return, resulting in venous stasis and inflammation of the cushion's epithelium.

Haemorrhoids are classified as either internal or external. This distinction is an anatomical one. Superior to the anal sphincter, there is an area known as the dentate line. At this junction epithelial cells change from squamous to columnar epithelial tissue. Above the dentate line haemorrhoids are classed as internal and below, external. Furthermore internal haemorrhoids are graded according to severity: grade I, do not prolapse out of the anal canal; grade II, prolapse on defecation but reduce spontaneously; grade III, require manual reduction; and grade IV, cannot be reduced.

Arriving at a differential diagnosis

In the first instance most patients with anorectal symptoms will self-diagnose haemorrhoids and often self-treat due to embarrassment about symptoms. Bleeding tends to cause the greatest concern and often instigates the patient to seek help. Invariably, rectal bleeding is of little consequence but should be thoroughly investigated to exclude sinister pathology. A number of haemorrhoid-specific questions should always be asked (Table 7.23).

Clinical features of haemorrhoids

Symptoms experienced by the patient are dependent on the severity or type of haemorrhoid and can include bleeding, perianal itching, mucous discharge and pain. Often patients are asymptomatic until the haemorrhoid prolapses. Any blood associated is bright red and is most commonly seen as spotting around the toilet pan, streaking on toilet tissue or visible on the surface of the stool. Symptoms are often intermittent and each episode usually lasts from a few days to a few weeks.

	Table 7.23
	Specific questions to ask the patient: Haemorrhoids
Question	**Relevance**
Duration	Patients with haemorrhoids tend to have had symptoms for some time before requesting advice. However, patients with symptoms that have been constantly present for more 3 weeks should be referred
Pain	Pain, if experienced, with haemorrhoids tends to occur on defecation. It can occur at other times, for example when sitting. Pain is usually described as a dull ache
	Sharp or stabbing pain at the time of defecation can suggest an anal fissure or tear
Rectal bleeding	Slight rectal bleeding is often associated with haemorrhoids. Blood appears bright red and might be visible in the toilet bowl or on the surface of the stool. The presence of blood is usually a direct referral sign but if the cause is haemorrhoids this could be treated unless the patient is unduly anxious in which case referral is appropriate
	Blood mixed in the stool has to be referred to eliminate a GI bleed
	Large volumes of blood or blood loss not associated with defecation must be referred to eliminate possible carcinoma
Associated symptoms	Symptoms associated with haemorrhoids are usually localised, for example anal itching. Other symptoms such as nausea, vomiting, loss of appetite and altered bowel habit should be viewed with caution and underlying pathology suspected. Referral would be needed
Diet	A lack of dietary fibre that leads to constipation is a contributory factor to haemorrhoids. The passage of hard stools and straining during defecation can cause haemorrhoids. Find out about the patient's diet and current bowel habits

Internal haemorrhoids are rarely painful, whereas external haemorrhoids can cause pain due to the cushion becoming thrombosed. Pain is described as a dull ache that increases in severity when the patient defecates, leading to patients ignoring the urge to defecate. This can then lead to constipation, which in turn will lead to more difficulty in passing stools and further increase the pain associated with defecation.

Conditions to eliminate

Dermatitis–related conditions

Localised anal itching can result from dermatitis or even threadworm infection. If pruritus is the major presenting symptom, then the most likely cause is contact dermatitis often caused by toiletries.

Medication

As constipation is a contributory factor in the manifestation of haemorrhoids, those medicines that are prone to causing constipation should, if possible, be avoided. Table 7.19 lists those medicines that are commonly known to cause constipation.

Conditions causing rectal bleeding

A number of conditions can present with varying degrees of rectal bleeding. However, other symptoms should be present which will allow them to be excluded.

Anal fissure

Anal fissures are common, with the 20- to 30-year-old age group most affected. Symptoms often follow a period of constipation and are normally caused by straining at stool. Pain, which can be severe, is always experienced on defecation and pain can last for a number of hours after defecation. Bright red blood is commonly seen. Non-urgent referral is necessary for confirmation of the diagnosis. In the meantime the patient should be instructed to eat more fibre and increase their fluid intake.

Ulcerative colitis and Crohn's disease

Other symptoms besides blood in the stool are usually present with ulcerative colitis and Crohn's disease. These symptoms tend to be as follows: stools that are watery, abdominal pain in the lower left quadrant, weight loss and fever. Patients will appear unwell and also find that they have urgency, nocturnal diarrhoea and early morning rushes. In the acute phase patients will have malaise.

Upper GI bleeds

Erosion of the stomach wall or upper intestine is normally responsible for GI bleeds and is often associated with NSAID intake. The colour of the stool is related to the rate of bleeding. Stools from GI bleeds can be tarry (indicating a bleed of 100–200 mL of blood) or black (indicating a bleed of 400–500 mL of blood). Urgent referral is needed.

Colorectal cancer

Approximately 40,000 new cases of colorectal cancer are registered each year in the UK and represent the second most common cause of cancer death in the UK. Occurrence is strongly related to age, with almost three-quarters of cases occurring in people aged 65 or over. It is characterised by rectal bleeding, a change in bowel habit and tenesmus. Rectal bleeding tends to be persistent and steady though slight for all tumours. Colorectal bleeds depend on the site of the tumour, for example, sigmoid tumours lead to bright red blood in or around the stool. Any patient over 40 years of age with persistent rectal bleeding and a change of bowel habit must be urgently referred. If over 60 years of age, then persistent rectal bleeding alone is sufficient to refer. NICE have produced referral guidelines for doctors for suspected cases of colorectal cancer (https://www.nice.org.uk/guidance/cg131?unlid=692190992016215111223).

Fig. 7.14 will aid the differentiation of haemorrhoids.

> ⓘ **TRIGGER POINTS indicative of referral: Haemorrhoids**
>
> | Symptoms/signs | Possible danger/reason for referral |
> | --- | --- |
> | Persistent change in bowel habit in patients over 40 years of age Unexplained rectal bleeding | Sinister pathology? |
> | Patients who have to reduce their haemorrhoids manually | OTC treatment will not help |
> | Severe pain associated with defecation | Anal fissure? |
> | Blood mixed in the stool Fever | Suspect GI bleeds or inflammatory bowel disease |

Evidence base for over-the-counter medication

Diet

Reviews by Alonso-Coelle et al. (2005, 2006) have concluded that general measures to prevent constipation will help decrease straining during defecation, ease the symptoms of haemorrhoids and reduce recurrence. Patients should therefore be asked about their normal diet to determine fibre intake. Those with diets low in fibre should be encouraged to increase their fibre and fluid intake, as this will help produce softer stools and reduce constipation. Patients should try to eat more fruit, vegetables, bran and wholemeal bread. If this is not possible, then fibre supplementation with a bulk-forming laxative could be recommended. Bulk-forming laxatives will take 2 to 3 days to relieve constipation and may take up to 6 weeks to improve symptoms of haemorrhoids.

Pharmacological intervention

Numerous products are marketed for the relief and treatment of haemorrhoids. These include a wide range of therapeutic agents and commonly include anaesthetics, astringents, anti-inflammatories and protectorants. Most products contain a combination of these agents.

The inclusion of such a diverse range of chemical entities appears to be based largely on theoretical grounds rather than any evidence base. Extensive literature searching found only one published trial regarding the efficacy of any marketed product (Ledward, 1980); however, this trial suffered from serious methodological flaws.

Anaesthetics (lidocaine, benzocaine and cinchocaine)

No trials appear to have been conducted using local anaesthetics in the treatment and relief of symptoms for haemorrhoids. However, anaesthetics have proven efficacy when used on other mucosal surfaces; their use could therefore be justifiably recommended. Their action is short lived and will produce temporary relief from perianal itching and pain. They require frequent application and might therefore cause skin sensitisation.

Astringents (allantoin, bismuth, zinc, Peru balsam)

Astringents are included in haemorrhoid preparations on the theoretical basis that they precipitate surface proteins thus producing a protective coat over the haemorrhoid. There appears to be no evidence to support this theory. Certain proprietary products only contain astringents and at best will provide a placebo effect.

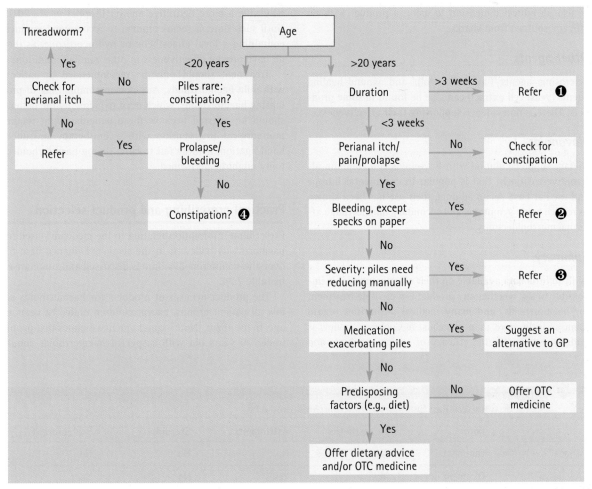

Fig. 7.14 Primer for differential diagnosis of haemorrhoids.

❶ Duration
Patients with long-standing symptoms that have not been seen previously by the GP should be referred to eliminate any underlying pathology. In the vast majority of cases no sinister findings will result.

❷ Rectal bleeding
In the majority of cases rectal bleeding is a sign of referral. However, in cases where sinister pathology has been excluded and only mild local bleeding has occurred, the pharmacist could instigate treatment.

❸ Severity
Medication is unlikely to help any patient who has to manually reduce haemorrhoids. Referral for other treatments is recommended.

❹ Constipation
See Fig. 7.12.

Anti-inflammatory drugs (hydrocortisone)

Steroids have proven effectiveness in reducing inflammation and would therefore be useful in reducing haemorrhoidal swelling; however, trials with OTC products containing hydrocortisone appear not to have taken place.

Protectorants (e.g., shark liver oil)

Protectorants are claimed to provide a protective coating over the skin and thus produce temporary relief from pain and perianal itch. These claims cannot be substantiated and as with astringents any benefit conveyed by a protectorant is probably a placebo effect. In addition, there is also an ethical dimension to using a product with no efficacy sourced from sharks.

Other agents

Sclerosing agents (lauromacrogol), and wound-healing agents (yeast cell extract) can also be found in some products. There is no evidence supporting their effectiveness.

Flavonoids

Dietary supplementation with flavonoids is a common alternative treatment that is popular in continental Europe and the Far East. As an adjunct, their use has been shown to reduce acute symptoms and secondary haemorrhage after haemorrhoidectomy.

Summary

With so little data available on their effectiveness, it is impossible to say whether any product is a credible treatment for haemorrhoids, and many medical authorities regard them as little more than placebos. A Cochrane review is underway to assess the efficacy of topical products and

may give a more definitive answer (Kopljar et al., 2011). Until such time, it seems prudent to recommend products containing a local anaesthetic or hydrocortisone, as they do have proven effectiveness in other similar conditions.

Treatment should only be recommended to patients with mild haemorrhoids. Any person complaining of prolapsing haemorrhoids, which need reducing by the patient, should be referred because these patients might require non-surgical intervention with sclerotherapy or rubber band ligation. If these fail to cure, then a haemorrhoidectomy might be performed.

Practical prescribing and product selection

Prescribing information relating to the medicines used for haemorrhoids reviewed in the section 'Evidence base for over-the-counter medication' is discussed and summarised in Table 7.24.

The product licenses of products for haemorrhoids allow all patient groups, except children under 12 years of age, to use them. (Note – good practice dictates that people under 20 years old with suspected haemorrhoids should

Table 7.24
Practical prescribing: Summary of haemorrhoid products

	Form	Anaesthetics	Astringents	Steroids	Protectorant
Anacal*	Ointment	No	No	No	No
Anodesyn	Ointment or suppository	Yes	Yes	No	No
Anusol	Cream, ointment or suppository	No	Yes	No	No
Anusol Plus HC; Anusol Soothing Relief	Ointment or suppository	No	Yes	Yes	No
Germoloids	Cream, ointment or suppository	Yes	Yes	No	No
Germoloids HC	Spray	Yes	No	Yes	No
Hemocane	Cream	Yes	No	No	No
Perinal	Spray	Yes	No	Yes	No
Preparation H**	Ointment	No	No	No	Yes
Preparation H	Gel	No	Yes	No	No

*contains a sclerosing agent.
** contains yeast cell extract.

7

be referred.) They do not interact with any other medicines and can be used in pregnancy and breastfeeding. The standard dose for any formulation is twice daily, plus application after each bowel movement. Minimal side effects have been reported and are usually limited to slight irritation. Products that contain hydrocortisone are subject to several licensing restrictions: they are restricted to use in patients over a certain age (Perinal spray 14 years, Germoloids spray 16 years and Anusol range18 years); no longer than a week's duration and not for use in pregnant or lactating women.

References

Alonso-Coello P, Guyatt GH, Heels-Ansdell D, et al. Laxatives for the treatment of hemorrhoids. Cochrane Database of Systematic Reviews 2005, Issue 4. Art. No.: CD004649. http://dx.doi.org/10.1002/14651858. CD004649.pub2.

Alonso-Coello P, Mills E, Heels-Ansdell D, et al. Fiber for the treatment of hemorrhoids complications: a systematic review and meta-analysis. Am J Gastroenterol 2006;101:181–8.

Alonso-Coello P, Zhou Q, Martinez-Zapeta MJ, et al. Meta-analysis of flavonoids for the treatment of haemorrhoids. Br J Surg 2006;93(8):909–20.

Ledward RS. The management of puerperal haemorrhoids: A double blind clinical trial of Anacal rectal ointment. The Practitioner 1980;224:660–1.

Further reading

Nisar PJ, Scholefield JH. Managing haemorrhoids. Br Med J2003:327;847–51.

Sneider EB, Maykel JA. Diagnosis and management of symptomatic hemorrhoids. Surg Clin North Am2010;90(1):17–32.

Abdominal pain

Background

Abdominal pain is a symptom of many different conditions, ranging from acute self-limiting problems to life-threatening conditions such as ruptured appendicitis and bowel obstruction. However, the overwhelming majority of cases will be of a non-serious nature, self-limiting and not require medical referral. The most common conditions that present to community pharmacies are dyspepsia affecting the upper abdomen, primary dysmenorrhoea and IBS affecting the lower abdomen. These are covered in more detail on pages 165 and 187. However, other conditions will present with abdominal pain (Table 7.25), and these are more thoroughly covered in this section. This book takes a 'four quadrant' approach to describing the location of signs and symptoms (Fig. 7.15).

Prevalence and epidemiology

The prevalence and epidemiology of abdominal pain within the population is determined by those conditions that cause it. As so many conditions can give rise to abdominal pain, it is likely that the majority of the population will, at some point, suffer from abdominal pain. For example, one study found that 40% of the UK population had suffered from dyspepsia during the previous 12 months and gastroenteritis, which is associated with abdominal pain, is extremely common.

Aetiology

Abdominal pain does not only arise from the GI tract but also from the cardiovascular and musculoskeletal system. Therefore the aetiology of abdominal pain is dependent on its cause. GI

Table 7.25
Causes of abdominal pain

Probability	Cause		
	Upper abdomen	Lower abdomen	Diffuse
Most likely	Dyspepsia	Irritable bowel syndrome, primary dysmenorrhoea	Gastroenteritis
Likely	Peptic ulcers	Diverticulitis (elderly)	Not applicable
Unlikely	Cholecystitis, cholelithiasis, renal colic	Appendicitis, endometriosis, renal colic	Not applicable
Very unlikely	Splenic enlargement, hepatitis, myocardial infarction	Ectopic pregnancy, salpingitis, intestinal obstruction	Pancreatitis, peritonitis

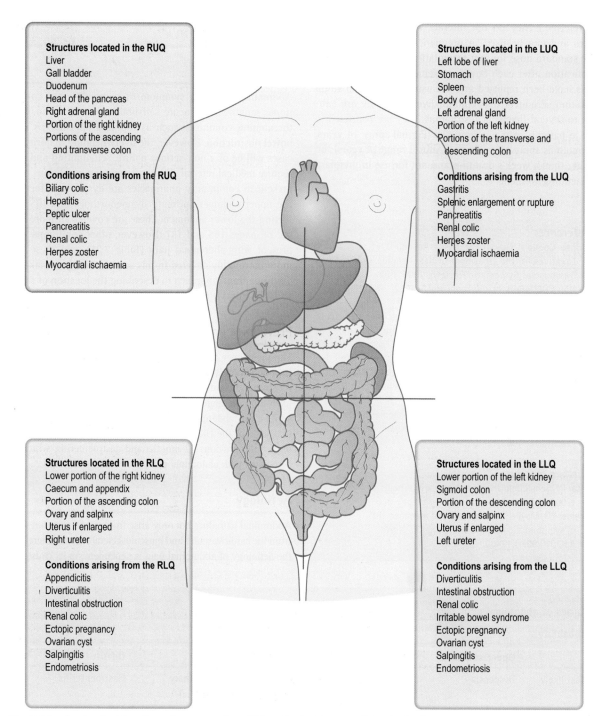

Structures located in the RUQ
Liver
Gall bladder
Duodenum
Head of the pancreas
Right adrenal gland
Portion of the right kidney
Portions of the ascending
  and transverse colon

Conditions arising from the RUQ
Biliary colic
Hepatitis
Peptic ulcer
Pancreatitis
Renal colic
Herpes zoster
Myocardial ischaemia

Structures located in the LUQ
Left lobe of liver
Stomach
Spleen
Body of the pancreas
Left adrenal gland
Portion of the left kidney
Portions of the transverse and
  descending colon

Conditions arising from the LUQ
Gastritis
Splenic enlargement or rupture
Pancreatitis
Renal colic
Herpes zoster
Myocardial ischaemia

Structures located in the RLQ
Lower portion of the right kidney
Caecum and appendix
Portion of the ascending colon
Ovary and salpinx
Uterus if enlarged
Right ureter

Conditions arising from the RLQ
Appendicitis
Diverticulitis
Intestinal obstruction
Renal colic
Ectopic pregnancy
Ovarian cyst
Salpingitis
Endometriosis

Structures located in the LLQ
Lower portion of the left kidney
Sigmoid colon
Portion of the descending colon
Ovary and salpinx
Uterus if enlarged
Left ureter

Conditions arising from the LLQ
Diverticulitis
Intestinal obstruction
Renal colic
Irritable bowel syndrome
Ectopic pregnancy
Ovarian cyst
Salpingitis
Endometriosis

Fig. 7.15   Anatomical location of organs and conditions that can cause abdominal pain.

tract causes include poor muscle tone leading to reflux (e.g., lower oesophageal sphincter incompetence), infections that cause peptic ulcers (from *H. pylori*) and mechanical blockages causing renal and biliary colic. Cardiovascular causes include angina and myocardial infarction whereas musculoskeletal problems often involve tearing of abdominal muscles.

Arriving at a differential diagnosis

The main role of the community pharmacist is to identify symptoms in patients that suggest more serious pathology so that patients can be further evaluated. This is not easy, as many abdominal conditions do not present with classic textbook symptoms, and patients tend to present to the pharmacist early in the course of the disease, often before the presenting symptoms have assumed the more usual textbook description. The low prevalence of serious disease and overlapping symptoms with minor illness makes the task even more difficult. Single symptoms are poor predictors of final diagnosis (except for reflux oesophagitis, in which the presence of heartburn is highly suggestive). It is therefore important to look for 'symptom clusters' and to use knowledge of the incidence and prevalence of conditions to determine whether referral is needed. This necessitates taking a very careful history and not relying on a single symptom to label a patient with a particular problem. Specific questions relating to abdominal pain should be asked (Table 7.26).

Table 7.26
Specific questions to ask the patient: Abdominal pain

Question	Relevance
Location of pain	Knowing the anatomical location of abdominal structures is extremely helpful in differential diagnosis of abdominal pain (see Fig. 7.13)
Presence only of abdominal pain/discomfort	In general, patients without other symptoms rarely have serious pathology. The symptoms are usually self-limiting and often no cause can be determined
Nature of the pain	Heartburn is classically associated with a retrosternal burning sensation Cramp-like pain is seen in diverticulitis, IBS, salpingitis and gastroenteritis Colicky pain (pain that comes and goes) has been used to describe the pain of appendicitis, biliary and renal colic and intestinal obstruction Gnawing pain is associated with pancreatitis and pancreatic cancer and boring pain with ulceration
Radiating pain	Abdominal pain that moves from its original site should be viewed with caution Pain that radiates to the jaw, face and arm could be cardiovascular in origin Pain that moves from a central location to the right lower quadrant could suggest appendicitis Pain radiating to the back may suggest peptic ulcer or pancreatitis
Severity of pain	Non-serious causes of abdominal pain generally do not give rise to severe pain. Pain scores should be used to try and quantify severity. For example 0 indicates no pain and 10 the worst pain imaginable. Scores higher than 6 suggest a high degree of pain and need to be referred
Age of patient	With increasing age, abdominal pain is more likely to have an identifiable and serious organic cause. Appendicitis is the only serious abdominal condition that is much more common in young patients
Onset & duration	In general, if no identifiable cause can be found, abdominal pain with sudden onset is generally a symptom of more serious conditions. For example, peritonitis, appendicitis, ectopic pregnancy, renal and biliary colic Pain that lasts more than 6 hours is suggestive of underlying pathology
Aggravating or ameliorating factors	Biliary colic can be aggravated by fatty foods Vomiting tends to relieve pain in gastric ulcers Pain in duodenal ulcer is relieved after ingestion of food Pain in salpingitis and appendicitis are often made worse by movement
Associated symptoms	Vomiting, weight loss, melaena, altered bowel habit and haematemesis are all symptoms that suggest more serious pathology and require referral

Conditions affecting the upper abdomen

Left upper quadrant pain

Dyspepsia/gastritis

Patients with dyspepsia present with a range of symptoms that commonly involve vague abdominal discomfort (aching) above the umbilicus (Fig. 7.16) associated with belching, bloating, flatulence, feeling of fullness and heartburn. It is normally relieved by antacids and aggravated by spicy foods or excessive caffeine. Vomiting is unusual. For further information on dyspepsia see page 165.

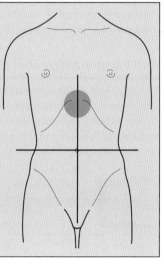

Fig. 7.16 The position of pain in gastritis and dyspepsia.

Splenic enlargement or rupture

If the spleen is enlarged, generalised left upper quadrant pain associated with abdominal fullness and early feeding satiety is observed (Fig. 7.17). Referred pain to the left shoulder is sometimes seen. The condition is rare and is nearly always secondary to another primary cause, which might be an infection, a result of inflammation or haematological in origin.

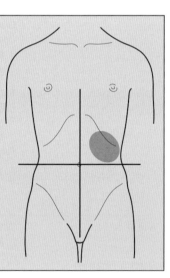

Fig. 7.17 The position of pain associated with splenic enlargement.

7

Right upper quadrant pain

Acute cholecystitis and cholelithiasis

Cholelithiasis (presence of gall stones in the bile ducts, also called biliary colic) is the more common presentation. (Fig. 7.18) Typically, the pain lasts for more than 30 minutes, but less than 8 hours, is colicky in nature and often severe. Nausea and vomiting are often present. Classically, the onset is sudden, starts a few hours after a meal and frequently awakens the patient in the early hours of the morning. In acute cholecystitis (inflammation of the gall bladder) symptoms are similar but also associated with fever and abdominal tenderness. The pain may radiate to the tip of the right scapula. The incidence of both increases with increasing age and is most common in people aged over 50. It is also more prevalent in women than in men.

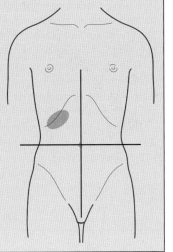

Fig. 7.18   The position of pain associated with acute cholecystitis and cholelithiasis.

Hepatitis

Liver enlargement from any type of hepatitis will cause discomfort or dull pain around the right rib cage (Fig. 7.19). Associated early symptoms are general malaise, tiredness, skin rash (pruritus) and nausea. On examination there is normally hepatic tenderness.

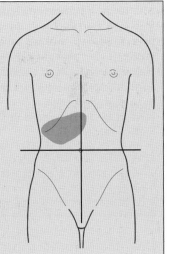

Fig. 7.19   The position of pain associated with hepatitis.

Ulcers

Ulcers are classed as either gastric or duodenal. They occur most commonly in patients aged 30 to 50 years old and are more common in men than in women. Symptoms are variable but typically the patient will have localised mid-epigastric pain (Fig. 7.20) described as 'constant', 'annoying' or 'gnawing/boring'.

With gastric ulcers, symptoms are inconsistent but the pain usually comes on whenever the stomach is empty – usually 15 to 30 minutes after eating – and is generally relieved by antacids or food and aggravated by alcohol and caffeine. NSAID use is associated with a three- to fourfold increase in gastric ulcers.

Duodenal ulcers tend to be more consistent in symptom presentation. Pain occurs 2 to 3 hours after eating, and pain that awakens a person at night is highly suggestive of duodenal ulcer.

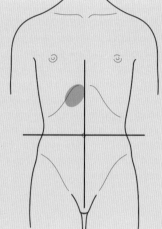

Fig. 7.20 The position of pain associated with ulcers.

Pain affecting both right and left upper quadrants

Acute pancreatitis

Pain of pancreatitis develops suddenly and is described as agonising and constant with the pain being centrally located (epigastric) that often radiates into the back (Fig. 7.21). Pain reaches its maximum intensity within minutes and can last hours or days. Vomiting is common but does not relieve the pain. Early in the attack patients might get relief from the pain by sitting forwards. It is commonly seen in those that misuse alcohol (25% of cases) or suffer from gallstones (50% of cases). Patients are very unlikely to present in a community pharmacy due to the severity of the pain but a mild attack could present with steady epigastric pain that is sometimes centred close to the umbilicus and can be difficult to distinguish between other causes of upper quadrant pain.

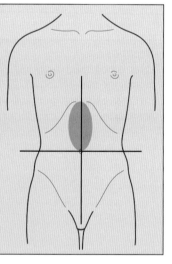

Fig. 7.21 The position of pain associated with pancreatitis.

Renal colic

Urinary calculi (stones) can occur anywhere in the urinary tract, although most frequently stones get lodged in the ureter. Pain begins in the loin, radiating around the flank into the groin and sometimes down the inner side of the thigh (Fig. 7.22). Pain is very severe and colicky in nature. Attacks are spasmodic and tend to last minutes to hours and often leave the person prostrate with pain. The person is restless and cannot lie still. Symptoms of nausea and vomiting might also be present. It is twice as common in men than in women and usually occurs between the ages of 40 and 60 years old.

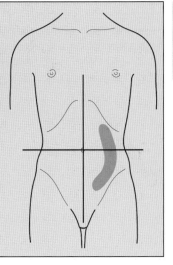

Fig. 7.22 The position of pain in renal colic.

Myocardial ischaemia

Angina and myocardial infarction (MI) cause chest pain that can be difficult to distinguish initially from epigastric/retrosternal pain caused by dyspepsia (Fig. 7.23). However, pain of cardiovascular origin often radiates to the neck, jaw and inner aspect of the left arm. Typically, angina pain is precipitated by exertion and subsides after a few minutes once at rest. Pain associated with MI will present with characteristic deep crushing pain. The patient will appear pale, display weakness and be tachycardic. Cardiovascular pain should respond to sublingual glyceryl trinitrate therapy.

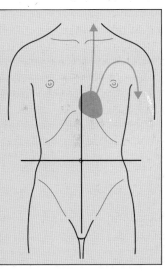

Fig. 7.23 The position of pain associated with myocardial ischaemia.

Herpes zoster (shingles)

Pain associated with herpes zoster typically occurs once the rash has erupted, although symptoms can precede the rash by several days. Pain that precedes the rash and is right sided can be confused with appendicitis (Fig. 7.24).

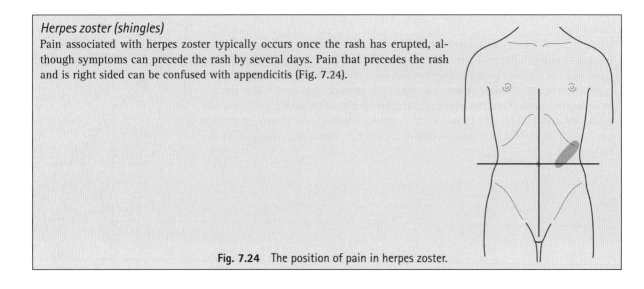

Fig. 7.24 The position of pain in herpes zoster.

Conditions affecting the lower abdomen

The most common causes of lower abdominal pain are muscle strains, IBS, appendicitis and dysmenorrhoea in women. Apart from appendicitis, all these conditions can present in either quadrant.

Irritable bowel syndrome

Pain is most often observed in the left lower quadrant (Fig. 7.25); however, the discomfort can be vague and diffuse and about one-third of patients exhibit upper abdominal pain. The pain is described as 'cramp-like' and is recurrent. Alternating diarrhoea and constipation and mucous coating the stools is also often present. For further information on IBS see page 187.

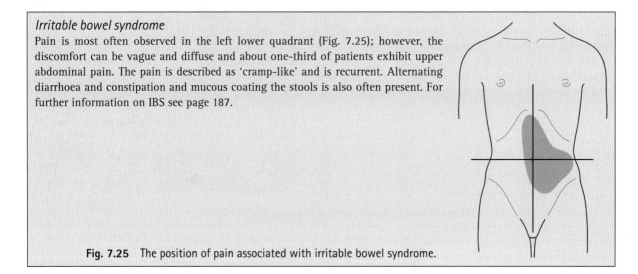

Fig. 7.25 The position of pain associated with irritable bowel syndrome.

Diverticulitis

The incidence of diverticulitis increases with increasing age. It is most prevalent in the elderly and is characterised by constant pain and local tenderness with associated fever. Pain is more commonly seen in the left lower quadrant (Fig. 7.26) but can be suprapubic and occasionally located in the right lower quadrant. Pain tends to be cramp-like in nature. Altered bowel habit is usual with diarrhoea more common than constipation.

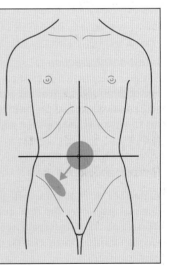

Fig. 7.26 The position of pain associated with diverticulitis.

Appendicitis

Classically, the pain starts in the mid-abdomen region, around the umbilicus, before migrating to the right lower quadrant after a few hours (Fig. 7.27), although right-sided pain is experienced from the outset in about 50% of patients. The pain of appendicitis is described as colicky or cramp-like but after a few hours becomes constant. Movement tends to aggravate the pain and vomiting might also be present. Appendicitis is most common in young adults, especially in young men.

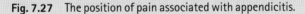

Fig. 7.27 The position of pain associated with appendicitis.

Conditions affecting women (other than period pain)

Generalised lower abdominal pain (Fig. 7.28) can be experienced in a number of gynaecological conditions:

- Ectopic pregnancy: these are usually experienced between weeks 5 and 14 of the pregnancy. Patients suffer from persistent moderate to severe pain that is sudden in onset. Referred pain to the tip of the scapula is possible. Most patients (80%) experience bleeding that ranges from spotting to the equivalent of a menstrual period. Diarrhoea and vomiting is often also present.
- Salpingitis (inflammation of the fallopian tubes): occurs predominantly in young, sexually active women, especially those fitted with an IUD. Pain is usually bi-lateral, low and cramping. Pain starts shortly after menstruation and can worsen with movement. Malaise and fever are common.
- Endometriosis: patients experience lower abdominal aching pain that usually starts 5 to 7 days before menstruation begins and can be constant and severe. The pain often worsens at the onset of menstruation. Referred pain into the back and down the thighs is also possible.

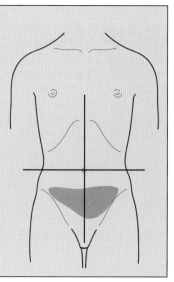

Fig. 7.28 The position of pain associated with women's conditions.

Intestinal obstruction

Intestinal obstruction is most prevalent in people over the age of 50. It has sudden and acute onset. The pain is described as colicky and can be experienced anywhere in the lower abdomen. Constipation and vomiting are prominent features.

Diffuse abdominal pain

A number of conditions will present with diffuse abdominal pain over the four quadrants. The most common cause of diffuse pain seen by the pharmacist is gastroenteritis. Other causes include peritonitis (and pancreatitis).

Gastroenteritis

Other symptoms of nausea, vomiting and diarrhoea will be more prominent in gastroenteritis than abdominal pain. The patient might also have a fever and suffer from general malaise.

Peritonitis

Severe pain in the upper abdomen is present. This is accompanied by intense rigidity of the abdominal wall producing a 'board like' appearance; fever and vomiting might also be present. Urgent referral is required due to associated complications.

Fig. 7.29 will aid in the differentiation of the different types of abdominal pain.

> **! TRIGGER POINTS indicative of referral: Abdominal pain**
>
> | Symptoms/signs | Possible danger/reason for referral |
> | --- | --- |
> | Abdominal pain with fever | Suggests potential diverticulitis, peritonitis, biliary colic or salpingitis |
> | Pregnancy or suspected pregnancy | Eliminate pain relating to pregnancy or ectopic pregnancy |
> | Abdominal pain associated with trauma | May indicate damage to organs |
> | Severe pain or pain that radiates | Suggests more sinister causes such as potential myocardial infarction or significant inflammation of the GI tract |
> | Elderly | Diverticulitis and obstruction more common |
> | Vomiting | Suggests conditions such as peritonitis, pancreatitis, appendicitis or renal or biliary colic |

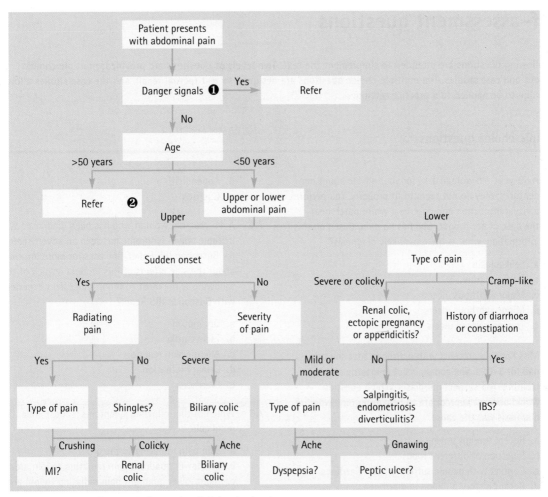

Fig. 7.29 Primer for differential diagnosis of abdominal pain.

❶ Danger signals are vomiting and fever.

❷ Organic disease is more likely to be the cause of abdominal pain in patients over 50 years of age, especially if symptoms are new or more severe than normal.

Evidence base for over-the-counter medication and practical prescribing and product selection

The three conditions that have abdominal pain/discomfort as one of the major presenting symptoms and can be treated OTC are dyspepsia, IBS and dysmenorrhoea. For further information on products used to treat these conditions, please refer to pages 132, 165 and 187.

Further reading
Bagshaw EJ. Abdominal pain protocol: right upper quadrant pain. Lippincotts Prim Care Pract 1999;3:486–92.
Guthrie E, Thompson D. Abdominal pain and functional gastrointestinal disorders. Br Med J 2002;325:701–3.
Kalloo AN, Kantsevoy SV. Gallstones and biliary disease. Prim Care 2001;28:591–606.

Lucenti MJ, Nadel ES, Brown DF. Right lower quadrant pain. J Emerg Med 2001;21:431–4.
Miller SK, Alpert PT. Assessment and differential diagnosis of abdominal pain. Nurse Pract 2006 Jul;31(7):38–45, 47.

Websites
The Pancreatitis Supporters' Network: http://www.pancreatitis.org.uk/

Self-assessment questions

The following questions are intended to supplement the text. Two levels of questions are provided: multiple choice questions and case studies. The multiple choice questions are designed to test factual recall, and the case studies allow knowledge to be applied to a practice setting.

Multiple choice questions

7.1 A 69-year-old woman asks for your advice about her dentures; they do not seem to fit properly. You perform a visual inspection and observe a white patch near the base of her tongue. She has no pain. Based on this information, what is the most likely diagnosis?

 a. Leukoplakia
 b. Lichen planus
 c. Major aphthous ulcers
 d. Minor aphthous ulcers
 e. Trauma-related ulcers

7.2 Miss Kandola presents with diarrhoea that she has had for 3 days. She complains of epigastric pain and bloating. You suspect giardiasis. Which question would be most appropriate to help determine whether giardiasis was the cause?

 a. Recent foreign travel
 b. Ingestion of different food
 c. Contact with people suffering from diarrhoea
 d. Recent history of blood in diarrhoea
 e. Diarrhoea in the early morning

7.3 Mr Mole, aged 48 years, wants something for indigestion. He has generalised epigastric pain but no other symptoms. He takes no medication but is borderline hypertensive. Which product would be the most suitable choice to relieve his symptoms?

 a. Ranitidine
 b. Omeprazole
 c. Calcium carbonate
 d. Aluminium hydroxide
 e. Magnesium trisilicate mixture

7.4 An adult patient presents with symptoms of abdominal pain and discomfort in the epigastric area. Based on the location of the symptoms, which of the following conditions is the least likely cause?

 a. Oesophagitis
 b. Duodenal ulcer
 c. Gastric ulcer

 d. Appendicitis
 e. Gastritis

7.5 A 41-year-old woman who has been diagnosed with irritable bowel syndrome has seen an advertisement for Buscopan IBS Relief. She asks for more information about the side effects of this product. Which of the following is the most common side effect experienced with Buscopan IBS Relief?

 a. Dry mouth
 b. Tachycardia
 c. Allergic skin reaction
 d. Urinary retention
 e. Diarrhoea

7.6 Which of the following symptoms is most indicative of renal colic?

 a. Loin pain radiating to the groin
 b. Left lower quadrant pain radiating to loin area
 c. Right lower quadrant pain radiating to loin area
 d. Back pain radiating to loin area
 e. Localised loin pain only

7.7 Which of the following patient groups are most likely to suffer from oral thrush?

 a. Denture wearers
 b. Well-controlled diabetics
 c. Middle-aged adults
 d. Young children
 e. Asthmatics using low dose corticosteroids

7.8 Mr Singh asks for an indigestion remedy. He says he has been getting discomfort (points towards the area in the mid chest) over the last few days. He has not noticed any other symptoms apart from a bit of wind. What would be the most likely diagnosis?

 a. Reflux
 b. Gastric ulcer
 c. Duodenal ulcer
 d. Angina
 e. Irritable bowel syndrome

Questions 7.9 to 7.14 concern the following conditions:

A. Irritable bowel syndrome
B. Giardiasis
C. Pyelonephritis
D. Haemorrhoids
E. Reflux
F. Ulcerative colitis
G. Constipation
H. Appendicitis
I. Dyspepsia
J. Diarrhoea

Select, from A to J, which of the above is most associated with the following statements:

7.9 Nocturnal diarrhoea is sometimes seen

7.10 Tenderness is felt in the loin area

7.11 Is associated with epigastric pain

7.12 Is associated with right lower quadrant pain

7.13 Is associated with left lower quadrant pain

7.14 Pain usually starts centrally then moves to the right lower quadrant

Questions 7.15 to 7.17: for each of these questions *one or more* of the responses is (are) correct. Decide which of the responses is (are) correct. Then choose:

A. If a, b and c are correct
B. If a and b only are correct
C. If b and c only are correct
D. If a only is correct
E. If c only is correct

Directions summarised

A	B	C	D	E
a, b and c	a and b only	b and c only	a only	c only

7.15 Gingivitis is most commonly associated with:

a. Swelling of the gums
b. Gums that bleed easily with trauma
c. Halitosis

7.16 Which of the following symptoms would indicate the need for direct referral to the general practitioner in a patient seeking advice for nausea and gastrointestinal upset?

a. Feeling of impending vomiting

b. Loss of appetite over the last 24 hours
c. Dark-coloured vomit

7.17 A common presentation of minor aphthous ulcers is:

a. Pain
b. Ulcers on the buccal mucosa and tongue
c. Crops of between 1 and 5

Questions 7.18 to 7.20: these questions consist of a statement in the left-hand column, followed by a statement in the right-hand column. You need to:

● decide whether the first statement is true or false
● decide whether the second statement is true or false

Then choose:

A. If both statements are true, and the second statement is a correct explanation of the first statement
B. If both statements are true, but the second statement is NOT a correct explanation of the first statement
C. If the first statement is true, but the second statement is false
D. If the first statement is false, but the second statement is true
E. If both statements are false

Directions summarised

	1st statement	2nd statement	
A	True	True	2nd explanation is a correct explanation of the first
B	True	True	2nd statement is not a correct explanation of the first
C	True	False	
D	False	True	
E	False	False	

	First statement	*Second statement*
7.18	Anal fissures cause pain	Pain on defecation causes patients to suppress defactory reflex
7.19	Diverticulitis is associated with fever	It is more common in young adults
7.20	Constipation is a prominent symptom in hypothyroidism	Sedentary lifestyle due to fatigue is the cause of constipation

Case study

Mrs SJ, a 28-year-old woman, asks to speak to the pharmacist because she wants something for her stomach ache. You find out that the pain is located in the lower and upper left quadrant, but mainly the upper quadrant.

a. From which conditions might she be suffering?

Reflux, non-ulcer dyspepsia, gastritis, primary dysmenorrhoea, endometriosis, irritable bowel syndrome, pancreatitis, renal colic, MI and herpes zoster.

Further questioning reveals Mrs SJ to be suffering with pain she describes as 'an ache'.

b. Name the likely conditions from which she could be suffering?

The use of the word 'ache' means you can rule out those conditions that present with severe, stabbing, burning or gnawing pain:

- *pancreatitis, renal colic: severe*
- *reflux: burning*
- *herpes zoster: severe, lancing*

But it could still be any of these: non-ulcer dyspepsia, gastritis, primary dysmenorrhoea, irritable bowel syndrome, endometriosis and MI.

However, as the pain is primarily upper quadrant, this makes primary dysmenorrhoea, endometriosis and irritable bowel syndrome less likely.

This leaves non-ulcer dyspepsia, gastritis and MI as possibilities.

c. Which questions would now allow you to differentiate between these conditions?

MI is the most unlikely of the three conditions and one would expect the patient to have more severe symptoms. Questions asking about radiation of pain, previous history of similar symptoms and precipitating/relieving factors should be asked.

You reach the differential diagnosis of non-ulcer dyspepsia but before you make any recommendations, you ask if she takes any medication from the GP, her response is as follows:

- *Paracetamol prn: She has taken this for 6 months for knee pain*
- *Atorvastatin 40 mg od: She has taken for the last 3 years for familial hyperlipidaemia*
- *Naproxen 500 mg bd prn: She has taken this for 6 months for knee pain*

d. Which of these medications, if any, do you consider are contributing to Mrs SJ's pain? Explain your rationale.

Of the three medicines that Mrs SJ is taking, the one most likely to cause GI irritation is naproxen. However, she has been taking this for the last 6 months and you would expect that dyspepsia symptoms would have been experienced already if she was going to have a reaction to naproxen. It is then unlikely that naproxen has caused the problem, unless the dose has recently been changed. Atorvastatin can also cause GI side effects but has been taken for the last 3 years and is therefore almost certainly not the cause of the symptoms. Paracetamol is not known to cause GI irritation so can also be ruled out. In conclusion it is likely that none of the medicines have caused Mrs SJ's symptoms.

CASE STUDY 7.2

Mr LR, a male patient (approximately 50 years old), presents to the pharmacy at lunch time asking for something for diarrhoea. The following questions are asked, and responses received.

Information gathering	Data generated
Describe symptoms	Going to the toilet 3 or 4 times a day. Normal habit is once or twice.
Nature of movements	Very watery
Duration	4 or 5 days
Other symptoms	Generally feels a bit rough. Headache and has a temperature. Been getting some cramping pains
Blood noticed	No
Has patient eaten anything different in a day or so before diarrhoea appeared?	No
Additional questions	No foreign travel Does not seem to be worse at any time of day
Previous history of presenting complaint	Has had the odd bout of diarrhoea before but usually clears up after a couple days

Information gathering	Data generated
Past medical history	RA, HT, mild stroke 2 years ago
Drugs (OTC, Rx, compliance)	Ibuprofen 600 mg tds; aspirin 75 mg od; Dipyridamole 200 mg bd; atenolol 25 mg od No change to medicines for last 6–9 months
Allergies	None known
Social history	Of little relevance in this case
Family history	No one in family with similar symptoms
On examination	General appearance is of a healthy person. No obvious signs of dehydration. Pinch test normal

Diagnostic pointers with regard to symptom presentation

The expected findings for questions when related to the different conditions that can be seen by community pharmacists are summarised below.

CASE STUDY 7.2 (Continued)

	Age	Acute or chronic	Timing	Periodicity	Weight loss	Blood in stools
Infection	Any	Acute	Any	Acute	No	Unusual
Medicines	Any	Acute or chronic	Any	No	No	No
IBS	<45 years	Acute	Mornings?	Recurs	No	No
Giardiasis	Any	Acute	Any	Acute	No	No
Faecal impaction	Elderly	Chronic	Any	No	No	No
Ulcerative colitis	Young adults	Acute	am and pm	Recurs	No	Yes
Crohn's disease	Young adults	Acute	am and pm	Recurs	No	Yes
Coeliac disease	Infants or middle-aged	Chronic	Any	No	Yes	No
Carcinoma	>50 years	Chronic	Any	No	Yes	Unusual

When this information is applied to that gained from our patient (see next table), we see that by the questions asked that the most likely cause of his symptoms is infection.

	Age	Acute or chronic	Timing	Periodicity	Blood in stools
Infection	✓	✓	✓	✓	✓
Medicines	✓	✓	✓	✗	✓
IBS	✗	✓	✗?	✓	✓
Giardiasis	✓	✓	✓	✓	✓
Faecal impaction	✗	✗	✓	✗	✓
Ulcerative colitis	✗	✓	✗	✓	✗
Crohn's disease	✗	✓	✗	✓	✗
Coeliac disease	✓	✗	✓	✗	✓
Carcinoma	✓	✗	✓	✗	✓?

Outcome:

Advise on restoring fluid intake and if needed loperamide could be sold.

7

CASE STUDY 7.3

Mrs RH, an elderly patient (about 75 years old), picks up her prescription and at the same time says she wants something to help get rid of a funny patch on the inside of her cheek. The following questions are asked, and responses received.

Information gathering	Data generated
Describe symptoms	White patch about the size of a 10-pence piece
How long has the patient had the symptoms?	Had for a couple of weeks
Type/severity of pain	Not really painful
Other symptoms	No other obvious symptoms
Additional questions	No systemic symptoms (e.g., fever, chills)
Previous history of presenting complaint	Had something similar a couple of years ago and the other chemist gave me some cream
Past medical history	RA, HT, stroke 2 years ago
Drugs (OTC, Rx, compliance)	Ibuprofen 600 mg tds; aspirin 75 mg od; Atenolol 25 mg od

Information gathering	Data generated
Allergies	None known
Social history Smoking Alcohol Drugs Employment Relationships	Lives on her own and watches TV most of the time–Loves quiz shows. Non-smoker and only occasionally drinks alcoholic beverages
Family history	
On examination	Discrete white patch. No underlying redness

Epidemiology dictates that the most likely cause of white patches in the oral cavity seen in primary care is thrush. However, given her age, other conditions are possible and include medicines, ill-fitting dentures, diabetes (undiagnosed) and leukoplakia.

Diagnostic pointers with regard to symptom presentation

The next table summarises the expected findings for questions when related to the different conditions that can be seen by community pharmacists.

	Number	Location	Size & shape	Age	Pain
Thrush	'Singular patch'	Anywhere	Irregular and variable size	Young and elderly	No
Minor ulcers	Up to 5 or so ulcers	Lips and inside cheeks	Less than 1 cm and round	10–40 years most common	Yes
Major ulcers	Numerous	Anywhere	Large (and of variable shape)	All ages	Yes
Herpetiform	Very numerous	Back of the mouth	Pinpoint and round	All ages	Yes
Herpes simplex	Numerous	Anywhere	Small	Children	Yes
Lichen planus	Diffuse	Tongue, cheek, gums	'Spiders web'	Adults	No
Leukoplakia	Singular patch	Tongue or cheek	Irregular and of variable size	Elderly	No
Carcinoma	Singular lesion	Tongue, mouth, lower lip	Irregular and of variable size	Elderly	No, but latter stages yes

When this information is applied to that gained from our patient (see next table), we see that from the questions asked the diagnosis could be thrush or leukoplakia. Although the woman is not really complaining of pain, there is a possibility that this 'white patch' has to be deemed potentially sinister, especially as she is of an age where leukoplakia is more likely. The positive smoking history would make leukoplakia more of a possibility. This person must be referred.

	Number	Location	Size & shape	Age	Pain
Thrush	✓	✓	✓	✓	✗
Minor ulcers	✗	✓	✗	✗	✗
Major ulcers	✗	✓	✗	✗?	✗
Herpetiform	✗	✗	✗	✓	✗
Herpes simplex	✗	✓	✗	✗	✗
Lichen planus	✓?	✓	✓	✓	✓?
Leukoplakia	✓	✓	✓	✓	✓
Carcinoma	✗?	✓	✓	✓	✓?

CASE STUDY 7.3 (Continued)

Activity

In cases 7.2 and 7.3 tables have been constructed to summarise the signs/symptoms associated with diarrhoeal and oral lesion presentations. Below is a blank table for lower abdominal pain. Construct answers for each condition. Answers are shown on STUDENT CONSULT.

	Age affected	Sex affected	Nature of pain	Usual location	Other prominent features
IBS					
Diverticulitis					
Renal colic					
Appendicitis					
Intestinal obstruction					
Endometriosis					
Salpingitis					

Answers

1 = a	2 = a	3 = e	4 = c	5 = a	6 = a	7 = a	8 = a	9 = F	10 = C
11 = I	12 = H	13 = A	14 = H	15 = B	16 = E	17 = A	18 = B	19 = C	20 = E

Dermatology

In this chapter

Background

The skin is the largest organ of the body. It has a complex structure and performs many important functions. These include protecting underlying tissues from external injury and overexposure to ultraviolet light, barring entry to microorganisms and harmful chemicals, acting as a sensory organ for pressure, touch, temperature, pain and vibration, and maintaining the homeostatic balance of body temperature.

It has been reported that dermatological disorders account for up to 15% of the workload of UK family doctors, with similar findings reported from community pharmacy. It is therefore important that community pharmacists are able to differentiate between common dermatological conditions that can be managed appropriately without referral to a doctor and those that require further investigation or treatment with a prescription-only medicine.

General overview of skin anatomy

Principally the skin consists of two parts, the outer and thinner layer called the epidermis and an inner, thicker layer named the dermis. Beneath the dermis lies a subcutaneous layer, known as the hypodermis (Fig. 8.1).

The epidermis

The epidermis is the major protective layer of the skin and has four distinct layers when viewed under the microscope. The basal layer actively undergoes cell division, forcing new cells to move up through the epidermis and form the outer keratinised horny layer. This process is continual and takes approximately 35 days. Pathological changes in the epidermis produce a rash or a lesion with abnormal scale, loss of surface integrity or changes to pigmentation.

The dermis

The majority of the dermis is made of connective tissue; collagen for strength, and elastic fibres to allow stretch. It provides support to the epidermis as well as its blood and nerve supply. Also located in the dermis are the hair follicle, sebaceous and sweat glands and arrector pili muscle. Under cold conditions, the arrector pili muscle contracts, pulling the hair in to a vertical position to provide thermal protection and causing characteristic 'goosebumps'.

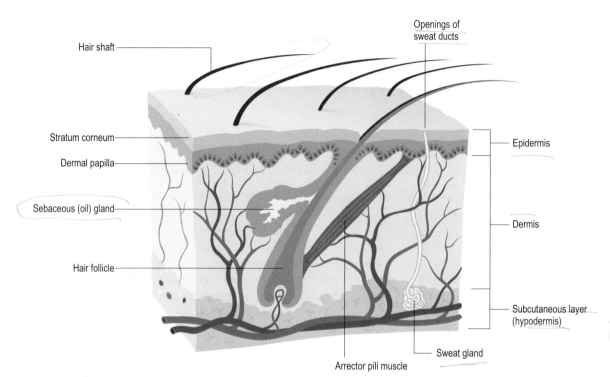

Fig. 8.1 The epidermis, dermis and associated structures.

Conditions of the dermis usually result in changes in the elevation of the skin, e.g., papules and nodules.

The hair

Each hair consists of a shaft, the visible part of the hair, and a root. Surrounding the root is the hair follicle, the base of which is enlarged into a bulb structure. The primary function of hair is one of protection.

Sebaceous glands

Sebaceous glands are found in large numbers on the face, chest and upper back. Their primary role is to produce sebum, which keeps hair supple and the skin soft. During puberty these glands become large and active due to hormonal changes. Frequently, sebum will accumulate in the sebaceous gland, and is one of the factors that lead to acne formation.

Sweat glands

These are the most numerous and important of the skin glands and are classed as apocrine or eccrine. Eccrine glands produce a transparent watery liquid (sweat) and are located all over the body and play a role in elimination of waste products and maintaining a constant core temperature. Apocrine sweat glands are mainly located in the axilla and begin to function at puberty and have no known biological function.

History taking

Unlike internal medicine, the majority of dermatological complaints presenting in community pharmacy can be seen. This affords the community pharmacist an excellent opportunity to base his or her differential diagnosis not only on questioning but also on physical examination. General questions that should be considered when dealing with dermatological conditions are listed in Table 8.1. Terminology describing skin lesions can be confusing and the more common terms used to describe their appearance are shown in Table 8.2.

Physical examination

A more accurate differential diagnosis will be made if the pharmacist actually sees the person's athlete's foot or 'rash' on the back. Providing adequate privacy can be obtained, there is no reason why the majority of skin complaints cannot

Table 8.1
Questions to consider when taking a dermatological history

Question	Relevance
Where did the problem first appear?	Certain skin problems start in one particular location before spreading to other parts of the body, e.g., impetigo usually starts on the face before spreading to the limbs Patients might need prompting to tell you where the problem started, as they are likely to want help for the most obvious or large skin lesion but neglect to tell you about smaller lesions that appeared first
Are there any other symptoms?	Many skin rashes are associated with itch and/or pain Mild itch is associated with many skin conditions including psoriasis and medicine eruptions Severe itch is associated with conditions such as scabies and atopic and contact dermatitis
Occupational history (relevant to adults only)	This is particularly pertinent for contact dermatitis, e.g., do symptoms improve when away from work?
General medical history	Many skin signs can be the first marker of internal disease, e.g., diabetes can manifest with pruritus; fungal or bacterial infection and thyroid disease can present with hair loss and pruritus
Travel	More people are taking holidays to non-Western countries and therefore have the potential to contract tropical diseases
Family and household contact history	Infections such as scabies can infect relatives and others with whom the patient is in close contact
The patient's thoughts on the cause of the problem	Ask for the patient's opinion. This might help with the diagnosis, or alternatively shed light on anxieties and theories as to the cause of the condition

be inspected. If examinations are performed, clearly explain the procedure you want to perform and gain the person's consent. Examinations should ideally be conducted in consultation rooms. It is worth remembering that many patients will be embarrassed by the appearance of skin conditions and the pharmacist needs to demonstrate empathy during the consultation. When performing an examination of the skin, a number of things should be looked for (Table 8.3). There is no substitute for experience when recognising skin problems. This is normally gained through seeing multiple similar cases and developing your pattern recognition skills (see page 4). A free image bank (http://www.dermnet.com/) is available where familiarity can be gained of different presentations of skin conditions.

Hyperproliferative disorders

Background

Hyperproliferative disorders are characterised by a combination of increased cell turnover rate and a shortening of the time it takes for cells to migrate from the basal layer to the outer horny layer. Typically, cell turnover rate is ten times faster than normal and cell migration takes 3 or 4 days rather than 35 days.

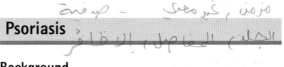

Psoriasis

Background

Psoriasis is a chronic relapsing inflammatory disorder characterised by a variety of morphological lesions that present in a number of forms. The most common form of psoriasis is plaque psoriasis, accounting for about 80–90% of cases (Table 8.4). Depending on the extent and severity of lesions, psoriasis can have a profound affect on the person's work and social life.

Prevalence and epidemiology

Psoriasis is a common skin disorder with an estimated worldwide prevalence between 1% and 3%. In the UK it has been reported to affect 1–2% of the population. However,

Table 8.2
Common terms used to describe skin lesions

Term	Description
Macule	A flat lesion which is less than 1 cm in diameter
Patch	A flat lesion which is greater than 1 cm in diameter
Papule	A raised, solid lesion less than 1 cm in diameter
Nodule	A raised, solid lesion greater than 1 cm in diameter
Vesicle	A clear, fluid-filled lesion lasting a few days which is less than 1 cm in diameter
Bulla	A clear, fluid-filled lesion lasting a few days which is greater than 1 cm in diameter
Pustule	A pus-filled lesion lasting a few days which is less than 1 cm in diameter
Comedone	A papule which is 'plugged' with keratin and sebum
Erythema	Redness due to dilated blood vessels that blanch when pressed
Excoriation	Localised damage to the skin due to scratching
Lichenification	Thickening of the epidermis with increased skin markings due to scratching

Table 8.3
Things to consider when performing a dermatological examination

Lesions	Relevance
Temperature	Use the backs of your fingers to make the assessment. This should enable you to identify generalised warmth or coolness of the skin and note the temperature of any red areas, e.g., generalised warmth can indicate infection, whereas localised warmth might indicate inflammation or cellulitis
Lesions	**Distribution** – many skin diseases have a 'typical' or 'classic' distribution Symmetrical – e.g., acne and psoriasis Asymmetrical – e.g., contact dermatitis Unilateral – e.g., shingles Localised – e.g., nappy rash **Arrangement** Discrete (with healthy skin in between) – e.g., psoriasis Coalescing (merging together) – e.g., eczema Grouped – e.g., insect bites **Feel of lesions** Smooth – e.g., urticaria Rough – e.g., actinic keratosis
Recent trauma	Is there any sign that individual lesions have developed on a site of trauma or injury such as a scratch? This is seen in a number of conditions such as psoriasis and viral warts

this is probably an underestimate, as many patients with mild psoriasis do not present to their doctor.

Psoriasis can present at any time in life, although it appears to be more prevalent in the second and fifth decade. It is rare in infants and uncommon in children. The sexes are equally affected, but it is more common in Caucasians.

Aetiology

The exact aetiology of psoriasis still remains unclear, but it is now recognised as an immune-mediated disorder with a genetic influence. Studies have identified a region on chromosome 6 as a contributor to psoriasis susceptibility (known as *PSORS1*) and this has been associated with at least 50% of psoriasis cases in several populations.

Table 8.4
Causes of psoriasis-like rash and their relative incidence in community pharmacy

Incidence	Cause
Most likely	Plaque psoriasis, scalp psoriasis
Likely	Seborrhoeic dermatitis, medicine-induced/exacerbated psoriasis
Unlikely	Guttate and flexural psoriasis, tinea corporis, lichen planus, pityriasis rosea
Very unlikely	Pustular psoriasis, erythrodermic psoriasis

However, genetic predisposition to psoriasis does not necessarily mean disease expression. Studies in twins also suggest that environmental factors might be needed for clinical expression of the disease because only 70% of genetically identical twins both develop the condition.

Psoriasis lesions also develop at sites of skin trauma, such as sunburn and cuts (known as the Koebner phenomenon), after streptococcal throat infection and during periods of stress.

Arriving at a differential diagnosis

Psoriasis can be located on various parts of the body (Fig. 8.2) and presents in a variety of different forms. Plaque and scalp psoriasis are the only forms of the condition that can be managed by the community pharmacist. It is therefore necessary that other forms of psoriasis, and conditions that look like psoriasis, can be recognised and distinguished. Asking symptom-specific questions will help the pharmacist establish a differential diagnosis (Table 8.5).

Clinical features of plaque psoriasis

Plaque psoriasis classically presents with characteristic salmon-pink lesions with slivery-white scales and well-defined boundaries (Fig. 8.3). On darker skin this

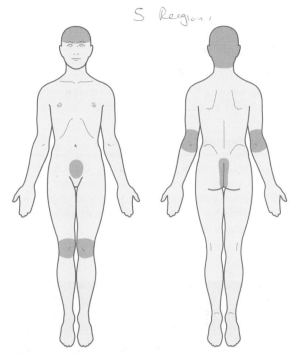

Fig. 8.2 Typical distribution of psoriatic plaques.

Table 8.5 Specific questions to ask the patient: Psoriasis	
Question	**Relevance**
Onset	Psoriasis can develop in patients of any age, although it first occurs most commonly in early adult life. However, in young and elderly patients the lesions tend to be atypical, which can make the diagnosis more difficult
Distribution of rash	Psoriasis often presents in a symmetrical distribution and most commonly involves the scalp and extensor aspects of the elbows and knees. The gluteal cleft and umbilicus can also be affected (Fig. 8.2) Conditions that resemble psoriasis, such as lichen planus (often inside of the wrists) and pityriasis rosea (thighs and trunk) have a different distribution to psoriasis
Other symptoms	Itch is not normally the predominant feature of psoriasis, unlike other conditions such as dermatitis and fungal infections Nail involvement in the form of pitting and onycholysis (separation of the nail plate from the nail bed) is often seen and can involve one or more of the nails. This is normally observed in patients with long-standing psoriasis
Look of rash	Scalp and plaque psoriasis usually show scaling as an obvious feature. This is not seen with other common skin conditions (e.g., dermatitis) or other forms of psoriasis When scalp involvement is mild, psoriasis can be impossible to distinguish from seborrhoeic dermatitis
Previous history of lesions	Psoriasis is a chronic relapsing and remitting disease, and it is likely that the patient will have had lesions in the past. Other skin diseases, such as fungal infections, are acute and patients do not normally have a history of the problem

characteristic colour is not apparent. Lesions can be single or multiple, and vary in size from pinpoint to covering extensive areas. If the scales on the surface of the plaque are gently removed and the lesion then rubbed, it reveals pinpoint bleeding from the superficial dilated capillaries. This is known as the Auspitz' sign and is diagnostic.

Clinical features of scalp psoriasis

Scalp psoriasis can be mild, exhibiting slight redness of the scalp, through to severe cases with total head involvement, marked inflammation and thick scaling (Fig. 8.4). The redness often extends beyond the hair margin and is commonly seen behind the ears.

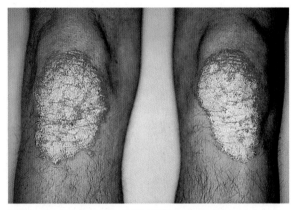

Fig. 8.3 Typical psoriatic plaques. Reproduced from DJ Gawkrodger, 2007, Dermatology: An Illustrated Colour Text, 4th edition, Churchill Livingstone, with permission.

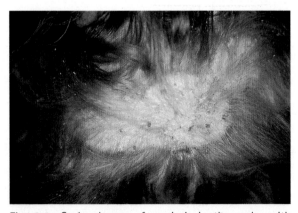

Fig. 8.4 Scaly plaques of psoriasis in the scalp, with localised hair loss. Reproduced from DJ Gawkrodger, 2007, Dermatology: An Illustrated Colour Text, 4th edition, Churchill Livingstone, with permission.

Conditions to eliminate

Likely causes

Seborrhoeic dermatitis

Mild scalp psoriasis can be very difficult to distinguish from seborrhoeic dermatitis. However, in practice this is rarely a problem since treatment for both conditions is often the same. For further information on seborrhoeic dermatitis see page 229.

Medication-exacerbated psoriasis

A number of medicines can precipitate, worsen or aggravate existing psoriasis. Medicines most commonly associated are lithium, antimalarials, beta-blockers, ACE inhibitors and NSAIDs. Other medicines with a reported association with psoriasis include digoxin, clonidine, amiodarone, gold, TNF-alpha inhibitors, fluoxetine, cimetidine, antibacterials (tetracycline and penicillin) and gemfibrozil (Kim & Del Rosso, 2010).

Unlikely causes

Guttate psoriasis (also known as raindrop psoriasis)

Guttate psoriasis is characterised by crops of scattered small lesions (less than 1 cm) covered with light flaky scales that often affects the trunk and proximal part of the limbs (Fig. 8.5). This form of psoriasis usually occurs

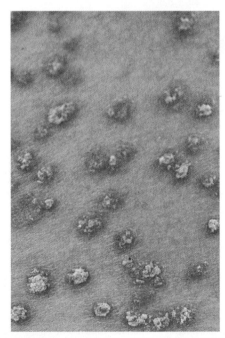

Fig. 8.5 Guttate psoriasis. Reproduced from J Wilkinson et al 2004, Dermatology in Focus, Churchill Livingstone, with permission.

in adolescents and often follows a streptococcal throat infection and in people genetically predisposed to psoriasis. The condition is usually self-limiting.

Flexural psoriasis

Flexural psoriasis refers to lesions that resemble plaque psoriasis but lack scaling and have atypical distribution: namely in the body folds, especially the groins and axillae. Itching, in this form, affects over 50% of people.

Tinea corporis

Tinea corporis can superficially look like plaque psoriasis. For further information on tinea infection see page 234.

Lichen planus

Lichen planus is an uncommon condition and is reported to only account for 0.2–0.8% of dermatological outpatient consultations. The lesions are similar in appearance to plaque psoriasis but are itchy and are normally located on the inner surfaces of the wrists and on the shins, an atypical distribution for psoriasis. Additionally, oral mucous membranes are normally affected with white, slightly raised lesions that look a little like a spider's web. The person will not have a family history of psoriasis.

Pityriasis rosea

The condition is characterised by erythematous scaling mainly on the trunk, but also on the thighs and upper arms. The colour of the rash tends to be a lighter pink colour than psoriasis and can be mildly itchy. A 'target' disc lesion normally appears first (herald patch), which is then followed approximately 1 week later with an extensive rash. It most commonly affects young adults. The condition usually remits spontaneously after 4 to 8 weeks. An accurate history will normally eliminate pityriasis rosea from psoriasis, as the condition is acute in onset and the patient can often identify the initial 'target' lesion.

Very unlikely causes

Pustular psoriasis
In this rare form of psoriasis sterile pustules are an obvious clinical feature. The pustules tend to be located on the advancing edge of the lesions and typically occur on the palms of the hands and soles of the feet (Fig. 8.6). It is much more common in women than in men (ratio of 9:1).

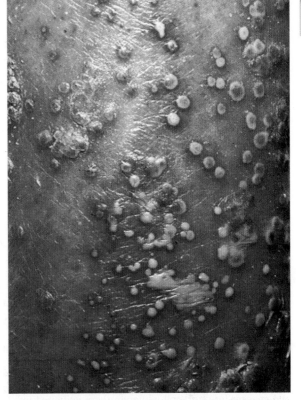

Fig. 8.6 Pustular psoriasis. Reproduced from J Wilkinson et al 2004, Dermatology in Focus, Churchill Livingstone, with permission.

Erythrodermic psoriasis

Erythrodermic psoriasis presents as an extensive erythema and shows very few classical lesions. It is therefore difficult to diagnose. Systemic symptoms can be severe and include fever, joint pain and diarrhoea. The condition is serious and can even be life threatening. Patients are extremely unlikely to present at a community pharmacy.

Tinea capitis (fungal infection of the scalp)

Tinea capitis is the most common infection in children worldwide but in Western nations it is rare. However, if the patient has scaling skin, broken hairs and a patch of alopecia, then a tinea infection should be considered.

Fig. 8.7 will aid in the differentiation of plaque psoriasis.

> ! **TRIGGER POINTS indicative of referral: Psoriasis**
>
> | Symptoms/signs | Possible danger/reason for referral |
> |---|---|
> | Lesions that are extensive, follow recent infection, have atypical psoriasis lesions or cause moderate-to-severe itching | Suggest more severe forms of psoriasis |
> | Precipitation or aggravation of lesions while taking medicines | If the medicine is suspected as the causative agent, re-assessment of therapy is required |

Evidence base for over-the-counter medication

Over-the-counter (OTC) remedies are effective in treating mild-to-moderate plaque psoriasis and scalp psoriasis. A patient who presents with severe plaque psoriasis or another form of psoriasis should be referred.

Any treatment recommended should also be in conjunction with patient education. Reassurance should be given about its benign, non-contagious nature, but emphasise that the condition is chronic and long-term, and has periods of remission and relapse.

Treatment is limited to the use of emollients, keratolytics and coal tar (or dithranol), although there is limited published literature supporting efficacy of these treatments.

Emollients

No published literature appears to have addressed either emollient efficacy or whether one emollient is superior to another in treating psoriasis. Subjective evidence over a long period of time has shown that emollients are useful and are an important aspect of psoriasis treatment. Emollients are used to help soften scaling and soothe the skin to reduce irritation, cracking and dryness. Patients might have to try several emollients before finding one that is most effective for their skin.

Keratolytics

Keratolytics, such as salicylic acid and lactic acid, have been incorporated into emollients to aid clearing scaliness. They are often used for scalp psoriasis where very thick scaling can occur. Although there appears to be no published evidence for their efficacy, clinical practice suggests that they should be used first when significant scaling is present before using other treatments.

Coal tar

Coal tar remained the mainstay of treatment until the introduction of dithranol, corticosteroids and, more recently, vitamin D and A analogues. A number of clinical studies have confirmed the beneficial effect coal tar has on psoriasis, although a major drawback in assessing the effectiveness of coal tar preparations is the variability in their composition, making meaningful comparisons between studies difficult. Comparisons between coal tar and other treatment regimens have been conducted. Tham et al. (1994) compared the effectiveness of calcipotriol 50 µg twice daily versus 15% coal tar solution each day. Both treatments were shown to be effective, although calcipotriol was significantly better than the coal tar solution. Harrington (1989) compared two commercially available OTC products at that time, Psorin and Alphosyl. Findings showed that both helped

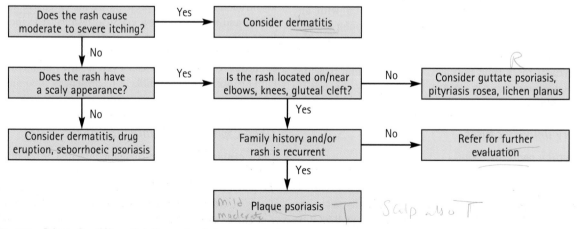

Fig. 8.7 Primer for differential diagnosis of plaque psoriasis.

in the treatment of psoriasis but Psorin (which includes 0.11% dithranol) was significantly more effective.

Dithranol

A systematic review in 2009 identified three placebo-controlled trials with dithranol, all demonstrating a statistically significant improvement over placebo (Mason et al., 2009). There appears to be no definitive answer as to which strength is most appropriate; however, current practice dictates starting on the lowest possible concentration and gradually increasing the concentration until improvement is noticed.

gradually ↑

Practical prescribing and product selection

Prescribing information relating to the medicines used to treat psoriasis discussed in the section 'Evidence base for over-the-counter medication' is summarised in Table 8.6; useful tips relating to patients presenting with psoriasis are given in 'Hints and Tips' in Box 8.1.

Emollients

All emollients should be regularly and liberally applied with no upper limit on how often they can be used. All are chemically inert and can therefore be safely used from birth onwards by all patients. They do not have any interactions with other medicines. For more information on emollients see page 266.

Tar-based products

All patient groups can safely use these products on either the skin or scalp. They have no drug interactions but can cause local skin or scalp irritation, and stain skin and clothes. There has been concern over topical tar products' association with an increased risk of skin cancer, although this appears to be unfounded (Roelofzen et al., 2010).

Dithranol (e.g., Dithrocream)

Dithranol should not be routinely recommended due to the high likelihood of skin irritation and/or burning. If used,

Table 8.6
Practical prescribing: Summary of tar-based products

	Scalp, skin or both	Salicylic acid	Sulphur	Other ingredients	Children	Application
Alphosyl 2-in-1 Shampoo	Scalp	No	No	No	All ages	Every 2–3 days
Capasal	Scalp	Yes	No	Coconut oil 1%	All ages	Daily
Cocois	Scalp	Yes	Yes	No	>6 years	Weekly
Exorex	Both	No	No	No	All ages	2–3 times a day
Polytar, Polytar Plus	Scalp	No	No	No	All ages	Once or twice weekly
Psoriderm	Both	No	No	No	All ages	Once or twice a day
SebCo	Scalp	Yes	Yes	No	>6 years	Daily when needed
T/Gel	Scalp	No	No	No	All ages	2–3 times a week

HINTS AND TIPS BOX 8.1: PSORIASIS

Problems with tar and dithranol products	Coal tar and dithranol share common problems of patient compliance. Both are messy to use, have an unpleasant odour and can stain skin and clothing
UV light	90% of patients with psoriasis improve when exposed to sunlight and most patients notice an improvement when they go on holiday
Emollient use	Remind patients that these should be used regularly and liberally
Emollient bath additives	Some bath additives, for example oilatum, will make the bath slippery and patients should be warned to exercise care when getting out of the bath

then the lowest strength should always be tried initially for at least 1 week and then increased to higher concentrations if needed. The aim should be to build up gradually over approximately 4 weeks to the highest tolerated strength that results in the best therapeutic effect.

↑ gradually.

References

Harrington Cl. Low concentration dithranol and coal tar (Psorin) in psoriasis: a comparison with alcoholic coal tar extract and allantoin (Alphosyl). Br J Clin Pract 1989;43:27–9.

Mason AR, Mason J, Cork M, et al. Topical treatments for chronic plaque psoriasis. Cochrane Database of Systematic Reviews 2009, Issue 2. Art. No.: CD005028. http://dx.doi.org/10.1002/14651858.CD005028.pub2.

Tham SN, Lun KC, Cheong WK. A comparative study of calcipotriol ointment and tar in chronic plaque psoriasis. Br J Dermatol 1994;131:673–7.

Further reading

Clark C. Psoriasis: first-line treatments. Pharm J 2004;274:623–6.

Dodd WA. Tars. Their role in the treatment of psoriasis. Dermatol Clin 1993;11:131–5.

Freeman K. Psoriasis: not just a skin disease. The Prescriber 2007;5th June:42–5, 49.

Gelfand JM, Weinstein R, Porter SB, et al. Prevalence and treatment of psoriasis in the United Kingdom: a population-based study. Arch Dermatol 2005;141:1537–41.

Kim GK, Del Rosso JQ. Drug-provoked psoriasis: is it drug induced or drug aggravated? Understanding pathophysiology and clinical relevance. J Clin Aesthet Dermatol 2010; 3(1): 32–38.

Leary MR, Rapp SR, Herbst KC, et al. Interpersonal concerns and psychological difficulties of psoriasis patients: effects of disease severity and fear of negative evaluation. Health Psychol 1998;17:530–6.

MacKie RM. Clinical dermatology. Hong Kong: Oxford University Press; 1999.

Nevitt GJ, Hutchinson PE. Psoriasis in the community: prevalence, severity and patients' beliefs and attitudes towards the disease. Br J Dermatol 1996;135(4):533–7.

Roelofzen JH, Aben KK, Olenhof UT et al. No increased risk of cancer after coal tar treatment in patients with psoriasis or eczema. J Invest Dermatol 2010; 130:953–61.

Scon P, Henning-Boehncke W. Psoriasis. N Engl J Med 2005;352:1899–912.

Tristani-Firouzi P, Kruegger CG. Efficacy and safety of treatment modalities for psoriasis. Cutis 1998;61:11–21.

Websites

National Psoriasis Foundation: https://www.psoriasis.org/

NICE guidance: www.nice.org.uk/cg153

Psoriatic Arthropathy Alliance: http://www.paalliance.org/

The Psoriasis Association: http://www.psoriasis-association.org.uk/

Dandruff (pityriasis capitis)

Background

Dandruff is a chronic, relapsing, non-inflammatory hyperproliferative skin condition that is often seen as socially unsightly and a source of embarrassment. It is a straightforward diagnosis with few other conditions from which to differentially diagnose it (Table 8.7).

Prevalence and epidemiology

Dandruff is very common and affects both sexes and all age groups, although it is unusual in prepubescent children. It has been estimated to affect 1–3% of the population (Gupta et al., 2004).

Aetiology

Increased cell turnover rate is responsible for dandruff, but the reason why cell turnover increases is unknown. Increasingly, research has focused on the role that microorganisms have on the pathogenesis of dandruff, and in particular the yeast *Malassezia* (previously known as *Pityrosporum ovale)*, although the evidence is inconclusive as to whether *Malassezia* is the primary cause of dandruff or is a contributory factor. It has been shown that *Malassezia* makes up more of the scalp flora of dandruff sufferers, which might explain why dandruff improves in the summer months (fungal organisms thrive in warm and moist environments that exist on the scalp due to the wearing of hats and caps). Further evidence to support a role of *Malassezia* in the aetiology of dandruff is the positive effect that antifungal therapy has on clearing dandruff.

Arriving at a differential diagnosis

Most patients will diagnose and treat dandruff without seeking medical help. However, for those patients

Table 8.7

Causes of scalp flaking and their relative incidence in community pharmacy

Incidence	Cause
Most likely	Dandruff
Likely	
Unlikely	Contact and seborrhoeic dermatitis
Very unlikely	Tinea capitis

?

Table 8.8
Specific questions to ask the patient: Dandruff

Question	Relevance
Presence of erythema	Dandruff is not associated with scalp redness unless the person has been scratching. Redness is characteristic of psoriasis and is common in adult seborrhoeic dermatitis
Itch	Dandruff tends to cause itching of the scalp unlike psoriasis and seborrhoeic dermatitis
Presence of other skin lesions	An adult with only scalp involvement is likely to have dandruff, especially in the absence of erythema Many patients who have scalp psoriasis also have plaque psoriasis affecting the arms, legs and the back

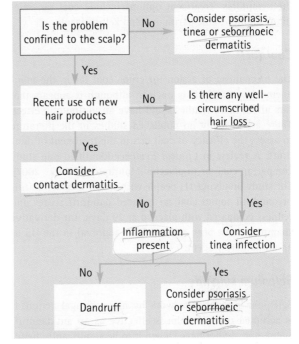

Fig. 8.8 Primer for differential diagnosis of dandruff.

that do ask for help and advice, it is important to differentiate dandruff from other scalp conditions. Asking symptom-specific questions will help the pharmacist determine whether referral is needed (Table 8.8).

Clinical features of dandruff

The scalp will be dry, itchy and flaky. Flakes of dead skin are usually visible in the hair close to the scalp, and are visible on the shoulders and collars of clothing.

Conditions to eliminate

Unlikely causes

Seborrhoeic dermatitis

Typically, seborrhoeic dermatitis will affect areas other than the scalp. In adults, the trunk is commonly involved, as are the eyebrows, eyelashes and external ear. If only scalp involvement is present, then the patient might complain of severe and persistent dandruff and the skin of the scalp will be red. For further information on seborrhoeic dermatitis see page 229.

Contact dermatitis

Ask about the use of new hair products such as dyes and perms. These can cause skin irritation and scaling. Avoidance of the irritant should see an improvement in the condition. If no improvement is seen after avoiding the

suspected irritant after 1 to 2 weeks, then a re-assessment of the symptoms is needed.

Very unlikely causes

Tinea capitis

If the problem is persistent and associated with hair loss, then fungal infection of the scalp should be considered.

Fig. 8.8 will aid the differentiation of dandruff from other scalp disorders.

TRIGGER POINTS indicative of referral: Dandruff

Symptoms/signs	Possible danger/reason for referral
OTC treatment failure with a 'medicated shampoo'	Suggests alternative diagnosis such as dermatitis or fungal infection
Suspected fungal infection	Needs confirmation before oral antifungal treatment

Evidence base for over-the-counter medication

The use of a hypoallergenic shampoo on a daily basis will usually control mild symptoms. In more persistent and severe cases a 'medicated' shampoo can be used to control the symptoms. Treatment options include coal tar, selenium sulphide, zinc pyrithione and ketoconazole.

Coal tar

The mechanism of action for crude coal tar in the management of dandruff is unclear, although it appears that tars affect DNA synthesis and have an antimitotic effect. There are virtually no published studies in the literature to assess the efficacy of coal tars in the treatment of dandruff. A review in *Clinical Evidence* identified one study comparing coal tar to placebo (Manriquez & Uribe, 2007). The study involving 111 people with seborrhoeic dermatitis or dandruff found coal tar reduced dandruff scores and redness compared with placebo at 29 days. Tar-derivative shampoos have been granted FDA approval in the US as an antidandruff agent.

Selenium sulphide

Selenium is thought to work by its antifungal action. It is accepted that selenium is effective as an antidandruff agent, and studies have shown it to be significantly better than placebo and nonmedicated shampoos.

Zinc pyrithione

Zinc pyrithione, like selenium, exhibits antifungal properties but also reduces cell turnover rates. It is believed that one or both of these properties confers its effectiveness in treating dandruff. Few trials have been conducted with

zinc pyrithione, although they have shown significant improvement in dandruff severity scores.

Ketoconazole

Ketoconazole inhibits *Malassezia* replication by interfering with cell membrane formation. It helps in controlling the itching and flaking associated with dandruff. Studies have shown it to be an effective treatment. It has been shown to be significantly better than zinc pyrithione and has similar efficacy to selenium (Sanfilippo & English, 2006). Ketoconazole has also been shown to act as a prophylactic agent in preventing relapse.

In addition, salicylic acid is included in some products (e.g., Capasal) for its keratolytic properties, although trials are lacking to substantiate its effect.

Practical prescribing and product selection

Prescribing information relating to the specific products used to treat dandruff and discussed in the section 'Evidence base for over-the-counter medication' is discussed and summarised in Table 8.9; useful tips relating to dandruff shampoo are given in 'Hints and Tips' in Box 8.2.

All antidandruff shampoos can cause local scalp irritation. If this is severe the product should be discontinued. Any patient group can use them, although some manufacturers state that these products should be avoided during pregnancy. However, there appear to be no data to substantiate this precaution.

Table 8.9
Practical prescribing: Summary of medicines for dandruff

Name of medicine	Use in children	Likely side effects	Drug interactions of note	Patients in which care is exercised	Pregnancy & breastfeeding
Coal tar products	All ages	Local irritation and dermatitis reported but rare	None	None	OK
Selenium	>5 years				Manufacturers state to avoid in pregnancy and while breastfeeding due to lack of safety data. However, safety data show it to be OK when used on small areas over a limited time. No evidence to say it would be absorbed into breast milk
Zinc pyrithione	All ages				OK
Ketoconazole	All ages				

HINTS AND TIPS BOX 8.2: DANDRUFF

Selsun Shampoo — Gold, silver and other metallic jewellery should be removed before use because it can be discoloured. It also has an unpleasant odour

Coal tar products

Products containing coal tar are discussed under practical prescribing for psoriasis. For further information on coal tar products see page 224.

Selenium sulphide (e.g., Selsun) ≃ ketoconazole

Adults and children over the age of 5 should use the product twice a week for the first 2 weeks and then once a week for the next 2 weeks. The hair should be thoroughly wet before applying the shampoo and left in contact with the scalp for 2 to 3 minutes before rinsing out. Selenium should be avoided if the patient has inflamed or broken skin because irritation can occur. Selenium can discolour hair and alter the colour of hair dyes.

Zinc pyrithione (e.g., Head & Shoulders)

Zinc-based products should be used on a daily basis until dandruff clears. Dermatitis has been reported with zinc pyrithione and should be borne in mind when treating patients with preexisting dermatitis.

Ketoconazole (Nizoral Dandruff and Nizoral Anti-Dandruff Shampoo) ≃ Selsun, better than head shoulders

This can be used to treat acute flare-ups of dandruff or as prophylaxis. To treat acute cases adults and children should wash the hair thoroughly, leaving the shampoo on for 3 to 5 minutes before rinsing it off. This should be repeated every 3 or 4 days (twice a week) for between 2 and 4 weeks. If used for prophylaxis, the shampoo should be used once every 1 to 2 weeks. It can cause local itching or a burning sensation on application and may rarely discolour hair.

References

Gupta AK, Batra R, Bluhm R, et al. Skin diseases associated with Malassezia species. J Am Acad Dermatol 2004;51:785–98.

Manríquez JJ & Uribe P 2007 Seborrhoeic dermatitis. BMJ Clin Evid 2007;2007:1713.

Sanfilippo A, English JC. An overview of medicated shampoos used in dandruff treatment. P & T Community 2006;31(7):396–400.

Further reading

Arrese JE, Pierard-Franchimont C, De-Doncker P, et al. Effect of ketoconazole-medicated shampoos on squamometry and Malassezia ovalis load in pityriasis capitis. Cutis 1996;58:235–7.

Danby FW, Maddin WS, Margesson LJ, et al. A randomized double-blind controlled trial of ketoconazole 2% shampoo versus selenium sulfide 2.5% shampoo in the treatment of moderate to severe dandruff. J Am Acad Dermatol 1993;29:1008–12.

Nigam PK, Tyagi S, Saxena AK, et al. Dermatitis from zinc pyrithione. Contact Dermatitis 1988;19:219.

Orentreich N. Comparative study of two antidandruff preparations. J Pharm Sci 1969;58:1279–84.

Peter RU, Richarz-Barthauer U. Successful treatment and prophylaxis of scalp seborrheic dermatitis and dandruff with 2% ketoconazole shampoo: Results of a multicentre, double blind, placebo-controlled trial. Br J Dermatol 1995;132:441–5.

Pereira F, Fernandes C, Dias M, et al. Allergic contact dermatitis from zinc pyrithione. Contact Dermatitis 1995;33:131.

Pierard-Franchimont C, Goffin V, Decroix J, et al. A multicenter randomized trial of ketoconazole 2% and zinc pyrithione 1% shampoos in severe dandruff and seborrheic dermatitis. Skin Pharmacol Appl Skin Physiol 2002;15(6):434–41.

Rigoni C, Toffolo P, Cantu A, et al. 1% econazole hair shampoo in the treatment of pityriasis capitis; a comparative study versus zinc pyrithione shampoo. G Ital Dermatol Venereol 1989;124:67–70.

Van Custem J, Van Gerven F, Fransen J, et al. The in vitro antifungal activity of ketoconazole, zinc pyrithione and selenium sulfide against Pityrosporum and their efficacy as a shampoo in the treatment of experimental pityrosporosis in guinea pigs. J Am Acad Dermatol 1990;22:993–8.

Seborrhoeic dermatitis — Infant form (cradle cap)

— Seborrhoeic dermatitis

Background

There are two distinct types of seborrhoeic dermatitis: an infantile form, often referred to as cradle cap, and an adult form. Seborrhoeic dermatitis can present with varying degrees of severity, ranging from mild dandruff to a severe and explosive form in acquired immune deficiency syndrome (AIDS) patients.

Prevalence and epidemiology

Estimates of the prevalence of clinically significant seborrhoeic dermatitis range from 1% to 5% of the population. Cradle cap is more prevalent than the adult form (Naldi & Rebora, 2009). Cradle cap usually starts in infancy, before the age of 6 months and is usually self-limiting; the adult form tends to be chronic and persistent. The adult form is more common in men than in women, and also more common in people with underlying neurological illness, for example, Parkinson's disease (Johnson & Nunley, 2000).

Aetiology

Despite its name, there appears to be no changes in sebum secretion. Like psoriasis and dandruff, seborrhoeic dermatitis is characterised by an increased cell turnover rate. The precise cause of seborrhoeic dermatitis remains unknown and several theories have been put forward, ranging from immunological, hormonal and nutritional mechanisms. Like dandruff, *Malassezia* plays an important role in the development of seborrhoeic dermatitis; however, it has not yet been established whether it has a primary or secondary role in the clinical presentation of seborrhoeic dermatitis.

Arriving at a differential diagnosis

The infantile form is relatively easy to recognise but can sometimes be confused with atopic dermatitis. Arriving at a differential diagnosis of the adult form is more problematic as the condition can affect different areas and present

Table 8.10
Causes of seborrhoeic dermatitis-like rash and their relative incidence in community pharmacy

Incidence	Cause
Most likely	Scalp involvement: Dandruff
Likely	Scalp involvement: Psoriasis rosea
Unlikely	Scalp involvement: Atopic dermatitis, contact dermatitis
Very unlikely	Medicines, pityriasis versicolor

with different degrees of severity. In mild cases it needs to be differentiated from dandruff and in more severe forms from allergic contact dermatitis, psoriasis and pityriasis versicolor (Table 8.10). Asking symptom-specific questions will help the pharmacist establish a differential diagnosis (Table 8.11).

Clinical features of seborrhoeic dermatitis

Cradle cap appears as large, yellow, greasy scales and crusts on the scalp. This can become thick and cover the whole scalp (Fig. 8.10). Other areas can be involved such as the face and napkin area.

Table 8.11
Specific questions to ask the patient: Seborrhoeic dermatitis

Question	Relevance
Itching	In cradle cap the rash does not itch. This is useful in differentiating cradle cap from atopic dermatitis as there is often overlap in the age at which they present.
Location	Infantile and adult forms of seborrhoeic dermatitis do present in different locations (Fig. 8.9). Additionally, the distribution in the adult form varies from other similar skin conditions (e.g., psoriasis – typically involves knees, elbows and sacral area).
Positive family history	Patients tend not to have a family history in seborrhoeic dermatitis. This is in contrast to patients with psoriasis or atopic dermatitis.
Other symptoms	Ear and eyelid problems are associated with seborrhoeic dermatitis. The general health of a child with seborrhoeic dermatitis will be unaffected. In contrast, a child who is fractious and miserable is more likely to have atopic dermatitis. Seborrhoeic dermatitis presents as usually a yellow, greasy scaliness to the skin, unlike psoriasis, which presents as a silvery scaliness to the skin.
Physical signs	If you run your fingers through the hair of someone with seborrhoeic dermatitis, little is felt. In psoriasis, accumulation of scales give the scalp an uneven, lumpy feel.

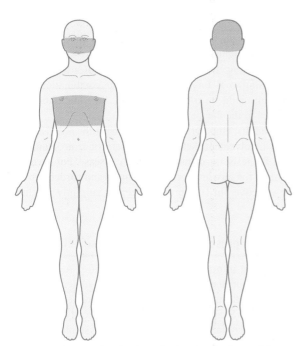

Fig. 8.9 Typical distribution of seborrhoeic dermatitis.

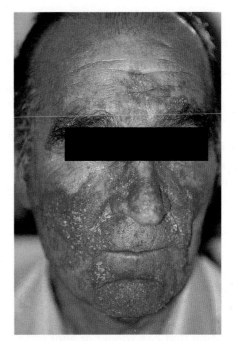

Fig. 8.11 Seborrhoeic dermatitis affecting the face. Reproduced from DJ Gawkrodger, 2007, Dermatology: An Illustrated Colour Text, 4th edition, Churchill Livingstone, with permission.

Conditions to eliminate

Likely causes

Psoriasis

Adults with scalp psoriasis can be confused with those patients who present with severe and persistent dandruff caused by seborrhoeic dermatitis. However, in scalp psoriasis the plaques tend to be crusty and extend away from the hairline, whereas seborrhoeic dermatitis causes scaling with underlying redness and affects the eyebrows and eyelids, unlike psoriasis.

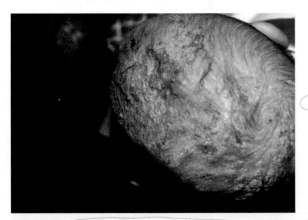

Fig. 8.10 Infantile seborrhoeic dermatitis. Reproduced from R Kliegman, RE Behrman, W Emerson Nelson and HB Jenson, 2007, Nelson Textbook of Pediatrics, Saunders Elsevier, with permission.

Rosacea

Rosacea predominately affects the face – an area usually involved in adult seborrhoeic dermatitis. For more information on rosacea see page 256 under the acne section.

Unlikely causes

Atopic dermatitis

In infants, atopic dermatitis usually presents as itchy lesions on the face and trunk. Scalp involvement is less common and the nappy area is usually spared. A positive personal or family history of the atopic triad of dermatitis, asthma or hay fever is common. For further information on differentiating atopic dermatitis from other conditions see page 313.

The adult form is characterised by a history of intermittent skin problems. The distribution of rash is synonymous with skin areas with high numbers of sebaceous glands, typically the central part of the face, scalp, eyebrows, eyelids, ears, nasolabial folds and mid-chest (Fig. 8.11). The rash is red with greasy-looking scales and is mildly itchy. Blepharitis and otitis externa are also common secondary complications.

Very unlikely causes

Pityriasis versicolor (meaning bran-like scaly rash of various colour)

Pityriasis versicolor, a yeast infection (90% of cases are caused by to *Malassezia* spp.), can be mistaken for adult seborrhoeic dermatitis because the lesions exhibit fine superficial scale and are located on the upper trunk. The lesions are usually small (less than 1 cm) but can join together to form larger plaques. The condition is associated with warm climates and most people will have acquired the infection when on holiday. The rash does not itch significantly, and the face is usually spared. It is most commonly seen in young adults. It can be treated with antifungal lotions and shampoos (see 'Dandruff', page 226), or imidazole creams for small numbers of lesions (see 'Fungal infections', page 237). Antifungal shampoos, such as ketoconazole and selenium sulphide (2.5%), are applied for 10 minutes and then washed off; this is repeated daily for 10 days. Imidazole creams are applied daily for 10 days.

Medication that can trigger or aggravate seborrhoeic dermatitis

A number of medicines are associated with triggering or aggravating existing seborrhoeic dermatitis. These include buspirone, cimetidine, gold, griseofulvin, haloperidol, interferon alfa, lithium, methyldopa and phenothiazines.

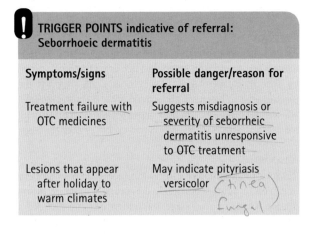

> **! TRIGGER POINTS indicative of referral: Seborrhoeic dermatitis**
>
> | Symptoms/signs | Possible danger/reason for referral |
> | --- | --- |
> | Treatment failure with OTC medicines | Suggests misdiagnosis or severity of seborrheic dermatitis unresponsive to OTC treatment |
> | Lesions that appear after holiday to warm climates | May indicate pityriasis versicolor (tinea) (fungal) |

Evidence base for over-the-counter medication

Treatment options for seborrhoeic dermatitis are the same as dandruff. Ketoconazole in a 2015 Cochrane review (Okokon et al., 2015) was shown to be effective compared with placebo.

For infants, simple measures, such as the daily use of a baby shampoo followed by gentle brushing, are usu-ally only required to improve the condition. If this fails, the scales can be removed by applying olive oil to the scalp overnight, followed by using a baby shampoo the next morning. If symptoms persist a medicated shampoo containing coal tar or keratolytic–tar combination (e.g., Capasal) could be tried. If this fails, the child should be referred to the doctor.

In adults, zinc pyrithione can be tried for mild cases of scalp involvement. Selenium and ketoconazole should be used for resistant or more moderate disease. For involvement on the face and torso, antifungals and corticosteroids are effective but OTC product licenses currently preclude their use.

Practical prescribing and product selection

Prescribing information relating to specific products used to treat seborrhoeic dermatitis is discussed under 'Dandruff' on page 228. In addition, at least one product (Dentinox Cradle Cap Shampoo) is marketed specifically for cradle cap. This contains sodium lauryl ether sulphosuccinate 6% and sodium lauryl ether sulphate 2.7%. The shampoo should be applied twice during each bath time until the scalp clears, after which it can be used when needed.

References

Johnson BA, Nunley JR. Treatment of seborrheic dermatitis. Am Fam Physician 2000;61:2703–10.

Naldi L, Rebora A. Seborrhoeic dermatitis. N Engl J Med 2009;360(4):387–96.

Okokon EO, Verbeek JH, Ruotsalainen JH, et al. Topical antifungals for seborrhoeic dermatitis. Cochrane Database of Systematic Reviews 2015, Issue 5. Art. No.: CD008138. http://dx.doi.org/10.1002/14651858.CD008138.pub3.

Further reading

Bergbrant IM, Faergemann J. The role of *Pityrosporum ovale* in seborrheic dermatitis. Semin Dermatol 1990;9:262–8.

Danby FW, Maddin WS, Margesson LJ, et al. A randomized double-blind controlled trial of ketoconazole 2% shampoo versus selenium sulfide 2.5% shampoo in the treatment of moderate to severe dandruff. J Am Acad Dermatol 1993;29:1008–12.

Go IH, Wientjens DP, Koster M. A double-blind trial of 1% ketoconazole shampoo versus placebo in the treatment of dandruff. Mycoses 1992;35:103–5.

Gupta AK, Bluhm R. Seborrhoeic dermatitis. J Eur Acad Dermatol Venereol 2004;18:13–26.

McGrath J, Murphy GM. The control of seborrhoeic dermatitis and dandruff by antipityrosporal drugs. Drugs 1991;41:178–84.

Fungal skin infections

Background

Two main groups of fungi infect man: *Candida* yeasts and dermatophytes. However, in this section only dermatophyte infections are considered. Dermatophyte skin infections are classed by anatomical location, for example: Athlete's foot (tinea pedis), groin infection (tinea cruris or 'jock itch'), ringworm of the skin (tinea corporis) and scalp ringworm (tinea capitis).

Prevalence and epidemiology

Globally, dermatophytic fungi are more prevalent in tropical and subtropical areas because fungal organisms prefer high temperatures and high humidity. Having said this, dermatophyte infections are commonly met in more temperate Western countries. Tinea pedis (athlete's foot) is the most common fungal infection, although prevalence rates vary depending on the population studied and whether diagnosis is made by clinical symptoms or culture confirmation. Athlete's foot is said to affect about 15% of the UK population and is common in people of all ages.

Other tinea infections such as tinea corporis and tinea cruris might present in the community pharmacy but are uncommon.

Aetiology

Dermatophyte infections are contagious and transmitted directly from one host to another. They invade the stratum corneum of the skin, hair and nails but do not generally infiltrate living tissues. The fungus then begins to grow and proliferate in the non-living cornified layer of keratinised tissue of the epidermis. Transmission of athlete's foot is thought to be commonly acquired from communal rooms (e.g., changing rooms), whereas infection of the groin can be acquired from contaminated towels and bed sheets, or by autoinoculation from an existing foot infection.

Arriving at a differential diagnosis

Dependent on the area affected, the infection will manifest itself in a variety of clinical presentations. Recognition of symptoms for each site affected (Fig. 8.12) will facilitate recognition and accurate diagnosis. All forms of tinea infection, perhaps with the exception of isolated lesions on the body, should be relatively easy to recognise but need to be differentially diagnosed from other similar skin lesions (Table 8.12).

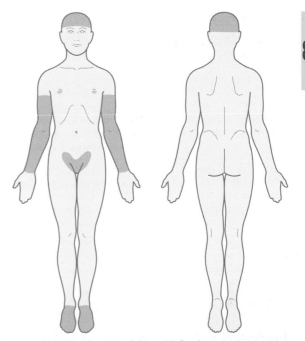

Fig. 8.12 Distribution of fungal infections.

Table 8.12
Causes of fungal-like rash and their relative incidence in community pharmacy

Incidence	Cause
Most likely	Athlete's foot, tinea corporis, psoriasis
Likely	Dermatitis, discoid eczema
Unlikely	Tinea cruris, pityriasis versicolor
Very unlikely	Pityriasis rosea, tinea faciei, tinea manuum

Patients with athlete's foot will often accurately self-diagnose the condition. However, the pharmacist should still confirm this self-diagnosis through a combination of questions (Table 8.13) and inspection of the feet. This is important, as it also provides an opportunity to check for fungal nail involvement.

Clinical features of tinea infections

Athlete's foot

Athlete's foot is characterised by itching, flaking and fissuring of the skin, and will appear white and 'soggy' due to maceration of the skin (Fig. 8.13). The feet often smell.

Table 8.13
Specific questions to ask the patient: Fungal infections

Question	Relevance
Age and sex of patient	Athlete's foot is most prevalent in adolescents and young adults, especially in males Nail involvement usually occurs in older adults Infection in the groin is much more common in men than in women
Presence of itch	Fungal infections usually cause itch, irritation or burning sensations. This usually eliminates conditions such as psoriasis but not dermatitis/eczema
Associated symptoms	Fungal lesions tend to be dry and scaly (except athlete's foot) and have a sharp margin between infected and non-infected skin
Previous and family history	Fungal infections are usually acute in onset with no previous episodes, although athlete's foot may become recurrent For lesions that do not show a classic textbook description, a positive family history of dermatitis or psoriasis might influence your differential diagnosis

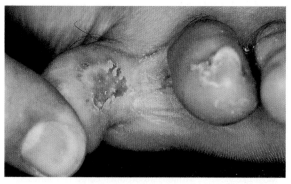

Fig. 8.13 Athlete's foot. Reproduced from AB Fleischer et al 2000, 20 Common Problems, with permission of the McGraw-Hill Companies.

The usual site of infection is in the toe webs, especially the fourth web space (web space next to the little toe).

Once acquired the infection can spread to other sites, including the sole and instep of the foot. Over time this can infect the nails (see 'fungal nail infection' on page 238). Cases of tinea infection where the plantar surface has become involved may be persistent and difficult to treat.

Tinea corporis

Tinea corporis is defined as an infection of the major skin surfaces that do not involve the face, hands, feet, groin or scalp. The usual clinical presentation is of itchy pink or red scaly slightly raised patches with a well-defined inflamed border (Fig. 8.14). Over time the lesions often show 'central clearing', as the central area is relatively resistant to colonisation. This appearance led to the term *ringworm*.

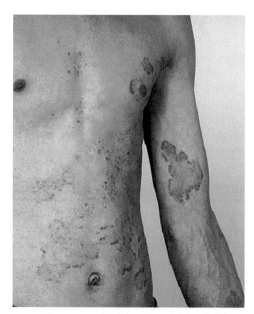

Fig. 8.14 Tinea corporis. Reproduced from P Buttaravoli, 2007, Minor Emergencies, 2nd edition, Elsevier Mosby with permission.

Lesions can occur singly, be numerous or overlap to produce a single large lesion and appear polycyclic (several overlapping circular lesions).

Conditions to eliminate

Most likely causes

Psoriasis
Isolated fungal body lesions can be difficult to distinguish from plaque psoriasis. However, if the patient has psoriasis

there will normally be a personal or family history of psoriasis. Lesions tend to be less itchy, exhibit more scaling and do not show central clearing.

Likely causes

Dermatitis – allergic and contact forms

Both fungal infections and dermatitis exhibit red itchy lesions, and therefore can be difficult to distinguish from one another. Patients with dermatitis will often have a personal history of dermatitis or be able to describe an event that triggered the onset of the rash. Misdiagnosis of a fungal infection for dermatitis and subsequent treatment with a steroid-based cream will diminish the itch, redness and scaling, but the infecting organism will proliferate. On withdrawal of the steroid cream the visible signs of the infection will return and be worse than before, often in a papular form (tinea incognito).

Discoid eczema

This presents as round, raised, coin-shaped lesions that particularly affect the arms and legs. It can itch and show superficial scale. It occurs mainly in middle-aged people.

Unlikely causes

Tinea cruris

The rash is usually isolated to the groin and inner thighs, but can spread to the buttocks. It is often bilateral and is normally intensely itchy, reddish brown and has a well-defined edge.

Pityriasis versicolor

Pityriasis versicolor presents with patchy, sharply demarcated macules with fine scale. The rash tends not to itch and shows less inflammation than in tinea corporis. It is most commonly seen in young adults. For further information on pityriasis versicolor see page 232.

Very unlikely causes

Tinea faciei

Fungal infections on the face are rare and are consequently often mistaken for other facial skin conditions. The lesions are similar in appearance to tinea corporis in that they will normally have a sharp, well-defined border, show scaling and be itchy. Conditions such as acne, rosacea and lupus need to be considered in its differential diagnosis.

Tinea manuum

Tinea manuum is often misdiagnosed as eczema or psoriasis due to its atypical tinea appearance. The patient usually suffers from chronic diffuse scaling of one palm. Often athlete's foot will be present, as the infection has spread to the hands from the feet due to the patient scratching their feet.

The condition is not common and if no foot involvement is implicated, then the diagnosis strongly points to dermatitis.

Pityriasis rosea

Initially a 'target' disc lesion (herald patch) appears approximately 1 week before the eruption of an extensive erythematous scaly rash that mainly affects the trunk but also thighs and upper arms. The herald patch is often misdiagnosed as tinea corporis.

❗ TRIGGER POINTS indicative of referral: Tinea infections

Symptoms/signs	Possible danger/reason for referral
Involvement of large areas of the trunk OTC treatment failure	Possible oral treatment needed
Suspected facial or hand involvement	Confirmation of diagnosis required, as both are rare causes of fungal infection

---

Evidence base for over-the-counter medication

Superficial dermatophyte infections can be treated effectively with topical OTC preparations. Six classes of medicines are available with varying levels of proven efficacy.

Allylamines

Terbinafine inhibits the biosynthesis of ergosterol – an essential component of fungal cell membranes. Reviews have shown terbinafine to have high cure rates, significantly better than placebo and comparable to imidazoles (El-Gohary et al., 2014).

Imidazoles

Imidazoles, like allylamines, act by inhibiting ergosterol production but at a later stage in the ergosterol biosynthesis pathway. They have largely replaced benzoic acid, undecenoates and tolnaftate because they have greater efficacy and an excellent safety record (Crawford & Hollis, 2007). There appear to be no clinically significant differences in cure rates between the different imidazoles, and the treatment choice will probably be driven by patient acceptability and cost.

Benzoic acid

Benzoic acid acts by lowering intracellular pH of dermatophytes and is combined with salicylic acid (Whitfield's ointment). There is insufficient evidence to determine its efficacy.

Griseofulvin

Griseofulvin (as a 1% spray) works by inhibiting cellular mitosis. It has proven effectiveness when taken orally but has only limited trial data as a topical formulation. One trial reported an 80% mycological cure rate after 4 weeks with once-daily application (Aly et al., 1994).

Tolnaftate

Tolnaftate is thought to work by distorting fungal hyphae but there are limited trial data to support its efficacy. Low patient numbers involved in the studies further compounds the difficulty in assessing its efficacy.

Undecenoates

The exact mechanism of action for undecenoates is not understood. They have been used to treat athlete's foot for over 30 years and is featured in the most recent United States Pharmacopoeia. In a Cochrane review, undecenoic acid was said to be efficacious in treating fungal infections for skin and nail infections of the foot (Crawford & Hollis, 2007).

Summary

On current evidence, an imidazole or terbinafine would be first-line treatment for superficial fungal infection. Both have similar mycological and symptom cure rates, although terbinafine might be preferred because it clears symptoms in a shorter space of time, although it is more expensive.

Practical prescribing and product selection

Prescribing information relating to specific products used to treat fungal infections and discussed in the section 'Evidence base for over-the-counter medication' is summarised in Table 8.14 and products available summarised in Table 8.15; useful tips relating to patients presenting with fungal infections are given in 'Hints and Tips' in Box 8.3.

Table 8.14
Practical prescribing: Summary of medicines for tinea infections

Name of medicine	Use in children	Likely side effects	Drug interactions of note	Patients in which care is exercised	Pregnancy & breastfeeding
Imidazoles					
Bifonazole	All ages	Mild burning or itching	None	None	OK
Clotrimazole					
Miconazole					
Ketoconazole					
Imidazole/steroid combination	>10 years				
Tolnaftate					
Scholl Athlete's Foot range	No lower age stated	None reported	None	None	OK
Undecenoates					
Mycota	No lower age stated	None reported	None	None	OK
Benzoic acid					
Whitfield's Ointment	No lower age stated	None reported	None	None	OK
Terbinafine					
Lamisil range & Scholl Advance Athlete's Foot Cream	>16 years (>18 yrs for Lamisil Once)	Redness, itching	None	None	OK
Griseofulvin (Grisol AF)	No lower age stated	Stinging	None	None	OK

Table 8.15
Summary of antifungal products and formulations

Active ingredient	Brand	Formulations
Bifonazole	Canesten Bifonazole Once Daily	Cream
Clotrimazole 1%	Canesten AF	Cream, spray
	Canesten	Cream, spray, solution
	Care	Cream
Clotrimazole 1% & hydrocortisone 1%	Canesten Hydrocortisone	Cream
Miconazole 2%	Daktarin Activ	Cream, spray, powder
	Daktarin	Cream and powder
Miconazole 2% & hydrocortisone 1%	Daktacort Hydrocortisone	Cream
Ketoconazole	Daktarin Gold	Cream
Terbinafine	Lamisil AT	Spray, cream, gel
	Lamisil Once	Solution
	Scholl Advance Athlete's Foot Cream	Cream
Tolnaftate	Scholl Athlete's Foot	Spray, powder
Undecenoic acid	Mycota	Cream, spray, powder

HINTS AND TIPS BOX 8.3: FUNGAL INFECTION

Reinfection and transmission	It is not known if improving foot hygiene or changing footwear can help cure athlete's foot but measures to reduce transmission include: 1. Dry the skin thoroughly after showering or having a bath. Keep a personal towel and do not share it to prevent the infection spreading from person to person 2. Wear cotton socks and change at least once a day 3. Avoid the use of occlusive non-breathable shoes 4. Dust shoes and socks with antifungal powder 5. Avoid scratching infected skin 6. Use flip-flops (or equivalent) when using communal changing rooms
Steroid-containing products	The license states that the maximum period of treatment is 7 days. This limits their usefulness, as many fungal infections will take longer to clear than 7 days, especially as products need to be used after the lesions have cleared to prevent reinfection. Therefore they are probably best used to control initial symptoms of redness and itch before switching to an imidazole-only product after the initial 7 days of treatment

Imidazoles

All topical imidazoles have excellent safety records and can be used by all patient groups. Side effects experienced are irritation on application. To prevent reinfection, imidazoles should be used after the lesions have cleared, although the length of time varies from product to product.

Clotrimazole (e.g., Canesten range)

Clotrimazole-containing products can be used for all dermatophyte and candida infections. All Canesten products should be applied two or three times a day, whereas Canesten hydrocortisone can only be used twice a day.

Bifonazole (Canesten Bifonazole Once Daily 1% w/w Cream)

Bifonazole is licensed for athlete's foot. For all patients the cream should be applied once daily.

Ketoconazole (Daktarin Gold, Daktarin Intensiv)

Ketoconazole has a license for athlete's foot, groin infection and candidal intertrigo. For athlete's foot the cream should be applied twice a day for 1 week. For groin infections and candidal intertrigo, the cream should be applied once or twice daily. If no improvement in symptoms is experienced after 4 weeks, then the patient should be referred to the doctor. For all conditions, treatment should be continued for 2 to 3 days after all signs of infection have disappeared to prevent relapse.

Miconazole (e.g., Daktarin range, Daktacort Hydrocortisone)

Products containing miconazole only are suitable for patients of all ages and should be applied twice a day. Treatment should continue for 10 days after all lesions have disappeared to prevent relapse. Daktacort hydrocortisone is suitable for children over 10 years of age and is licensed for candidal intertrigo and athlete's foot.

Tolnaftate (e.g., Scholl Athlete's Foot range)

Products containing tolnaftate have no interactions or side effects and can be used by all patients. They can be used for athlete's foot and infections of the groin, and should be used twice a day with treatment continuing for at least 1 week after the infection has cleared up.

Undecenoates (e.g., Mycota)

Products containing undecenoates have no interactions and can be used by all patients. They are licensed for athlete's foot, and should be used twice a day and treatment continued for at least 1 week after the infection has cleared up. Local irritation has been reported.

Benzoic acid (e.g., Whitfield's ointment)

Benzoic acid (in combination with salicylic acid) is now rarely used. However, it is a safe medicine and can be used by all patients.

Terbinafine (Lamisil range & Scholl Advance Athlete's Foot Cream)

Terbinafine can be used to treat athlete's foot, groin infection and tinea corporis. The cream should be applied once or twice a day whereas the spray and gel should be used only once daily. It has no interactions, has few reported side effects and can be used by all patients. All products are licensed for people over 16 years of age, except Lamisil Once, which is for use in people over 18 years of age.

Griseofulvin (Grisol AF spray)

Licensed for athlete's foot, Grisol should be applied to the area once daily. Each spray delivers 400 µg of griseofulvin with a maximum of three sprays in 24 hours for more extensive or severe infection. The spray should be used for 10 days after the lesions clear to prevent reinfection. It has few reported side effects and can be used by all patients.

References

Aly R, Bayles CI, Oakes RA, et al. Topical griseofulvin in the treatment of dermatophytoses. Clin Exp Dermatol 1994;19:43–6.

Crawford F, Hollis S. Topical treatments for fungal infections of the skin and nails of the foot. Cochrane Database of Systematic Reviews 2007, Issue 3. Art. No.: CD001434. http://dx.doi.org/10.1002/14651858.CD001434.pub2.

El-Gohary M, van Zuuren EJ, Fedorowicz Z, et al. Topical antifungal treatments for tinea cruris and tinea corporis. Cochrane Database of Systematic Reviews 2014, Issue 8. Art. No.: CD009992. http://dx.doi.org/10.1002/14651858.CD009992.pub2

Further reading

Drake LA, Dinehart SM, Farmer ER, et al. Guidelines of care for superficial mycotic infections of the skin: tinea corporis, tinea cruris, tinea faciei, tinea manuum, and tinea pedis. Guidelines/Outcomes Committee. American Academy of Dermatology. J Am Acad Dermatol 1996;34:282–6.

Elewski B. Tinea capitis. Dermatol Clin 1996;14:23–31.

Moriarty B, Hay R, Morris-Jones R. The diagnosis and management of tinea. Brit Med J 2012;345:e4380.

Fungal nail infection (onychomycosis)

Background

The deregulation of amorolfine in the UK and other Western countries (e.g., Australia) now makes it possible for community pharmacists to treat infection affecting the toenails. Onychomycosis is defined as a chronic fungal infection of the fingernails or toenails, although only infection of the toenail is covered. The infection is common but probably underreported because of patient embarrassment or ignorance that they have an infection. If left untreated it can lead to pain and discomfort, which can make wearing shoes difficult. Nails, over time, will disfigure and crumble away.

Prevalence and epidemiology

It is estimated that 5–10% of the general population suffer from onychomycosis (Thomas et al., 2010). The incidence of infection increases with increasing age and is particularly common in people over 70 years of age (e.g., estimated at up to 50%).

Aetiology

Over 90% of cases are caused by dermatophytes (*Trichophyton rubrum* and *T. interdigitale*), with the remainder caused by yeasts and moulds. In most cases predisposing factors can be determined in the development of nail infection: for example, an initial skin infection (tinea pedis), in immunocompromised patients, or poor peripheral circulation and neuropathies (e.g., diabetes).

Arriving at a differential diagnosis

There are a number of different types of onychomycosis and it is important to be able to differentiate between them because amorolfine is only licensed for the treatment of distal lateral subungual onychomycosis. Taking a history of the presenting symptom will be helpful, but a visual inspection of the toenails is strongly advocated.

Clinical features of distal lateral subungual onychomycosis (DLSO)

DLSO is usually asymptomatic and people often seek medical help because of concerns about the appearance of the nail. The nail takes on a dull opaque and yellow appearance. Over time the nail thickens and distorts, and as infection spreads and worsens, the nail becomes brittle

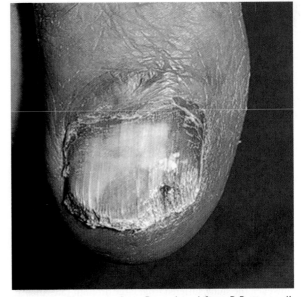

Fig. 8.15 Tinea unguium. Reproduced from P Buttaravoli, 2007, Minor Emergencies, 2nd edition, Elsevier Mosby with permission.

and crumbles away or falls off (Fig. 8.15). The key clinical symptoms that differentiate DLSO from other types of onychomycosis are summarised in Table 8.16.

Other conditions to eliminate

Psoriasis, eczema and trauma can affect the nail and need to be considered. In psoriasis nail pitting is visible; for trauma there should be an identifiable event that affected the nail; and in eczema and psoriasis the skin should be affected, either near and around the feet (eczema) or remotely (psoriasis plaques on areas such as knees and elbows).

Table 8.16
Main types of onychomycosis

Type	Key characteristics	Spread of infection
DLSO	Mainly big toe	Note yellowing starts at distal part of toe or side of nail
Proximal subungual onychomycosis (PCO)	Immunocompromised patients	Yellow spots appear at the base of the nail (i.e., in the half-moon area of the nail)
Superficial white onychomycosis	Often occurs in previously damaged nails. Chalky-white in appearance and can be scraped off the nail surface	Located on the surface of the nail

TRIGGER POINTS indicative of referral: DLSO

Symptoms/signs	Possible danger/reason for referral
Fungal infection other than DLSO	Requires medical confirmation and possible oral treatment
OTC treatment failure or suspected poor compliance	Suggests misdiagnosis or the need for oral treatment

HINTS AND TIPS BOX 8.4: CURANAIL

Why only two nails?	This is in line with UK guidance as more severe infections require systemic treatment (e.g., terbinafine)
Hygiene measures	• Keep the area clean • Change socks regularly • Avoid trauma to the nails • Avoid sharing towels

Evidence base for over-the-counter medication

Amorolfine is a broad-spectrum antifungal agent that works by inhibiting ergosterol synthesis. An open-labelled, non-randomised trial has shown it to be effective, producing clinical cure in 37% of toenail infections (Zaug, 1992). However, the study suffered from large dropout rates (nearly 30%), and there were no comparisons with other available topical antifungal treatments. A further trial comparing once- versus twice-weekly application of amorolfine reported similar cure rates (46%) with weekly application (Reinel, 1992). A Cochrane review found limited evidence for the efficacy of any topical treatments for nail infections, but suggested that cure rates may be better with amorolfine, although this suggestion was based on small trials (Crawford & Hollis, 2007). UK guidance (August 2015) advocates the use of amorolfine when the infection is mild and superficial.

Practical prescribing and product selection

Prescribing information relating to amorolfine is summarised in Table 8.17; useful tips relating to patients presenting with fungal nail infection are given in 'Hints and Tips' in Box 8.4.

Amorolfine (e.g., Loceryl Curanail)

Amorolfine is available as a 5% nail lacquer. It is used weekly and treatment lasts until the affected nail(s) have regrown and are clear of infection. This takes approximately 6 months for fingernails and 9 to 12 months for toenails. Each pack provides treatment for 3 months, which affords the pharmacist an opportunity to review treatment before further medication is given. The product license restricts use to no more than two nails in people over 18 years of age and who have no underlying medical conditions that predispose them to fungal infection (e.g., immunocompromised and diabetics). The manufacturer states it should not be used in pregnant or breastfeeding women. To apply amorolfine the nail must be first filed and cleaned. Files and cleaning pads are provided in the treatment pack and are not reusable. The lacquer should then be evenly applied and left to dry. Amorolfine is unlikely to cause side effects, but skin irritation has been reported.

References

Crawford F, Hollis S. Topical treatments for fungal infections of the skin and nails of the foot. Cochrane Database of Systematic Reviews 2007, Issue 3. Art. No.: CD001434. http://dx.doi.org/10.1002/14651858.CD001434.pub2.

Reinel D. Topical treatment of onychomycosis with amorolfine 5 per cent nail lacquer: comparative efficacy and tolerability of once and twice weekly use. Dermatology 1992;184(Suppl):21–4.

Thomas J, Jacobson GA, Narkowicz CK, et al. Toenail onychomycosis: an important global disease burden. J Clin Pharm Ther 2010;35(5):497–519.

Table 8.17
Practical prescribing: Summary of medicines for fungal nail infections

Name of medicine	Use in children	Likely side effects	Drug interactions of note	Patients in which care is exercised	Pregnancy & breastfeeding
Amorolfine	>18 years	Skin irritation (rare)	None	None	Manufacturers state to avoid, although evidence suggests it is safe to use

Zaug M, Bergstraesser M. Amorolfine in the treatment of
onychomycosis an dermatomycoses (an overview). Clin Exp
Dermatol 1992;179(Suppl. 1):61–70.

Further reading
Seebacher C, Brasch J, Abeck D, et al. Onychomycosis. JDDG
2007;1:61–6.
Finch JJ, Warshaw EM. Toenail onychomycosis: current
and future treatment options. Dermatol Ther
2007;20:31–46.

Website
For more images of fungal nail infection visit: http://www.
dermnetnz.org/fungal/onychomycosis.html

Hair loss (androgenetic alopecia)

Background

Each hair consists of a shaft made up of dead keratinised cells and a root (Fig. 8.1), and is found on most skin surfaces (palms of hands, soles of feet and lips being notable exceptions). Each hair follicle goes through a growth cycle, which consists of a long growing phase (anagen) followed by a short resting phase (telogen). At the end of the resting phase, the hair falls out (catagen) and a new hair starts growing in the follicle, beginning the cycle again. The hair cycle occurs randomly for each follicle so that normal hair loss from the adult scalp is approximately 100 hairs per day; where the rate is greater than this, clinical signs of hair loss can be observed. Hair loss affects both men and women, and is associated with strong emotional and psychological consequences. People have been socialised to link a full head of hair with youth and vitality, whereas baldness portrays a feeling of unattractiveness and loss of youth. Hair loss can be due to a number of aetiologies; however, this section concentrates on androgenetic alopecia (male-pattern baldness) because it is the most common cause of hair loss.

Prevalence and epidemiology

Men are more susceptible than women to androgenetic alopecia and usually experience more severe hair loss. Men tend to be affected from the second decade onwards (30% of men by 30 years old will be affected to some degree) and the prevalence of male pattern baldness in Caucasians who reach old age approaches 100%. Asian and Black men

are less prone to hair loss. In women the condition becomes more pronounced after menopause.

Patients usually have a positive family history. The nature and extent of hair loss will follow identical patterns to those seen in the patient's immediate parents and grandparents, which can be used as a predictor to the patient's potential hair-loss pattern.

Aetiology

Hair is classed as either terminal or vellus hair. Terminal hair is longer and thicker, and found on the scalp and eyebrows. Vellus hair covers the remainder of the body and is shorter and downy. In androgenetic alopecia terminal hair follicles transform into more vellus-like hair follicles as a result of preferential binding by dihydrotestosterone (produced from the conversion of androgen by 5-alpha-reductase) to hair follicle receptors. Eventually the follicle ceases activity completely, with resulting hair loss.

Arriving at a differential diagnosis

Hair loss is obviously easy to notice. Empathy and understanding towards the patient needs to be shown. Although androgenetic alopecia is the most common form of hair loss, other causes need to be eliminated (Table 8.18 and Fig. 8.16). Asking symptom-specific questions will help the pharmacist determine whether referral is needed (Table 8.19).

Clinical features of androgenetic alopecia

Men initially notice a thinning of the hair and a frontal receding hairline that might or might not be accompanied with hair loss at the crown. In women the frontal hairline is maintained with diffuse hair loss that is somewhat accentuated at the crown.

Table 8.18
Causes of hair loss and their relative incidence in community pharmacy

Incidence	Cause
Most likely	Androgenetic alopecia
Likely	Postpartum, stress, nutritional deficiency states, medicines
Unlikely	Alopecia areata, endocrine disorder
Very unlikely	Tinea capitis, traction alopecia, trichotillomania

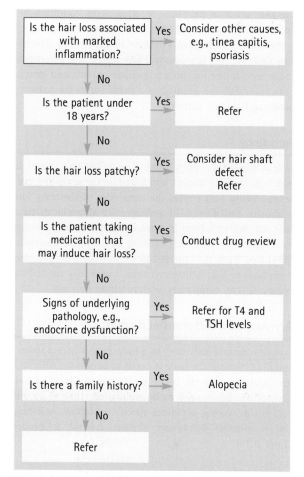

Fig. 8.16   Primer for differential diagnosis of hair loss.

Conditions to eliminate

Likely

Postpartum

During pregnancy, circulating levels of oestrogen increase, with a resulting rise in the number of follicles in anagen (growth phase); the hair therefore thickens. However, after delivery the hair follicles return to the resting phase and the hair is shed. Women might believe that they are experiencing hair loss when in reality the hair is returning to the normal pre-pregnancy state. Reassurance should be given that this is a temporary and self-limiting problem.

Stress

Stress is known to induce hair loss. The reason behind this is poorly understood. Enquiry to ascertain lifestyle factors that might have caused recent stress and anxiety to the patient should be explored.

Nutritional factors

Iron deficiency is associated with female hair loss. If iron deficiency is the cause, a 2-month course of iron supplementation should result in a thickening of the hair. If the patient fails to respond to treatment, then the patient should be reassessed.

Medicine-induced causes

Many medicines can interfere with the hair cycle and cause transient hair loss, cytotoxic medicines being one of the most obvious examples. However, many medicines have been associated with hair loss. Table 8.20 lists some of the more commonly implicated medicines. If medicines

---

Table 8.19
Specific questions to ask the patient: Hair loss

Question	Relevance
Hair loss accompanied with other symptoms	Androgenetic alopecia is not associated with other symptoms. Itch and/or erythema are indicators of another cause; e.g., fungal scalp infection, psoriasis or seborrhoeic dermatitis
Pattern of hair loss	In men hair loss begins at the front of the head and recedes backwards or at the crown. In women hair loss tends to be generalised and diffuse. Presentations that differ to this or are sudden in onset suggest another cause of hair loss
Medical and drug histories	There is now strong evidence that iron deficiency in women can cause hair loss. A number of endocrine conditions can cause hair loss, most notably thyroid disorders. A number of medicines can cause hair loss (Table 8.20)
Hair loss triggered by a specific event	Hair loss can be caused by a stressful event, or following surgery or after childbirth

Table 8.20
Medicines known to cause hair loss

Medicine or medicine class	Incidence of hair loss
Antineoplastics	Almost 100% (to varying degrees)
Anticoagulants	Telogen effluvium* in approximately 50%
Lithium carbonate	Telogen effluvium in approximately 10%
Interferons	Telogen effluvium in 20% to 30%
Oral contraceptives	Seen 2–3 months after stopping
Retinoids	Approximately 20% of patients
Colchicine, carbimazole	Rare

*Telogen effluvium – shift of more hairs into resting phase (telogen) of the hair cycle, which results in shedding of hair.

other than cytotoxics are suspected of causing hair loss, the prescriber should be contacted to discuss other possible treatment options.

Unlikely

Alopecia areata

Refers to hair loss of unknown origin, although there is often an association with atopy and autoimmune disease, and a positive family history is found in up to 25% of patients. It is relatively uncommon, affecting 0.1% to 0.2% of the UK population. Unlike androgenetic alopecia the hair loss is sudden and mainly affects children and adolescents (60% will have had their first episode before the age of 20). It is most commonly observed as patchy hair loss of sudden onset, although the whole scalp can be affected. The condition is usually self-limiting and regrowth of hair is often observed but repeated episodes are not unusual.

Underlying endocrine disorder

Hypothyroidism (and other endocrine disorders such as diabetes) can result in poor hair growth. In hypothyroidism the hair is thin and brittle, and the patient might be lethargic and have a history of recent weight gain. Referral to the doctor for blood tests should be considered.

Very unlikely causes

Fungal scalp infection (tinea capitis)

The first signs of infection are the appearance of a well-circumscribed round patch of alopecia that is associated with itch and scaling. Common areas of involvement include the occipital, parietal and crown regions. Inspection of the area might reveal erythema and 'black dots' on the scalp as a result of infected hairs.

Traction alopecia

Most commonly seen in women, traction alopecia refers to hair loss due to excess and sustained tension on the hair, usually as a result of styling hair with rollers or a particular type of hairstyle. It is reversible if the tension on the hair is removed.

Trichotillomania

Trichotillomania is a psychiatric disorder, which refers to patients who have an impulsive desire to twist and pull scalp hair, but often deny it. Hair loss is asymmetrical and an unusual shape. It would be very unusual for such patients to present to a community pharmacy.

! **TRIGGER POINTS indicative of referral: Hair loss**

Symptoms/signs	Possible danger/reason for referral
Patients under 18 years old Sudden onset	Unlikely to be androgenetic alopecia
Suspected iron deficiency anemia	Medical referral for blood test
Trichotillomania Fungal infection of the scalp Possible endocrine cause	All require further assessment and medical confirmation

Evidence base for over-the-counter medication

Currently, minoxidil is the only product marketed for androgenetic alopecia. It is available in 2% and 5% concentrations.

A number of clinical trials have investigated the efficacy and safety of minoxidil at both concentrations. The majority of these have been conducted on precisely the population that would respond the best to treatment; men between 18 to 50 years of age, with mild to moderate thinning of the hair at the vertex. Despite this, trial results are not totally convincing. Minoxidil is superior to placebo (although placebo does invoke a large initial response) and promotes a small increase in regrowth of vellus hair and increases the diameter of the hair shaft. However, longitudinal studies show that less than half of patients treated experience moderate to marked hair growth. Hair counts appear to be greatest after 12 months of treatment, but by 30 months hair counts have decreased (albeit still above baseline) and the bald area increases back in size to its initial diameter.

Minoxidil therefore appears to delay and slow down hair loss in less than half of its target patient population. Furthermore, if treatment is stopped, any hair growth achieved is lost within 6 to 8 weeks on discontinuation of therapy, and baldness returns to pretreatment levels.

The situation in women is not too dissimilar, although the 5% solution offers no advantage over the 2% solution and has therefore not been granted a product license at that strength.

Summary

Minoxidil will not significantly help the majority of balding individuals. It will promote hair growth in approximately 50% of minimally balding young men but, over time, the effect tails off. After 30 months the effect is still greater than baseline but, on the whole, will not achieve cosmetically acceptable hair growth. In other words, the use of minoxidil is useful for specific patients who want to 'buy' themselves time from the inevitable balding process.

Oral finasteride via the doctor (1 mg per day) can be used to treat androgenic alopecia in men, but currently there is no good-quality evidence that it is superior to minoxidil.

Practical prescribing and product selection

Prescribing information relating to minoxidil is discussed and summarised in Table 8.21; useful tips relating to the treatment of patients with minoxidil are given in 'Hints and Tips' in Box 8.5.

Minoxidil (e.g., Regaine range as either solution or foam)

The dose for minoxidil is 1 mL of solution (or 1 g of foam – equivalent to half a capful) applied to dry hair on the total affected areas of the scalp twice daily. If fingertips are used to facilitate drug application, hands should be washed afterwards. Although minoxidil is applied topically, absorption into the systemic circulation can occur and result in chest pain, rapid heartbeat, faintness or dizziness, although these are rare. If these occur the patient should stop using the product immediately. Other less important adverse effects associated with topical minoxidil are local irritation, redness and itching, but these appear to be related to the vehicle – propylene glycol – rather than minoxidil. Changes in blood pressure should not occur because the serum level of minoxidil after topical application is below the amount that is needed to cause changes to blood pressure; however, as a precaution minoxidil should be avoided in hypertensive patients if possible. Some patients also report a temporary increase in hair shedding 2 to 6 weeks after beginning treatment. This subsides and is most likely due to the action of minoxidil, shifting hairs from the resting telogen phase to the growing anagen phase.

Table 8.21
Practical prescribing: Summary of medicines for hair loss

Name of medicine	Use in children	Likely side effects (1% to 10% of patients)	Drug interactions of note	Patients in which care is exercised	Pregnancy & breastfeeding
Minoxidil (Regaine)	Not applicable	Skin irritation, headache	None	Avoid in patients with cardiovascular disease	Avoid

HINTS AND TIPS BOX 8.5: HAIR LOSS

Changes to hair colour and texture	Some patients have experienced changes in hair colour and/or texture with minoxidil use. The patient should be warned of this possible problem before using the product
How long should the patient use Regaine?	It can take 4 months or more before evidence of hair growth can be expected. Users should discontinue treatment if there is no improvement after 1 year

Further reading

Burke KE. Hair loss. What causes it and what can be done about it. Postgrad Med 1989;85:52–8, 67–73, 77.

Gilhar A, Etzioni, A, Paus R. Alopecia areata. N Engl J Med 2012;366:1515–25.

Katz HI, Hien NT, Prawer SE, et al. Long-term efficacy of topical minoxidil in male pattern baldness. J Am Acad Dermatol 1987;16:711–18.

Koperaki JA, Orenberg EK, Wilkinson DL. Topical minoxidil therapy for androgenetic alopecia: a 30 month study. Arch Dermatol 1987;123:1483–7.

Price VH, Menefee E, Strauss PC. Changes in hair weight and hair count in men with androgenetic alopecia, after application of 5% and 2% topical minoxidil, placebo, or no treatment. J Am Acad Dermatol 1999;41:717–21.

Rietschel RL, Duncan SH. Safety and efficacy of topical minoxidil in the management of androgenetic alopecia. J Am Acad Dermatol 1987;16:677–85.

Roberts JL. Androgenetic alopecia in men and women: an overview of cause and treatment. Dermatol Nurs 1997;9:379–88.

Tosti A, Misciali C, Piraccini BM, et al. Drug-induced hair loss and hair growth: incidence, management and avoidance. Drug Saf 1994;10:310–17.

van Zuuren EJ, Fedorowicz Z, Carter B, et al. Interventions for female pattern hair loss. Cochrane Database of Systematic Reviews 2012, Issue 5. Art. No.: CD007628. http://dx.doi.org/10.1002/14651858.CD007628.pub3.

Website

British Association of Dermatologists' guidelines for the management of alopecia areata. 2012. Available at: http://www.bad.org.uk/library-media%5Cdocuments%5CAlopecia_areata_guidelines_2012.pdf

Warts and verrucas

Background

Warts and verrucas are benign growths of the skin caused by the human papilloma virus (HPV). Certain types of HPV have an affinity for certain body locations, for example, the hands, face, anogenital region and feet. Spontaneous resolution is seen in 30% of people within 6 months and two-thirds of cases within 2 years. Despite their self-limiting nature they are cosmetically unacceptable to many patients and with nearly 60% of people trying an OTC treatment before visiting a doctor, the pharmacist has a major role to play in their management.

Prevalence and epidemiology

The prevalence of warts has not been accurately documented, and published prevalence data vary widely. Children are most affected, with 2–20% experiencing symptoms before the age of 16. Warts are uncommon in infants and in the elderly, and caution should be exercised if an elderly patient presents to the pharmacy with a self-diagnosed wart.

Aetiology

HPV gains entry to the host by epithelial defects in the epidermis. It is transmitted by direct skin-to-skin contact, although contact with an infected person's shed skin can also transmit the virus. Infection via the environment is more likely to occur if the skin is macerated and in contact with roughened surfaces, for example in swimming pools and communal washing areas. Once established in the epithelial cells, the virus stimulates basal cell division to produce the characteristic lesion.

Patients, especially children, should be warned not to pick, bite or scratch warts as this can allow viral particle shedding to penetrate skin breaks. This process is known as autoinoculation and is responsible for multiple lesions becoming established and transferred to other parts of the body.

Arriving at a differential diagnosis

Warts and verrucas are not difficult to diagnose. However, pharmacists must be able to recognise other similar conditions that superficially look like warts and verrucas (Table 8.22). Asking symptom-specific questions will help the pharmacist establish a differential diagnosis (Table 8.23). HPV infections involving the anogenital area are outside the remit of community pharmacists and must be referred.

Table 8.22
Causes of wart-like lesions and their relative incidence in community pharmacy

Incidence	Cause
Most likely	Common warts and verrucas
Likely	Corns, molluscum contagiosum
Unlikely	Plane warts, seborrhoeic keratosis
Very unlikely	Basal cell carcinoma

Table 8.23
Specific questions to ask the patient: Human papilloma virus

Question	Relevance
Age of patient	Warts are unusual in very young children, e.g., infants. Young children and adolescents are most likely to get warts but this is also the age group in which molluscum contagiosum is most prevalent The likelihood that nodular lesions are caused by seborrhoeic warts or carcinoma increases with increasing age
Location	Warts are common on the hands and knees; verrucas are usually on the weight-bearing parts of the sole Warts can occur on the face but so too can plane warts and carcinoma. Referral is always needed as all OTC treatments can cause scarring
Associated symptoms	Itching and bleeding is not associated with warts and verrucas, and must be viewed with suspicion, especially in older patients Pain on walking is often associated with verrucas
Colour/appearance	Typically warts have a 'cauliflower' appearance and are raised and pale Warts with a reddish hue or that change colour should be referred Lesions that are raised, smooth and have a central 'dimple' suggests molluscum contagiosum

Clinical features of warts and verrucas

Warts

Warts most often occur on the backs of the hands, fingers and knees, either singly or in crops. When examined the wart appears as a raised, hyperkeratotic papule with thrombosed, black vessels often visible as black dots within the wart. They tend to be rough textured, skin-coloured and are usually less than 1 cm in diameter (Fig. 8.17).

Verrucas

Verrucas are found on the soles of the feet, usually in weight-bearing areas, for example, on the metatarsal heads or heel. Owing to constant pressure imparted on the sole of the foot the normal outward expansion of the wart is thwarted and instead grows inward. Pressure on nerves can then cause considerable pain, and patients often complain of pain when walking. Inspection of the lesion will normally reveal tiny black dots (thrombosed capillaries) on the surface (Fig. 8.18). Owing to keratin build-up this characteristic sign might not be visible unless the hardened skin is first shaved away. Verrucas, like warts, are rarely larger than 1 cm in diameter and can occur singly or in crops. A number of closely located plantar warts can coalesce to form a large single plaque and is termed a 'mosaic wart'.

Conditions to eliminate

Likely causes

Molluscum contagiosum

Molluscum contagiosum primarily affects children under 5 years old. It is not particularly common and a doctor

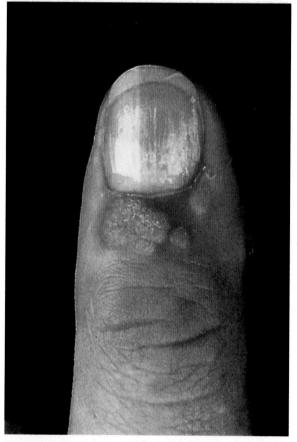

Fig. 8.17 Common wart. Reproduced from J Wilkinson et al 2004, Dermatology in Focus, Churchill Livingstone, with permission.

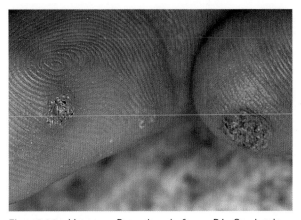

Fig. 8.18 Verruca. Reproduced from DJ Gawkrodger, 2007, Dermatology: An Illustrated Colour Text, 4th edition, Churchill Livingstone, with permission.

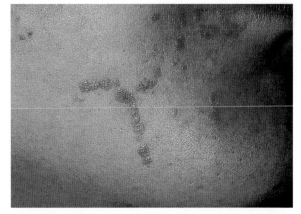

Fig. 8.19 Plane warts. Reproduced from DJ Gawkrodger, 2007, Dermatology: An Illustrated Colour Text, 4th edition, Churchill Livingstone, with permission.

with a list size of 2000 will probably see 5 new cases per year. It is caused by a pox virus and patients present with multiple lesions usually on the face and neck, although the trunk can be involved. The lesions resemble common warts but each raised papule tends to be smooth and have a central dimple, the latter is a useful diagnostic point (see Fig. 10.6, page 322). Lesions tend to be between 1 and 5 mm in diameter. The condition is self-limiting and will resolve without medical intervention. Patients should be told this, but if they believe treatment is necessary, referral to the doctor is advisable.

Corns

Corns and plantar warts can be confused. The reader is referred to page 251 on corns and calluses for information on differentiating corns from verrucas.

Unlikely causes

Plane warts (flat warts or verruca plana)

These most frequently occur in groups on the face and the back of the hands. They are small in size (1–5 mm in diameter), slightly raised and can take on the skin colour of the patient (Fig. 8.19). As drug treatment is destructive in nature, plane warts located on the face should be referred to avoid the risk of scarring.

Basal cell papilloma (seborrhoeic wart)

Basal cell papillomas are benign growths that are increasingly common with increasing age. They usually occur on the trunk and present as raised, often multiple lesions that have a superficial 'stuck on' or waxy appearance (Fig. 8.20). Lesions are usually brown but can range in colour from pink to black.

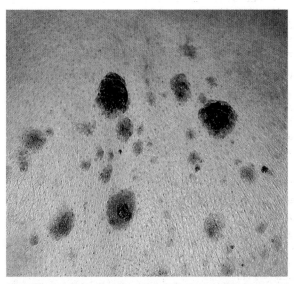

Fig. 8.20 Seborrhoeic wart. Reproduced from DJ Gawkrodger, 2007, Dermatology: An Illustrated Colour Text, 4th edition, Churchill Livingstone, with permission.

Very unlikely causes

Basal cell carcinoma

Basal cell carcinoma is the most common form of skin cancer and its incidence is related to sunlight exposure. It typically occurs in older people, especially where there is a history of prolonged skin exposure. Men are twice as likely to be affected. The usual site where lesions develop is the face. Any wart-like lesion that is itchy, has an irregular outline, is prone to bleeding and exhibits colour change should be referred to eliminate serious pathology. For more information on skin cancers see page 269.

> **TRIGGER POINTS indicative of referral: Warts and verrucae**
>
> | | |
> |---|---|
> | Anogenital warts | Outside scope of OTC treatment |
> | Multiple and widespread warts | |
> | Diabetic patients | Treatment options can cause skin damage |
> | Lesions on the face | |
> | Patients over 50 years of age presenting with a first-time wart | Potential sinister pathology |
> | Warts that itch or bleed without provocation | |
> | Warts that have grown and changed colour | |

Evidence base for over-the-counter medication

A number of ingredients are used to treat warts and verrucas, although salicylic acid is the most commonly used agent and can be found in many OTC treatments, both alone and combined with lactic acid.

A recent Cochrane review (Kwok et al., 2012) investigated topical treatments for treating non-genital warts. This review identified 85 trials that included a range of different treatments. Overall, the quality of the trials was low due to poor methodology and reporting. Those that investigated salicyclic acid showed it to be more effective than placebo and comparable to cryotherapy in treating verrucas.

Salicylic acid is often combined with other ingredients, in particular lactic acid. However, there is no evidence to support greater efficacy when lactic acid (or other ingredients) is added.

Other agents commercially available include formaldehyde, glutaraldehyde and silver nitrate pencils. Information regarding their effectiveness stems from small-scale or poorly designed studies, and they should not be routinely recommended.

Compliance with treatment has been identified as a limiting factor in the cure rate for warts and verrucas. One study that investigated Occlusal (salicyclic acid 50%) reported an 80% cure rate after only 2 weeks of therapy. This might be an alternative option for patients whose compliance could be questioned. However, the study suffered from poor design and had only a small number of patients, so the results must be viewed with caution.

Cryotherapy using liquid nitrogen has been used for many years as a treatment of recalcitrant or widespread warts. Trials comparing cryotherapy with salicylic acid show benefit of cryotherapy for hand warts but not verrucas (Kwok et al., 2012). It should be noted that this review did not consider OTC freezing treatments that contain dimethyl ether and propane (e.g., Wartner). It has been reported elsewhere that these are not as effective as liquid nitrogen, as they only achieve temperatures of around $-57\,°C$ compared with $-196\,°C$ (Lynch et al., 2014).

Summary

Any salicylic acid-based product should have modest success rates in clearing warts and verrucas after a 12-week treatment period, providing patient compliance is good. If treatment has been unsuccessful with salicylic acid, then a second-line medicine such as glutaraldehyde or formaldehyde could be tried. Cryotherapy should be performed through the doctor and OTC 'freezing' products avoided due to the adverse side effects associated with their use.

Practical prescribing and product selection

Prescribing information relating to specific products used to treat warts and verrucas in the section 'Evidence base for over-the-counter medication' is summarised in Table 8.24; useful tips relating to patients presenting with warts and verrucas are given in 'Hints and Tips' in Box 8.6.

As the majority of warts and verrucas will spontaneously resolve, treatment is not necessarily needed. Pharmacists should determine from the patient how much the wart or verruca affects day-to-day life and also what social impact the lesions have on the patient. It is also worth assessing patient motivation to comply with medication regimens because treatment is over a period of months, not days or weeks.

Salicylic acid products (e.g., Bazuka Extra Strength (26%), Occlusal (50%), Verrugon (50%)) & Salicylic acid/lactic acid combinations (Bazuka, Cuplex, Duofilm, Salactol, Salactac)

Before using a salicylic acid-based product, the affected area should be soaked in warm water and towelled dry. The surface of the wart or verruca should be rubbed with a pumice stone or emery board to remove any hard skin. This should be done at least once per week. A few drops of the product should be applied to the lesion, taking care to localise the application to the affected area. The procedure should be repeated daily. Salicylic acid can be recommended to most patients, although diabetics are a notable exception. Salicylic

Table 8.24
Practical prescribing: Summary of medicines for warts and verrucas

Name of medicine	Use in children	Likely side effects	Drug interactions of note	Patients in which care is exercised	Pregnancy & breastfeeding
Salicylic acid					
Compound W	>6 years	Local skin irritation	None	Avoid in diabetic patients	OK
Bazuka Extra Strength	>2 years				
Occlusal	No lower age stated				
Verrugon					
Wartex					
Salicylic acid and lactic acid					
Bazuka	>2 years	Local skin irritation	None	Avoid in diabetic patients	OK
Cuplex	No lower age stated				
Duofilm	>2 years				
Salactol	No lower age stated				
Salatac					
Glutaraldehyde					
Glutarol	No lower age stated	Local skin irritation. Skin will be stained brown	None	Avoid in diabetic patients	OK
Formaldehyde					
Veracur	No lower age stated	No local affects reported	None	Avoid in diabetic patients	Pregnancy Manufacturer advises avoidance, although there are no reports of teratogenicity Breastfeeding OK
Silver nitrate	No lower age stated	Local skin irritation	None	Avoid in diabetic patients	OK

acid does not interact with any medicines. It can cause local skin irritation and because of its destructive action should be kept away from unaffected skin.

Glutaraldehyde (Glutarol)

Application of glutaraldehyde is the same as salicylic acid but it should be used twice a day. It can cause skin irritation and stains the outer layer of the skin brown.

Formaldehyde (Veracur)

Veracur, like glutaraldehyde, is applied twice a day. In all other respects it has the same side effects and precautions for use as salicylic acid.

Silver nitrate (e.g., Avoca)

To use silver nitrate pencils the tip must be first moistened and then applied to the wart or verruca for 1 to 2 minutes.

HINTS AND TIPS BOX 8.6: VERRUCAS AND WARTS

Is it a verruca or a corn?	If diagnosis is uncertain, then removal of the top layer of skin from the lesion can be performed. If black spots are not visible this implies the lesion is a corn and not a verruca
Length of treatment	Patients should be told that it is a slow process. Treatment commonly lasts 3 months. If OTC medication has been unsuccessful after this time, then the patient could be referred to the GP
Cure rates	There is some evidence that resolution might be enhanced by soaking the wart or verruca before application and/or occlusion of the site (by use of plasters or collodion-like vehicle) to aid penetration
Bazuka and Bazuka Extra Strength	Do not be fooled into thinking the extra strength has better cure rates. It has a higher concentration of salicylic acid (26% as opposed to 12%), but this does not necessarily equate to a more efficacious product
Salatac gel	The gel forms an elastic film after application. This has to be removed each time before the gel can be reapplied

This should be repeated after 24 hours. It is recommended that three applications are used for warts and six applications for verrucas. Like other treatments the process is destructive and the surrounding skin should be protected.

References

Kwok CS, Gibbs S, Bennett C, et al. Topical treatments for cutaneous warts. Cochrane Database of Systematic Reviews 2012, Issue 9. Art. No.: CD001781. http://dx.doi.org/10.1002/14651858.CD001781.pub3.

Lynch MD, Cliffe J, Morris-Jones R. Management of cutaneous viral warts. Brit Med J 2014; 348 http://dx.doi.org/10.1136/bmj.g3339.

Further reading

Dall'oglio F, D'Amico V, Nasca MR, et al. Treatment of cutaneous warts: an evidence-based review. Am J Clin Dermatol 2012;13(2):73–96.

Hirose R, Hori M, Shukuwa T, et al. Topical treatment of resistant warts with glutaraldehyde. J Dermatol 1994;21:248–53.

Johnson LW. Communal showers and the risk of plantar warts. J Fam Pract 1995;40:136–8.

Steele K, Shirodaria P, O'Hare M, et al. Monochloroacetic acid and 60% salicylic acid as a treatment for simple plantar warts: effectiveness and mode of action. Br J Dermatol 1988;118:537–43.

Yazar S, Basaran E. Efficacy of silver nitrate pencils in the treatment of common warts. J Dermatol 1994;21:329–33.

Website

British Association of Dermatologists – information on cutaneous warts: http://www.bad.org.uk/library-media%5Cdocuments%5CWarts_2014.pdf

Corns and calluses

Background

Foot disorders can be broadly subdivided into either those that result from opportunistic infection or those that result from incorrect distribution of pressure. This section discusses the latter.

Prevalence and epidemiology

The exact prevalence of corns and calluses is not known. Surveys have indicated that up to 18% of working people complain of corns and calluses (Springett et al., 2003). Corns and calluses tend to more often be seen in older patients (useful tips relating to patients presenting with corns are given in 'Hints and Tips' in Box 8.7).

Aetiology

Corns form due to a combination of friction and intermittent pressure against one of the bony prominences of the feet (e.g., heel and metatarsal heads). Inappropriate footwear is frequently the cause. Continued pressure and

HINTS AND TIPS BOX 8.7: CORNS

Shoes to relieve pressure	Patients should be encouraged to wear open shoes such as sandals or thongs

friction results in hyperkeratoses (excessive skin growth of the keratinised layer), leaving even less space between the shoe and the foot, and therefore the corn is pressed even more firmly against the underlying soft tissues and bone.

Callus formation is also caused by constant friction and pressure. Calluses can be beneficial, providing a natural barrier to objects and protecting underlying tissues; however, when such a thickened mass of skin occurs in abnormal places (e.g., border of the big toe) pain is experienced.

Arriving at a differential diagnosis

Diagnosis of corns and calluses is best done by appearance. Pharmacists should therefore ask to inspect the person's feet.

Differential diagnosis should be straightforward and is usually between corns, calluses and verruca. Most patients will accurately self-diagnose and seek advice and help to remedy the situation. The pharmacist's role will be to confirm the self-diagnosis and give advice and/or treatment where appropriate. Asking symptom-specific questions will help the pharmacist determine the best course of action (Table 8.25).

Clinical features of corns

Corns (helomas) have been classified into a number of types, although only soft and hard corns are commonly met in practice. Hard corns (heloma durum) are generally located on the top of the toes. Corns exhibit a central core of hard grey skin surrounded by a painful, raised, yellow ring of inflammatory skin. Any of the toes can be affected but is most common on the second toe. Soft corns (heloma molle) form between the toes rather than on the tops of toes and are due to pressure exerted by one toe against another. They have a whitened appearance and remain soft due to moisture being present between the toes causing maceration of the corn. Soft corns are most common in the fourth web space.

Clinical features of calluses

Calluses, depending on the cause and site involved, can range in size from a few millimetres to centimetres. They appear as flattened, yellow–white thickened skin. In women the balls of the feet are a common site. Other sites that can be affected are the heel and lower border of the big toe. Patients frequently complain of a burning sensation, resulting from fissuring of the callus.

Conditions to eliminate

Verrucas

Verrucas can be mistaken for a corn or callus, although verrucas tend to have a spongy texture with the central area showing tiny black spots. They are also rarely located on or between the toes and commonly occur in younger patients than do corns and calluses. For further information see page 246.

Bunions

Bunions are 10 times more common in women than in men and are directly related to wearing tight shoes. Initially, irritation of skin by ill-fitting shoes causes bursitis of the big toe. Over time the inflamed area begins to harden and subsequently bursal fluid solidifies into a gelatinous

Table 8.25 Specific questions to ask the patient: Corn/callus	
Question	Relevance
Location	Lesions on the tops or between the toes suggest a corn compared with verrucas, which are on the plantar surface of the foot
Aggravating or relieving factors	Pain experienced with corns is a result of pressure between footwear and the toes. If footwear is taken off, then the pain is relieved Pain associated with verrucas will be felt irrespective if footwear is worn
Appearance	Corns and calluses appear as white or yellow hyperkeratinised areas of skin unlike verrucas, which show black thrombosed capillaries seen as black dots on the surface of the verruca
Previous history	Patients with corns will often have a previous history of foot problems. The cause is usually due to poorly fitting shoes, such as high heels. Prolonged wear of such footwear can lead to calluses and permanent deformity of bunions

mass. The result will be a bunion joint (the first meta-tarsal phalangeal joint). Patients often complain of pain and have difficulty in walking and while wearing normal shoes. Referral to a podiatrist is recommended.

> ⚠ **TRIGGER POINTS indicative of referral: Corns and calluses**

Symptoms/signs	Possible danger/reason for referral
Discomfort/pain is causing difficulty in walking	Better assessed and managed by a podiatrist
There is impaired peripheral circulation, e.g., diabetes	
Soft corns are present	
There is treatment failure	

Evidence base for over-the-counter medication

Corns and calluses are due to friction and pressure. Removal of the precipitating factors will result in resolution of the problem. Therefore preventative measures should form the mainstay of treatment. Correctly fitting shoes are essential to help prevent corn and callus formation. If pressure and friction still persist when correctly fitted shoes are worn, then patients can obtain relief by shielding or padding. Moleskin or thin podiatry felt placed around the corn allows pressure to be transferred from the corn to the padding. Specific proprietary products are available for such purposes. In callus formation a 'shock absorbing' insert such as a metatarsal pad is useful to relieve weight off the callus and so reduces stress on the plantar skin.

Treatment should be avoided if possible but if deemed appropriate keratolytics can be used, although there is no evidence to suggest that they are effective.

Practical prescribing and product selection

Products used to treat corns and calluses are exactly the same as those used for warts and verrucas. Prescribing information relating to specific products used to treat corns and calluses is therefore discussed in the section 'Evidence base for over-the-counter medication for warts and verrucas' on page 248. However, a number of proprietary products are marketed for sufferers with corns and calluses, for example, products in the Carnation and Scholl range. These products contain high concentrations of salicylic acid (usually 50%) that are surrounded by a non-medicated self-adhesive ring.

Reference
Springett K, Whiting M, Marriott C. Epidemiology of plantar forefoot corns and callus, and the influence of dominant side. The Foot 2003;13:5–9.

Further reading
Robbins JM. Recognizing, treating and preventing common foot problems. Cleve Clin Jnl Med 2000;67:45–56.
Silfverskiold JP. Common foot problems. Relieving the pain of bunions, keratoses, corns and calluses. Postgrad Med 1991;89:183–8.

Scabies

Background

Scabies can be defined as a pruritic skin condition caused by the mite *Sarcoptes scabiei*. It is easily missed or mis-diagnosed as dermatitis. The diagnostic burrows are small and scratching often makes them difficult to see.

Prevalence and epidemiology

The incidence of scabies in the UK is low (0.1% of the population) but epidemics can occur on a cyclical basis approximately every 15 to 20 years. Outbreaks in schools and care homes are not uncommon. In temperate climates (e.g., the UK), it appears to be more prevalent in urban areas and in the winter months.

Aetiology

The mite is transmitted by direct physical contact (e.g., holding hands, hugging or sexual contact). Mating occurs on the skin surface after which the female mite burrows into the stratum corneum to lay eggs. The faecal pellets she leaves in the burrow cause a local hypersensitivity reaction and is assumed to cause the release of inflammatory mediators that trigger an allergic reaction invoking intense itching. This normally takes 15 to 20 days in a primary infestation but can take up to 6 weeks to develop. In subsequent infestations this hypersensitivity reaction develops much more quickly. During the asymptomatic period the mite can be passed onto others unknowingly. The eggs hatch and mature in 14 days after which the cycle can begin again.

Arriving at a differential diagnosis

A definitive diagnosis of scabies is confirmed by extraction of the mite from its burrow, although in primary care this is rarely performed and a differential diagnosis is made

Table 8.26
Causes of scabies-like rash and their relative incidence in community pharmacy

Incidence	Cause
Most likely	Insect bites, allergic contact dermatitis
Likely	Scabies
Unlikely	Pompholyx
Very unlikely	Dermatitis herpetiformis

Table 8.27
Specific questions to ask the patient: Scabies

Question	Relevance
Visible signs of the mite	Burrows, which are up to 1 cm long and blue–grey in colour, might be visible although in practice this characteristic is often not present. For the pharmacist who will only see a limited number of cases, it is best to concentrate on other clinical signs rather than attempt to look for signs of burrows
Location of rash	Scabies classically affects the finger webs, the sides of the fingers and wrists
History of presenting complaint	If contact dermatitis is suspected, then questioning should reveal a past history of similar skin lesions Often people with scabies will be care workers looking after institutionalised people A positive history in other family members increases the likelihood that the patient has scabies

on clinical appearance, patient history and symptoms reported by close family. Confusion can arise from mistaking scabies for other pruritic skin disorders (Table 8.26). Asking symptom-specific questions will help the pharmacist establish a differential diagnosis (Table 8.27).

Clinical features of scabies

Severe pruritus, especially at night, is the hallmark symptom of scabies. Besides the classic location of lesions, in men the penile and scrotal skin, and in women beneath the breasts and nipples can be affected. Infants who are not

yet walking may have marked sole involvement. The rash is usually made up of small red papules that can change into vesicles over time.

Conditions to eliminate

Likely cause

Insect bites
A host of insects, fleas and mites can inflict a bite or sting. This usually results in an itchy papule that can become firm and last several days. Occasionally, the rash can become blistered, normally as a result of scratching, and secondary bacterial infection can occur. Bites often tend to be in groups and are asymmetrical. See page 345 for further information.

Allergic contact dermatitis
The condition presents as an area of inflamed, itchy skin with either papules or vesicles being present. However, enquiry in to the patient's history should reveal a past history of similar lesions in allergic contact dermatitis. For further information on dermatitis see page 262.

Unlikely cause

Dyshidrotic eczema (pompholyx)
Pompholyx simply means bubble, and refers to the presence of intensely itchy vesicles or blisters on the palms of the hands (and occasionally on the soles of the feet). Stress and heat are known to precipitate the condition.

Very unlikely cause

Dermatitis herpetiformis
Dermatitis herpetiformis is a condition characterised by intense itchy clusters of papules and vesicles. It is more often seen in middle-aged people, especially in men. It commonly involves the buttocks, elbows, knees and sacral region, with hand involvement being rare. The lesions usually exhibit a symmetrical distribution. On investigation up to 90% of patients are found to have a gluten enteropathy.

! TRIGGER POINTS indicative of referral: Scabies

Symptoms/signs	Possible danger/ reason for referral
Secondary infection of the skin	May require antibiotics
Severe and extensive symptoms Institutional outbreaks Suspected dermatitis herpetiformis	Outside scope of community pharmacy

Evidence base for over-the-counter medication

The efficacy and safety of scabicidal agents is difficult to determine due to limited trial data. Benzyl benzoate, crotamiton, permethrin and malathion have all been used. A Cochrane review (Strong & Johnstone, 2007) found permethrin to have high cure rates and be more effective than any other scabicidal agent.

The efficacy of malathion is questionable, as no randomised controlled trials appear to have been conducted. However, case reports have suggested malathion is effective in curing scabies, with a cure rate of approximately 80%.

Benzyl benzoate has been used to treat scabies for many years. However, its efficacy has not been demonstrated in randomised controlled trials. In uncontrolled trials benzyl benzoate has been shown to provide cure rates of approximately 50%.

Practical prescribing and product selection

Prescribing information relating to specific products used to treat scabies in the section 'Evidence base for over-the-counter medication' is discussed and summarised in Table 8.28; useful tips relating to patients presenting with scabies are given in 'Hints and Tips' in Box 8.8.

It is important that all people in the same household and in close contact with the affected are treated at the same time to prevent reinfection, even though they might be asymptomatic (latent period before itch develops). **Permethrin is the drug of choice**, although all products used to treat scabies can be given to all patient groups and have no drug interactions.

Permethrin (Lyclear Dermal Cream)

General guidance for application of Lyclear is that adults and children over 12 should use up to a full tube as a single application. Some adults might need to use more than one tube to ensure total body coverage, but a maximum of two tubes (60 g in total) is recommended for a single application. For children under 12 years of age the manufacturers suggest the following: ¼ tube for those 2 months to 5 years of age and ½ tube for those between 6 and 12 years of age. The whole body should be washed thoroughly 8 to 12 hours after treatment. Treatment should be repeated after 7 days.

Malathion (Derbac M)

The liquid can be used on adults and children over 6 months old and is left on for 24 hours. If hands or any other parts of the body must be washed during this period,

Table 8.28
Practical prescribing: Summary of medicines for scabies

Name of medicine	Use in children	Likely side effects	Drug interactions of note	Patients in which care is exercised	Pregnancy & breastfeeding
Permethrin	>2 years	Burning, stinging or tingling	None	None	OK
Benzyl benzoate	>12 years	Burning, irritation			
Malathion	>6 months	Skin irritation but rare			

HINTS AND TIPS BOX 8.8: SCABIES

Application	UK guidelines state that treatment should be applied to the whole body including the scalp, neck, face and ears. This is at odds with some manufacturer's data
Itching after treatment	Pruritus can persist for 2–3 weeks after treatment and the patient might benefit from crotamiton. Antihistamines appear to have a limited role in relieving itch but their sedative effect (e.g., chlorphenamine) might be useful for temporary help in aiding sleep
Hygiene measures	Clothes, towels and bed linen should be machine washed (at 50 °C or above) at the time of the first application of treatment to prevent reinfestation and transmission to others
Bathing	Treatment should not be applied after a hot bath because this increases systemic absorption and removes the drug from its treatment site

the treatment must be reapplied to those areas immediately. Treatment should be repeated after 7 days.

Benzyl benzoate

Benzyl benzoate should not be routinely recommended but if used it is for adult use only. Dosing (as per BNF 70) is that it should be applied to the whole body and repeated the following day. A third application may be required in some cases. It causes skin irritation and a transient burning sensation in approximately 25% of patients. This is usually mild but can occasionally be severe in sensitive individuals. In the event of a severe skin reaction the preparation should be washed off using soap and warm water. It is also irritating to the eyes, which should be protected if it is applied to the scalp.

Reference

Strong M, Johnstone P. Interventions for treating scabies. Cochrane Database of Systematic Reviews 2007, Issue 3. Art. No.: CD000320. http://dx.doi.org/10.1002/14651858. CD000320.pub2.

Further reading

Angarano DW, Parish LC. Comparative dermatology: parasitic disorders. Clin Dermatol 1994;12:543–50.
Buffet M, Dupin N. Current treatments for scabies. Fundam Clin Pharmacol 2003;17:217–25.
Burgess I, Robinson R, Robinson J, et al. Aqueous malathion 0.5% as a scabicide: clinical trial. Br Med J 1986;292:1172.
Chosidow O. Clinical practices. Scabies. N Engl J Med 2006;354:1718–27.
FitzGerald D, Grainger RJ, Reid A. Interventions for preventing the spread of infestation in close contacts of people with scabies. Cochrane Database of Systematic Reviews 2014, Issue 2. Art. No.: CD009943. http://dx.doi.org/10.1002/14651858.CD009943.pub2.
Glaziou P, Cartel JL, Alzieu P, et al. Comparison of ivermectin and benzyl benzoate for treatment of scabies. Trop Med Parasitol 1993;44:331–2.
Hanna NF, Clay JC, Harris JR. Sarcoptes scabiei infestation treated with malathion liquid. Br J Vener Dis 1978;54:354.
Heukelbach J, Feldmeier H. Scabies. Lancet 2006;367:1767–74.
Johnston G, Sladden M. Scabies: diagnosis and treatment. Br Med J 2005;331:619–22.

Acne vulgaris

Background

Acne can be defined as an inflammatory disease of the pilosebaceous follicles, causing comedones, papules and pustules on the face (99% of cases), chest (60%) and upper back (15%). It affects approximately 80% of adolescents. Diagnosis is usually straightforward and most patients presenting in the community pharmacy will generally be seeking appropriate advice on correct product selection rather than wanting someone to put a name to their rash. The majority of cases seen in the pharmacy setting will be mild and can be managed appropriately without referral to the doctor. However, more persistent and severe cases need referral for more potent topical or systemic treatment. Acne often causes significant psychological impact such as lack of confidence, low self-esteem and depression.

Prevalence and epidemiology

Acne lesions develop at the onset of puberty. Girls therefore tend to develop acne at an earlier age than boys. The peak incidence for girls is between the ages of 14 and 17, compared with 15 to 19 years of age for boys. Recent evidence shows that the average age when acne develops has decreased by 1 year over the last 30 years from 15.8 years old in 1979 to 15 in 2007 (Goldberg et al., 2011). Although acne is closely associated with adolescence, up to 12% of women and 3% of men aged 25 to 40 either continue to get facial acne or develop acne (late-onset acne) after adolescence. Acne persists in a very small proportion of patients (5% of women and 1% of men) into their forties. There might be a familial tendency to acne, and it is slightly more common in boys, who also experience more severe involvement. In addition, white patients are more likely to experience moderate to severe acne than black patients, although black skin is prone to worse scarring.

Aetiology

At the onset of puberty a cascade of events takes place resulting in the formation of noninflammatory and inflammatory lesions. In response to increased testosterone levels, the pilosebaceous gland begins to produce sebum (if the sebaceous glands become oversensitive to testosterone, they produce excess oil and the skin becomes greasy; a hallmark of acne). At the same time epithelial cells lining the follicle undergo change. Before puberty dead cells are shed smoothly out of the ductal opening but at puberty this process is disrupted, and in patients with acne these cells develop abnormal cohesion and partially block the opening and effectively reduce sebum outflow. Over time the opening of the duct becomes blocked, trapping oil in the hair follicle. Bacteria, particularly *Propionibacterium acnes*, proliferate in the stagnant oil, stimulating cytokine production, which in turn produces local inflammation, leading to the appearance of a spot. In response to the proliferation of bacteria, white blood cells infiltrate the area to kill the bacteria and in turn die leading to pus formation. The pustule eventually bursts on the skin surface, carrying the plug away. The whole process can then start again.

Arriving at a differential diagnosis

Only about 30% of people with acne consult their doctor – the pharmacist therefore plays an important role in the management of patients with acne. The first step in the management of acne is to assess severity, as this will shape management decisions. Several rating scales have been developed with the aim of trying to grade the severity of an individual's condition. None have gained universal acceptance, although most dermatology texts simply grade the severity of acne into mild, moderate or severe. Table 8.29 describes mild, moderate and severe acne presentations. OTC treatment should be limited to those patients with mild to moderate acne.

Clinical features of mild acne vulgaris

Patients suffering from mild acne characteristically have predominately open and closed comedones with a small number of active lesions normally confined to the face (Fig. 8.21). Acne can sometimes consist predominately of blackheads and whiteheads with very few inflammatory lesions. This is termed comedonal acne and occurs most commonly in Asian and Afro-Caribbean patients. Certain jobs can also predispose patients to acne-like lesions and are commonly associated with long-term contact with oils.

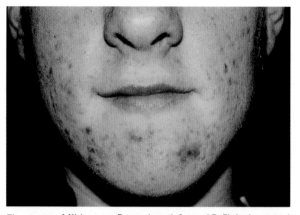

Fig. 8.21 Mild acne. Reproduced from AB Fleischer et al 2000, 20 Common Problems in Dermatology, with permission of the McGraw-Hill Companies.

Conditions to eliminate

Rosacea

Rosacea is an inflammatory disease of the skin follicles. It is uncertain what causes rosacea, although successful treatment with antibiotics suggests that bacterial pathogens play a significant role in the disease. It is normally seen in patients over 40 years of age and is more common in women than in men. It is classically characterised by recurrent flushing and blushing of the central face, especially the nose and medial cheeks. Crops of inflammatory papules and pustules are also a common feature, although comedones are not present (Fig. 8.22). Eye irritation and blepharitis is present in about 20% of patients.

Medicines causing acne-like skin eruptions

A number of medicines can produce acne-like lesions. Steroids (oral or topical) are commonly implicated. Other medicines associated include lithium, oral contraceptives (especially those with high progestogen levels), phenytoin, azathioprine and rifampicin.

Perioral dermatitis

Perioral dermatitis tends to affect young women between 25 and 40 years of age, and exhibits an acne-like rash generally around the mouth and nasolabial folds (Fig. 8.23). Itching and burning can also be present, and the rash can take on a dermatitis-like quality.

Polycystic ovary syndrome

A clinical manifestation of this condition can be acne vulgaris. Any women that has menstrual irregularity (infrequent

Table 8.29
Grading of Acne
Mild acne consists mainly of non-inflammatory comedones with few inflammatory (papulopustular) lesions mainly confined to the face
Moderate acne can be described as having many inflammatory lesions that are not confined to the face. Lesions are sometimes painful and there is a possibility of mild scarring
Severe acne has all the characteristics of moderate acne plus the development of nodules and cysts. Lesions are often widespread, involving the upper back and chest. Scarring will usually result Acne of any severity which is causing psychological upset should be classed as severe

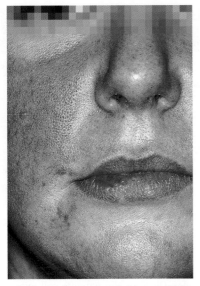

Fig. 8.22 Rosacea. Reproduced from J Wilkinson et al 2004, Dermatology in Focus, Churchill Livingstone, with permission.

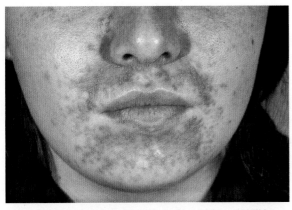

Fig. 8.23 Perioral dermatitis. Reproduced from J Wilkinson et al 2004, Dermatology in Focus, Churchill Livingstone, with permission.

❗ TRIGGER POINTS indicative of referral: Acne

Symptoms/signs	Possible danger/reason for referral
Moderate or severe acne OTC treatment failure Suspected rosacea	Generally require antibiotic therapy
Prepubertal or older people	Acne is uncommon in these age groups

---

or no periods) and also exhibits hirsutism and/or is over-weight must be referred for further investigation.

Evidence base for over-the-counter medication

The aim of treatment must be to clear the lesions and prevent scarring. Mild acne can be managed OTC but it is important to show understanding and empathy when advising patients. Acne is predominantly a condition that affects adolescents; a time when appearance is all-important. It is worth taking a few minutes to counsel patients about their condition, allay fears and make sure their expectations of treatment are realistic.

OTC acne treatments contain either benzoyl peroxide, salicylic acid, sulphur, nicotinamide or an antibacterial.

Benzoyl peroxide

Benzoyl peroxide exerts its main effect by reducing the concentration of *Propionibacterium acnes* by releasing oxygen into the anaerobic micro-environment. Bacteria cannot develop resistance to this mode of action. Many studies have investigated the efficacy of benzoyl peroxide. It has been proven to be effective, especially in mild to moderate acne. However, there is no evidence to suggest that 10% benzoyl peroxide is more effective than lower strengths.

A variety of other agents have been compared against or in combination with benzoyl peroxide. None of these products have been shown to be significantly better than benzoyl peroxide alone. For example, the addition of miconazole 2% (Acnidazil – now discontinued in the UK) was shown to be no more effective than benzoyl peroxide. Likewise, when Quinoderm was compared with Quinoderm HC (benzoyl peroxide and hydrocortisone) no significant differences in efficacy were observed.

Evidence of efficacy for salicylic acid and sulphur is poor. Both agents have been used for many years on the basis of their keratolytic action, but on current evidence they are best avoided. Nicotinamide is a more recent addition to the OTC market. Data suggest it is as effective as clindamycin 1% gel; however, no randomised controlled trials seem to have been conducted to support this finding.

Complementary treatments

Evidence is lacking to support the use of complementary treatments. A 2015 Cochrane review (Cao et al., 2015) found some low-quality evidence for reduction in acne lesions using bee venom, tee tree oil and those following a low glycaemic load diet. However, these data were drawn from single trials of varying methodological quality.

Summary

First line treatment of acne should be benzoyl peroxide 2.5% or 5%. Patients should see an improvement in their symptoms after 6 weeks. If the patient's symptoms fail to improve in this time, then referral to a doctor would be appropriate. However, if beneficial, treatment should be continued for at least 4 to 6 months.

Practical prescribing and product selection

Prescribing information is discussed and summarised in Table 8.30; useful tips relating to patients presenting with acne are given in 'Hints and Tips' in Box 8.9.

Benzoyl peroxide

Benzoyl peroxide is licensed for use in adults and children (for products, see Table 8.31). Benzoyl peroxide is usually applied once or twice daily depending on patient response, although once-daily application is often sufficient. It should be applied to all areas of the skin where acne occurs and not just to the active lesions. It can cause drying, burning and peeling on initial application. If this occurs the patient should be told to stop using the product for a day or two before starting again. Patients should therefore start on the lowest strength commercially available,

especially if the patient suffers from sensitive skin or has fair skin color. Occasionally patients will experience contact dermatitis, although it has been reported to affect only 1% to 2% of patients. Apart from local adverse effects, benzoyl peroxide is safe.

Nicotinamide (Freederm, Nicam)

Nicotinamide should be applied to the affected area twice daily after the skin has been washed. Enough gel should

Table 8.31
Products available in the UK containing benzoyl peroxide

Name	Form	Strength	Other ingredients
Acnecide	Gel & wash	5%	
Brevoxyl	Cream	4%	
PanOxyl	Aquagel	10%	
Quinoderm	Cream	5%, 10%	Antimicrobial hydroxyquinoline sulphate 0.5%

Table 8.30
Practical prescribing: Summary of medicines for acne

Name of medicine	Use in children	Likely side effects	Drug interactions of note	Patients in which care is exercised	Pregnancy & breastfeeding
Benzoyl peroxide	Not appropriate	Skin irritation, burning or peeling	None	None	OK
Nicotinamide	Not appropriate	Dry skin, pruritus, erythema, burning, irritation	None	None	OK

HINTS AND TIPS BOX 8.9: ACNE

Myths surrounding acne	Sunshine helps reduce acne – there is no convincing evidence that this is the case Chocolate causes spots. There is no proof that any food causes acne Stress causes acne. Stress cannot cause acne although it can make it worse
Applying benzoyl peroxide	Benzoyl peroxide has a potent bleaching effect. It has the ability to permanently bleach clothing and bed linen. Patients should be advised to always wash their hands after applying the product

be used to cover the affected area. Like benzoyl peroxide, drying of the skin is the main side effect. If this occurs, then the dose should be reduced to once daily.

References

Cao H, Yang G, Wang Y, et al. Complementary therapies for acne vulgaris. Cochrane Database of Systematic Reviews 2015, Issue 1. Art. No.: CD009436. http://dx.doi. org/10.1002/14651858.CD009436.pub2.

Further reading

Burke B, Eady EA, Cunliffe WJ. Benzoyl peroxide versus topical erythromycin in the treatment of acne vulgaris. Br J Dermatol 1983;108:199–204.

Fluckiger R, Furrer HJ, Rufli T. Efficacy and tolerance of a miconazole-benzoyl peroxide cream combination versus a benzoyl peroxide gel in the topical treatment of acne vulgaris. Dermatologica 1988;177:109–14.

Goldberg JL, Dabade TS, Davis SA, et al. Changing age of acne vulgaris visits: Another sign of earlier puberty? Pediatr Dermatol 2011;28(6):645–8.

Hunt MJ, Barnetson RS. A comparative study of gluconolactone versus benzoyl peroxide in the treatment of acne. Aust J Dermatol 1992;33:131–4.

Johnson BA, Nunley JR. Topical therapy for acne vulgaris. How do you choose the best drug for each patient? Postgrad Med 2000;107:69–70, 73–76, 79–80.

Kligman AM. Acne vulgaris: tricks and treatments. Part II: The benzoyl peroxide saga. Cutis 1995;56:260–1.

Magin P, Pond D, Smith W, et al. A systematic review of the evidence for 'myths and misconceptions' in acne management: diet, face washing and sunlight. Fam Pract 2005;22:62–70.

Marks R. The enigma of rosacea. J Dermatol Treat 2007;18(6):326–8.

Purdy S, de Berker D. Clinical review: Acne. Br Med J 2006;333:949–53.

Sagransky M, Yentzer BA, Feldman SR. Benzoyl peroxide: a review of its current use in the treatment of acne vulgaris. Exp Opin Pharmacother 2009;10(15):2555–62.

Shalita AR, Smith JG, Parish LC, et al. Topical nicotinamide compared with clindamycin gel in the treatment of inflammatory acne vulgaris. Int J Dermatol 1995;34:434–7.

Cold sores (Herpes simplex labialis)

Background

A cold sore is an infection caused by the herpes simplex virus (HSV). There are two main subtypes of the virus: HSV1 and HSV2. Cold sores are caused by HSV1, whereas HSV2 is most commonly implicated in genital lesions.

Prevalence and epidemiology

Herpes simplex virus infection is one of the most commonly encountered human viral infections. It is estimated that more than 50% of adults in the Western world show serologic evidence of having been infected by HSV1, although this might not manifest as symptoms. It is reported that 20–50% of people will experience a cold sore at some time. Most people with recurrent cold sores will have fewer than two episodes per year, but 5–10% of affected people have a minimum of six recurrences per year.

Aetiology

Infection is spread by viral shedding into saliva and results from direct mucous membrane contact (e.g., kissing) at sites of abraded skin between an infected and an uninfected individual. The virus then infects epidermal and dermal cells, causing skin vesicles. After primary infection the virus travels to the sensory ganglia where it lies dormant in the dorsal root ganglia of the trigeminal nerve until reactivation. Once reactivated (often triggered by some known stimulus, Table 8.32) the virus migrates from these sensory ganglia to the outer layer of the skin of lips and forms cold sore lesions again. When first contracted, the virus is known as the primary infection and is often asymptomatic. It is most commonly contracted by preschool children.

Arriving at a differential diagnosis

Cold sores should not be too difficult to diagnose, although conditions such as impetigo can look similar to cold sores. Asking symptom-specific questions will help the pharmacist establish a differential diagnosis (Table 8.32).

Clinical features of cold sores

Patients typically experience prodromal symptoms of itching, burning, pain or tingling symptoms before vesicle eruption. These symptoms might be noticed from a few hours to a couple of days before the lesions develop. The lesions appear as blisters and vesicles with associated redness on the outer lip (Fig. 8.24). These crust over – usually within 24 hours – and tend to be itchy and painful and might bleed. Lesions spontaneously resolve in 7 to 10 days, therefore most outbreaks last 14 days from the recognition of prodromal symptoms to the resolution of lesions.

Many patients can identify a cause of their cold sore, with sunlight (UV light) reported to induce cold sores in 20% of sufferers. Recurrence is common and lesions tend

<table>
<tr><td colspan="2">(?) Table 8.32
Specific questions to ask the patient: Cold sores</td></tr>
<tr><td>**Question**</td><td>**Relevance**</td></tr>
<tr><td>Appearance</td><td>Patients with cold sores will often experience prodromal symptoms before the skin eruption whereas no 'warning' symptoms are present with impetigo or angular cheilitis</td></tr>
<tr><td>Location</td><td>Cold sores typically occur around the mouth and for this reason are known as herpes simplex labialis. They can also occur around and inside the nose, but this is less common
Impetigo also occurs in the same areas but is more prone to spread to other areas of the face or move to other parts of the body, for example the arms
Angular cheilitis occurs at the corners of the mouth and can be mistaken for cold sores due to their similar locations</td></tr>
<tr><td>Trigger factors</td><td>Stress, ill health, sunlight, viral infection (e.g., the common cold) and menstruation are all implicated in triggering cold sore attacks. These triggers are not associated with other similar conditions and the patient should be asked if they can identify what brought on the lesions</td></tr>
</table>

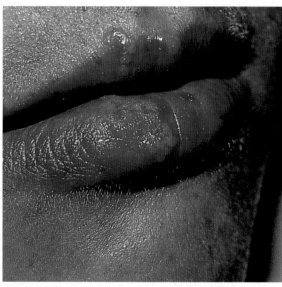

Fig. 8.24 Cold sore. Reproduced from G White, 2004, Color Atlas of Dermatology 3rd edition, Churchill Livingstone, with permission.

to occur in the same location. Immunocompromised patients or patients taking immunosuppressive medication can experience severe symptoms and should be referred.

Conditions to eliminate

Impetigo

Impetigo usually starts as a small, red, itchy patch of inflamed skin that quickly develops into vesicles that rupture and weep. The exudate dries to a brownish-yellow sticky crust. The area around the mouth and nose is most commonly affected rather than the lip itself (Fig. 10.7). Currently, referral is needed for either topical (e.g., fusidic acid) or systemic (flucloxacillin) therapy.

Angular cheilitis

Angular cheilitis can occur at any age. It is more common in patients who wear dentures. The corners of the mouth become cracked, fissured and red. The lesions can become boggy and macerated, and are slow to heal because movement of the mouth hinders healing of the lesions (Fig. 8.25). It is painful but generally does not itch or crust over, as is typical with cold sores.

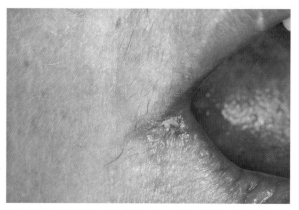

Fig. 8.25 Angular cheilitis. Reproduced from R Cawson et al 2002, Essentials of Oral Pathology and Oral Medicine, Churchill Livingstone, with permission.

Aphthous ulcers

These can occur on the lip but tend to be on the inside rather than the outer part of the lip. For further information see page 152.

⚠ TRIGGER POINTS indicative of referral: Cold sores

Symptoms/signs	Possible danger/reason for referral
Duration longer than 14 days	Unlikely to be cold sores
Cold sores located within the mouth	Outside scope of community pharmacy
Severe and widespread lesions	
Patients who are immunocompromised or take immunosuppressive medicines	
Lesions that spread away from the lips and onto the face	Impetigo more likely

---

Evidence base for over-the-counter medication

A number of products are marketed for the relief and treatment of cold sores. None have shown conclusively to be effective in both its prevention and treatment. Products containing ammonia, zinc and phenol appear to have no evidence of efficacy. However, they might be useful in drying lesions and preventing secondary bacterial infections. Local anaesthetics (e.g., lidocaine) and choline salicylate might also be useful for mildly painful lesions. For information on these products see page 156.

Only the antivirals aciclovir and penciclovir – which work by inhibiting the herpes virus DNA polymerase – have demonstrated clinical effectiveness against the herpes virus. Orally, antivirals such as aciclovir are highly effective, but the evidence for topical administration is less conclusive. Trial data have shown topical antivirals not to have a preventative effect (Chi et al., 2015). With regard to speeding up the resolution of established cold sores (when using aciclovir), if applied in the prodromal stage the total healing time of subsequent lesions is reduced by a ½ to 1 day (Worall, 2009).

A hydrocolloid patch is available for the treatment of cold sores (Compeed Cold Sore Patch). Hydrocolloid dressings are available for wounds and enhance healing by providing a moist environment. A study comparing Compeed patch with aciclovir 5% cream found similar efficacy in terms of self-reported global assessment of efficacy and time until healing (7.57 days for Compeed vs 7.03 days for aciclovir; $p = 0.37$) (Karlsmark et al., 2008). However, the study was not blinded for the primary outcome (self-reported global assessment), casting some doubts on the findings. Further, the study was not set up as an equivalence study, and therefore the lack of difference in the outcomes could be due to too small a sample size. Given the uncertainty in the benefit of aciclovir, the small additional healing time seen with Compeed in this trial (approximately ½ a day) could mean Compeed is no better than placebo.

Summary

Aciclovir and penciclovir are first-line therapy for the treatment and prevention of cold sores. However, they should be used as soon as the patient experiences symptoms for them to have any effect.

Practical prescribing and product selection

Prescribing information relating to antivirals is discussed and summarised in Table 8.33. For completeness the table also contains some of the other commonly used cold sore products; useful tips relating to patients presenting with cold sores are given in 'Hints and Tips' in Box 8.10.

Aciclovir (e.g., Cymex Ultra, Virasorb, Zovirax)

Aciclovir can be used topically by all patient groups, including pregnant and breastfeeding women, although manufacturers advise caution because of limited data regarding the exposure of pregnant women to aciclovir. It has no drug interactions and causes only transient stinging after first application in the minority of patients. Aciclovir should be applied five times daily at approximately 4-hourly intervals and treatment should be continued for 5 days.

Penciclovir (Fenistil cold sore cream)

Penciclovir, like aciclovir, has the same side effect profile, cautions and contraindications, although the manufacturers advise consulting a doctor before use in pregnancy and breastfeeding, presumably on lack of safety data. However, there appears to be no evidence to suggest it causes any problems in these groups. For people over 12 years of age it should be applied every 2 hours and treatment continued for 4 days.

Table 8.33
Practical prescribing: Summary of medicines for cold sores

Name of medicine	Use in children	Likely side effects	Drug interactions of note	Patients in which care is exercised	Pregnancy & breastfeeding
Aciclovir	All state can be used in children but no lower age limit stated	Stinging	None	OK	OK
Cymex Ultra					
Virasorb					
Zovirax					
Penciclovir (Fenistil)	>12 years	None	None	None	Manufacturers recommend use under medical supervision
Ammonia & phenol (Blistex Relief Cream)	Yes, but no lower age stated	None	None	None	OK
Zinc & lidocaine (Lypsyl Cold Sore Gel)	>12 years	Stinging	None	None	OK
Urea (Cymex)	Yes, but no lower age stated	None	None	None	OK

HINTS AND TIPS BOX 8.10: COLD SORES

Sun-induced cold sores	For those patients in whom the sun triggers cold sores, a sun block would be the most effective prophylactic measure
Applying products	Patients should be encouraged to use a separate towel and wash their hands after applying products because viral particles are shed from the cold sore and can be transferred to others
Decrease transmission	Risk of transmission is highest during the first 1–4 days of symptoms and people should be advised not to kiss others

References

Chi CC, Wang SH, Delamere FM, et al. Interventions for prevention of herpes simplex labialis (cold sores on the lips). Cochrane Database of Systematic Reviews 2015, Issue 8. Art. No.: CD010095. http://dx.doi.org/10.1002/14651858. CD010095.pub2.

Karlsmark T, Goodman JJ, Drouault Y, et al. Randomized clinical study comparing Compeed cold sore patch to acyclovir cream 5% in the treatment of herpes simplex labialis. J Eur Acad Dermatol Venereol 2008:22(10);1184–1192.

Worrall G. Herpes labialis. BMJ Clin. Evid 2009. Available at: http://clinicalevidence.bmj.com/x/systematic-review/1704/overview.html

Further reading

Emmert DH. Treatment of common cutaneous herpes simplex virus infections. Am Fam Physician 2000;61:1697–704.

Whitley RJ, Kimberlin DW, Roizman B. Herpes simplex viruses. Clin Infect Dis 1998;26:541–55.

Eczema and dermatitis

Background

The terms 'eczema' and 'dermatitis' are often used interchangeably. Dermatitis simply means inflammation of the skin, whereas eczema has no universally agreed definition but in some countries indicates a more acute condition. Many authorities subdivide eczema and dermatitis into either exogenous (due to an obvious external cause) or endogenous (assumed to be of a genetic cause); however, the distinction is not clear. The condition is also referred to as either acute – a single exposure to an irritant, or chronic – repeated exposure. In this section, for consistency, the term dermatitis will be used.

Dermatitis is characterised by sore, red, itching skin. In primary care, the two most common forms of dermatitis are irritant and allergic dermatitis.

Prevalence and epidemiology

The exact prevalence of irritant and allergic contact dermatitis (ICD and ACD) is unclear, although ICD is much more common than ACD and has been reported to account for 80% of all occupational skin disorders. ACD is said to affect 1–2% of the population with certain patient groups, such as patients with leg ulcers who are at higher risk of developing ACD.

Aetiology

Different physiological mechanisms are responsible for ICD and ACD. In ICD an agent must penetrate the outer layer of skin – the stratum corneum – to invoke a physiological response. The type of irritant, the concentration, quantity involved and length of exposure will affect the severity of reaction. This can occur with a single exposure, or more commonly, with frequent exposures when the irritant accumulates in the stratum corneum. For example, strong acids and alkaline substances can produce ulceration on a single exposure, whereas other agents (e.g., zinc oxide tape) potentially require multiple exposure and tend to invoke a weaker reaction and cause a prickly heat type of dermatitis.

ACD first requires sensitisation to occur. This leads to specific cell-mediated sensitisation. Once the skin has become sensitised to an allergen, re-exposure to the allergen triggers memory T cells to initiate an inflammatory response 24 to 48 hours after re-exposure. Because these T cells are distributed throughout the body, the reaction is not limited to the site of exposure and explains why lesions are seen away from the site of exposure. The risk of sensitisation can depend on the individual's susceptibility as well as the particular allergen's concentration and quantity. Re-exposure can occur days and sometimes years after initial exposure. A list of common irritants and allergens is shown in Table 8.34.

Table 8.34
Irritants and allergens known to precipitate dermatitis

Irritants that can precipitate ICD	Allergens that can precipitate ACD
Detergents and soaps	Nickel (especially in jewellery) Chromate in cement
Solvents and abrasives	Topical corticosteroids (5% of patients)
Oils	Cosmetics – particularly fragrances, hair dyes, preservatives, and nail varnish resin
Acids and alkalis, including cement	Rubber, including latex
Reducing agents and oxidizing agents	Dyes, formaldehyde and epoxy resins

Arriving at a differential diagnosis

Many causes of dermatitis are related to occupations that include beauticians, construction workers, hairdressers and mechanics. Questions about exposure to irritants and allergens at work can often identify the cause of symptoms.

Gaining an accurate diagnosis can be difficult as clinical features of similar conditions overlap (Table 8.35). Asking symptom-specific questions will help the pharmacist establish a differential diagnosis (Table 8.36).

Clinical features of ACD and ICD

All forms of dermatitis cause redness, drying of the skin and irritation/pruritus to varying degrees, and might show papules and vesicles. Itching is a prominent feature and

Table 8.35
Causes of dermatitis-like rash and their relative incidence in community pharmacy

Incidence	Cause
Most likely	Irritant contact dermatitis
Likely	Urticaria, allergic contact dermatitis, psoriasis
Unlikely	Fungal infection, discoid dermatitis
Very unlikely	Pompholyx

Table 8.36 **Specific questions to ask the patient: Dermatitis**	
Question	Relevance
Location	The distribution of rash for contact dermatitis is closely associated with clothing and jewellery (Fig. 8.26)
Exposure	A history of when the rash occurs gives a useful indication as to the cause, e.g., a construction worker might complain of sore hands while at work but when on holiday the condition improves only for it to worsen when they go back to work

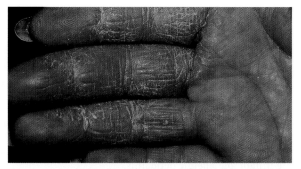

Fig. 8.27 Irritant dermatitis. Reproduced from G White, 2004, Color Atlas of Dermatology, 3rd edition, Churchill Livingstone, with permission.

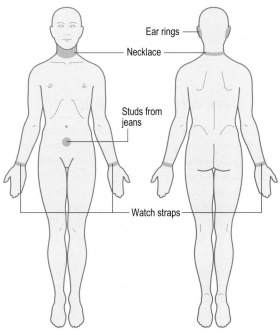

Fig. 8.26 Distribution of contact dermatitis.

often causes the patient to scratch, which results in broken skin with subsequent weeping. In chronic exposure, the skin becomes dry, scaly and can crack and fissure (Fig. 8.27). In both cases rash develops at the site of exposure. In the acute phase, lesions appear rapidly – within 6 to 12 hours – of contact. The rash in ICD tends to be well demarcated. In ACD, the rash tends to be less well defined; milder involvement away from the site of exposure is seen on repeated exposure and can reactivate at previously exposed sites. It is estimated that 75% of all cases of contact dermatitis and 80–90% of occupational dermatitis involve the hands.

Conditions to eliminate

Likely causes

Urticaria

Urticarial rashes can result from many causes, most notably due to food allergies, food additives (Table 8.37) and medicines. Like dermatitis, the rash is itchy and red but resembles the rash seen when stung by a stinging nettle (Fig. 8.28). Weals can be red or white, and are itchy and surrounded by an area of redness. The rash appears suddenly and tends to fade and disappear after 24 hours. In addition, the skin can be oedematous and blanches when pressed. Urticarial reactions often respond well to systemic antihistamines.

Psoriasis

Isolated lesions of psoriasis can be superficially similar to dermatitis; they appear red and scaly, although a key difference is the lack of prominent itch in psoriasis. The distribution of lesions is also usually different, and psoriasis is not precipitated by exposure to certain irritants or allergens. For further information on psoriasis see page 219.

Unlikely causes

Fungal infections

Fungal infections exhibit the classical dermatitis-type symptoms of itchy red rash and can therefore be easily confused. Very clear lesion demarcation along with differing location and central clearing all point towards fungal infection. For further information on fungal infections see page 233.

Discoid dermatitis   Raised coin shaped lesion, Round

This differs from other forms of eczema as the lesions have clearly demarcated edges and are circular or oval.

Table 8.37
Food additives known to cause allergic reaction

Sulphites (E220–E227)	Sulphites are used to preserve smoked and processed meats, dried fruit (apricots) and salads. They are commonly found in liquid form in cold drinks and fruit juice concentrates, and wine and sprayed onto foods to keep them fresh and prevent discolouration or browning.
Benzoic acid and parabens (E210–E219)	Benzoates and parabens have antibacterial and antifungal properties for prevention of food spoilage. These agents are added to pharmaceutical and food products, and occur naturally in prunes, cinnamon, tea and berries.
Antioxidants (E320–E321)	Fat and oils in food turn rancid when exposed to air. Synthetic phenolic antioxidants butylated hydroxyanisole and butylated hydroxytoluene prevent this spoilage from happening but can trigger asthma, rhinitis and urticaria.
Flavour enhancers (E620–E635)	These are used to enhance food palatability, most notably aspartame, which can trigger urticaria and swelling, and monosodium glutamate (E620), which can trigger the 'Chinese restaurant syndrome' of headache and burning plus tightness in the chest, neck and face.
Colourings (E100–E180)	Colourings are used to make food visually more attractive; the azo dyes (Tartrazine, E102, Sunset Yellow, E110) and non-azo dyes (erythrocine) have been associated with triggering urticaria, asthma and generalised allergic reactions.

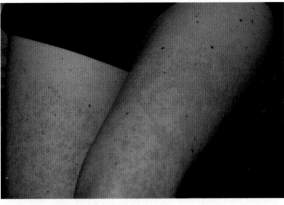

Fig. 8.28 Urticarial reaction to grass.

Lesions tend to affect the arms and legs, and are often distributed symmetrically. It is more common in middle-aged people.

Very unlikely causes

Dyshidrotic eczema (pompholyx)
Pompholyx simply means 'bubble' and refers to the presence of intensely itchy vesicles or blisters on the palms of the hands and occasionally on the soles of the feet. Stress and heat are known to precipitate the condition.

Fig. 8.29 will aid the differentiation of dermatitis.

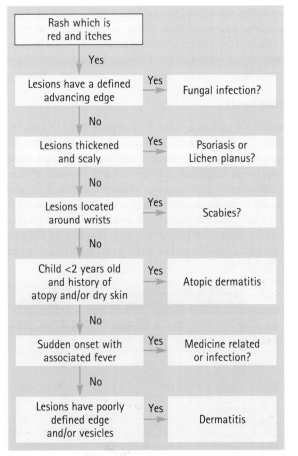

Fig. 8.29 Primer for differential diagnosis of dermatitis.

! TRIGGER POINTS indicative of referral: Dermatitis

Symptoms/signs	Possible danger/reason for referral
Children under age 10 in need of corticosteroids	Steroid use outside current OTC product licenses
Lesions on the face, unresponsive to emollients	
Widespread or severe dermatitis	Need for medical intervention
OTC treatment failure	

Evidence base for over-the-counter medication

Treatment should include three steps: avoiding irritants, managing the itch and maintaining skin integrity.

Non-pharmacological interventions include avoidance of the causative agent; however, determining the cause is often difficult and avoidance is sometimes impractical. Sweating intensifies the itching so strategies to keep the person cool will help; cotton and loose-fitting clothing can be worn.

Pharmacological treatment of dermatitis should be managed with a combination of emollients and steroid-based products.

Emollients

Emollients should be used on a regular basis to keep the condition under control and flare-ups can then be treated with corticosteroids. Choosing the most efficacious emollient for an individual is difficult due to the lack of comparative trial data between products and the variable nature of patient response. In general, patients respond to a thicker emollient rather than an elegant cosmetic brand because these allow greater retention of water, for example 50% liquid paraffin and 50% white soft paraffin. However,

patient acceptability of such products needs to be considered. Cream formulations rather than ointments tend to be more readily accepted by patients, as they are easier and less messy to use. In general, skin which is moderately dry to very dry will respond best to an ointment and skin which is mildly dry will respond best to a cream. If the skin is broken or weeping, then a water-soluble cream can be useful. To avoid the drying effects of soap, a soap substitute should be used.

Steroids

In the UK, hydrocortisone (classed as mild potency) and clobetasone (moderately potent) are available. Both have proven efficacy in treating dermatitis and should be considered first-line treatment for acute dermatitis. The choice between hydrocortisone and clobetasone is based on the severity of the dermatitis and where the dermatitis is, with hydrocortisone being best for areas that have thin skin (e.g., flexures), and clobetasone possibly better for other areas (e.g., hands and palms) or where hydrocortisone has failed to control symptoms.

Practical prescribing and product selection

Prescribing information relating to specific products used to treat dermatitis discussed in the section 'Evidence base for over-the-counter medication' is summarised in Table 8.38; useful tips relating to using products to treat dermatitis are given in 'Hints and Tips' in Box 8.11.

Emollients

There are a large number of emollients on the market. They come in a range of formulations to suit all skin types and patient preference (Table 8.39). Patients should be instructed to apply emollients both liberally and whenever needed. They are pharmacologically inactive, and so can be used by all patients regardless of age or medical status. A number of ingredients incorporated into emollients do

Table 8.38
Practical prescribing: Summary of medicines for dermatitis

Name of medicine	Use in children	Likely side effects	Drug interactions of note	Patients in which care is exercised	Pregnancy & breastfeeding
Emollients	From birth onwards	None	None	None	OK
Corticosteroids Hydrocortisone	>10 years	None	None	None	OK
Clobetasone	>12 years				

HINTS AND TIPS BOX 8.11: DERMATITIS

Patch testing	If the rash persists despite avoiding likely irritants and allergens, then patch testing could be tried
How much to apply?	Patients should be instructed to use a fingertip unit. This is the distance from the tip of the adult index finger to the first crease. One unit is sufficient to cover an area twice the size of an adult flat hand
Quantity required?	The BNF gives the following guidance for a week's use: Both hands, 15–30 g Both arms, 30–60 g Both legs or trunk, 100 g
When to apply emollients and corticosteroids?	After using a corticosteroid an emollient can be applied to the same area 30 minutes later

Table 8.39
Summary of proprietary emollient products

Product name	Formulation	Combination product	Contains potential sensitising agents
Aquamax	Cream, wash		Yes
Aveeno	Cream, bath oil, wash, lotion		Yes
Aquadrate	Cream	Urea	No
Aquamol	Cream		Yes
Balneum	Bath oil, cream	Urea (cream)	Yes
Balneun Plus	Bath oil, cream	Urea (cream)	Yes
Calmurid	Cream	Urea, lactic acid	No
Cetraben	Cream, bath oil, ointment		Yes
Dermalex	Cream		
Dermamist	Spray		No
Dermalo	Bath oil		No
Dermol	Cream, lotion, shower and bath emollient, wash emulsion	Antimicrobials	Yes
Diprobase	Cream, ointment, lotion		Yes (cream)
Doublebase	Bath oil, gel, shower gel		No
Eczmol	Cream	Antimicrobials	
E45	Cream, lotion, emollient wash cream		Yes (cream and lotion only)
E45 Itch relief	Cream	Urea	Yes
Emollin	Spray		No
Emulsiderm	Bath emulsion	Antimicrobials	Yes

(Continued)

Table 8.39
Summary of proprietary emollient products (Continued)

Product name	Formulation	Combination product	Contains potential sensitising agents
Epaderm	Cream, ointment		Yes
Eucerin	Cream, lotion	Urea	Yes
Eumocream	Cream	Glycerol	Yes
Flexitol		Urea	Yes
Hewletts	Cream		Yes
Hydromol Intensive	Cream	Urea	No
Hydromol	Cream, ointment, bath and shower emollient		Yes (cream and ointment)
Lipobase	Cream		Yes
Lotil Cream	Cream		Yes
Nutraplus	Cream	Urea	Yes
Oilatum	Cream, gel, junior, shower gel, bath oil		Yes
Oilatum Plus	Bath oil	Antimicrobials	Yes
QV	Cream, ointment, lotion, wash, bath oil		Yes (except oil)
Ultrabase	Cream		Yes
Unguentum M	Cream		Yes
Vaseline Dermacare	Cream, lotion		Yes
ZeroAQS	Cream		Yes
Zerobase	Cream		Yes
Zerocream	Cream		Yes
Zeroderm	Ointment		Cetostearyl alcohol, polysorbate 60
Zerodouble Gel	Gel		Yes
Zeroguent	Cream		Yes
Zerolatum	Bath oil		No
Zeroneum	Bath oil		Yes

have the potential to sensitise skin, and patients should be advised to patch test the product on the back of the hand before starting to routinely use it.

Corticosteroids

Although corticosteroids can be sold to patients OTC, there are a number of restrictions to their sale. In the UK these are:

- the patient must be over 10 years of age for hydrocortisone (over 2 years of age in Australia) and over 12 years of age for clobetasone;
- duration of treatment is limited to a maximum of 1 week;
- a maximum of 15 g can be sold at any one time;
- they cannot be used on facial skin, the anogenital region, or broken or infected skin.

In the opinion of the author, these restrictions limit their usefulness and mean that many patients, who could be otherwise treated successfully if the product licenses were not so prohibitive, must be referred to a doctor. For example, 1% hydrocortisone cream, if used short term, is an ideal steroid to use on the face with no adverse events; also, 15 g of product is often insufficient for surface areas, such as limbs and the body, even if used only for a week.

Hydrocortisone

Hydrocortisone can either be bought alone (e.g., Hc45, Lanacort) or in combination with other ingredients (e.g., Eurax HC, Canesten Hydrocortisone). It is prudent to use products solely containing hydrocortisone for dermatitis, applying them twice. If secondary infection is suspected, for example with a fungal infection, then products such as Canesten Hydrocortisone can be used.

Clobetasone (Eumovate eczema and dermatitis cream)

Like hydrocortisone, it should be applied twice a day.

Further reading

Bellingham C. Proper use of topical corticosteroids. Pharm J 2001;267:377.
Clark C, Hoare C. Making the most of emollients. Pharm J 2001;266:277–9.
Cunliffe B. Eczema. Pharm J 2001;267:855–6.

Websites

National Eczema Society: http://www.eczema.org/
National Eczema Association: http://www.nationaleczema.org/

Sun exposure and melanoma risk

Background

The ultraviolet spectrum is subdivided into three regions: UVA (320–400 nm); UVB (290–320 nm); and UVC (200–290 nm). Light from the UVA spectrum causes skin tanning and UVB light causes sunburn, whereas UVC light is effectively filtered out by the ozone layer. It is now well recognised that excessive or prolonged exposure to the sun's rays and inadequate skin protection can result in pre-cancerous and cancerous neoplasms. There are many types of skin cancer, but three types are associated with sun exposure – squamous cell carcinoma (SCC), basal cell carcinoma (BCC) and malignant melanoma (MM) – and are responsible for more than 95% of all skin cancers. SCC and BCC result from chronic long-term exposure to sunlight whereas MM is associated with acute, intense, and intermittent blistering sunburns. BCC and SCC are often grouped together as non-melanoma skin cancer (NMSC).

Prevalence and epidemiology

The incidence of cancers related to skin damage has dramatically increased since the 1980s, and are greatest in Caucasian people living in equatorial regions. In 2011 there were just over 13 000 new cases of MM in the UK. MMs are slightly more common in women, although the incidence in both sexes has been steadily increasing. Affluent women appear to be at highest risk of developing MM, whereas men from lower socioeconomic groups are at greatest risk of developing NMSC.

Aetiology

The body's response to the effects of UVA and UVB light is protective. On exposure to ultraviolet light melanocytes increase production of melanin, thus causing a darkening of the skin, the all-important suntan! Melanin absorbs both UVA and UVB, and effectively protects the skin from damage; however, melanin synthesis is slow and skin damage might well have already occurred manifesting as sunburn. Sunburn is an inflammatory response to excessive exposure to ultraviolet light whereby an increase in inflammatory mediators results in capillary vasodilatation and increased capillary permeability. In addition to melanin production, epidermal hyperplasia occurs, causing the skin to thicken; this provides further protection against the skin.

Arriving at a differential diagnosis

Pharmacists have a major role to play in dealing with patients who have been exposed to excessive amounts of sunlight. They can promote sun safety messages, both passively and actively (when dealing with requests regarding sunburn) and make appropriate referrals with regard to suspicious lesions. Pharmacists must be able to recognise suspicious lesions, especially those resembling MM because it has the highest mortality of skin cancers, but if treated early is curable.

Clinical features of malignant melanoma

MM is one of the few cancers that is associated with young adults, although it is more common in older people. It can appear on all body sites yet their distribution between men and women does differ (Fig. 8.30). In the UK population the most common site is the lower leg in women, and on

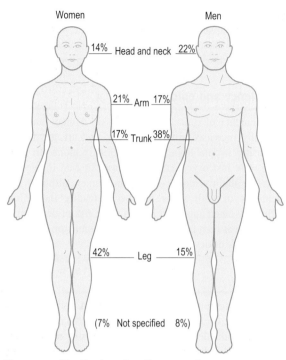

Fig. 8.30 Distribution of malignant melanoma.

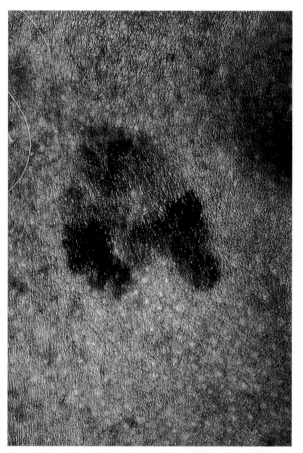

Fig. 8.31 Superficial spreading melanoma. Irregular in colour and shape. Reproduced from J Wilkinson et al 2004, Dermatology in Focus, Churchill Livingstone, with permission.

the back in men. Risk factors include early childhood sun exposure, people with multiple moles and those with susceptible sunburn skin types. The first sign of melanoma is often a change in the size, shape, or colour of a mole, although melanoma can also appear on the body as a new mole (Fig. 8.31). Early identification is essential and two commonly used checklists are used to aid diagnosis; the '7 point' checklist and the 'ABCDE' list.

1 The 7 point list

This checklist consists of 3 major and 4 minor points:

Major (scores 2)

1. Change in shape
2. Change in size
3. Change in colour

Minor (scores 1)

1. Largest diameter 7 mm or more
2. Inflammation
3. Oozing
4. Change in sensation (e.g., itch or irritation)

Any lesion should be suspected as MM with a score of 3 or more.

2 The ABCDE Rule

This checklist consists of 5 points:

- Asymmetry – Ordinary moles are usually symmetrical in shape. Melanomas are likely to be irregular or asymmetrical.
- Border – Moles usually have a well-defined, regular border. Melanomas are more likely to have an irregular border with jagged edges.
- Colour – Moles are usually a uniform brown. Melanomas tend to have more than one colour. They may be varying shades of brown mixed with black, red, pink, white or a bluish tint.
- Diameter – Moles are normally no bigger than the blunt end of a pencil (about 6 mm across). Melanomas are usually more than 7 mm in diameter.
- Evolution – the symmetry, border, colour, or diameter of a mole has changed over time.

It is likely that patients will ask for advice and reassurance on skin lesions that they are concerned could be melanoma. It is essential that these people are given information, ideally both orally and written, regarding the changes that might subsequently suggest MM and be instructed to seek medical help as soon as they notice changes.

NMSC

NMSCs are the most common cancers in the UK. They are associated with older people, with the average age of diagnosis in the early 70s. The cancers are rarely fatal but can cause substantial morbidity. Both cancers commonly occur on skin surfaces that are exposed to a lifetime accumulation of UV radiation such as the hands, face and scalp. They are more common in people who have worked outdoors, in fair-skinned people, and those living in tropical and subtropical climates. BCC and SCC vary in their appearance. SCC initially presents as raised lesions that exhibit a horny or scaly appearance that later become non-healing lesions often larger than 1 cm which can ulcerate; BCC starts as a small translucent papule with a rolled edge and obvious telangiectasia over the surface. Over time (growth can be very slow) the size of the papule increases and can ulcerate and crust over.

Conditions to eliminate

Actinic keratosis

Actinic keratosis is the most common pre-malignant skin condition and affects the same group of people as SCC, with approximately 1 in 1000 cases progressing to SCC. Lesions occur on parts of the body that are exposed to long-term sun exposure (e.g., head, forearms, hands). They begin as small rough spots. Roughness is a key feature – often referred to as feeling like rubbing sandpaper. They are generally flat and brown, and have well demarcated edges. Symptoms of actinic keratosis include tenderness, itchiness and burning. Over a period of years, they enlarge and often become red and scaly.

Seborrhoeic keratosis (also known as seborrhoeic warts or basal cell papillomas)

These are benign, flat or raised lesions that vary in colour. Initially, they take on the colour of the person's skin but gradually darken. They range in colour from light brown to jet black and have a 'stuck on' appearance (Fig. 8.20). They are more usual on the trunk and increase in incidence from 40 years onwards. Over time they can become wart-like. Occasionally, they can become inflamed, itchy or bleed but this is normally because they have been caught on clothing.

> **! TRIGGER POINTS indicative of referral: Sunburn/damage**
>
> | Symptoms/signs | Possible danger/reason for referral |
> | --- | --- |
> | Facial lesions, especially in people over 60 | Suggests actinic keratosis or SCC/BCC |
> | Lesions that have become itchy, irritated or are prone to bleeding
Moles that have changed in size, shape or colour | Suggests potential melanoma |

Evidence base for over-the-counter medication

Avoidance measures

The most effective strategy for preventing skin damage/sunburn and reducing the chance of developing cancers is avoidance of UV light. Cancer research UK has promoted a Sun SMART campaign which highlights the key sun avoidance measures that should be promoted to the public:

S Spend time in the shade between 11 am and 3 pm

M Make sure you never burn

A Aim to cover up with a T-shirt, hat and sunglasses

R Remember to take extra care with children

T Then use factor 15 + sunscreen and four stars

The SunSmart programme (www.sunsmart.com.au) also has public guidance on how to avoid sun damage called: Slip! Slop! Slap! Seek! Slide!

1. **Slip** on sun-protective clothing that covers as much of your body as possible.
2. **Slop** on SPF 30 + broad-spectrum sunscreen liberally to dry skin, at least 20 minutes before sun exposure. Reapply every 2 hours when outdoors.
3. **Slap** on a broad-brimmed hat that shades your face, neck and ears.
4. **Seek** shade, particularly between the hours of 10 am and 2 pm (and 11 am and 3 pm during daylight savings).
5. **Slide** on sunglasses.

Sunscreens

Although sunscreens play an important role in sunburn protection, they should never replace minimising sun exposure. Sunscreens use the sun protection factor (SPF) system to indicate the level of protection against UV radiation. It is a measure of the protection from UVB radiation. This is calculated under experimental conditions using four times the amount of sunscreen usually applied by consumers. It is important that patients and consumers do not assume a linear increase in protection as the SPF increases. For example, a sunscreen with an SPF of 15 blocks 93% of UVB, whereas a doubling to SPF 30 only increases protection by 4% to 97%.

In the UK a star rating also exists to indicate the level of protection offered against UVA relative to protection against UVB. A five-star rating indicates the product has a balanced amount of UVA and UVB protection. The lower the star rating, the greater the protection offered against UVB compared with UVA.

Practical prescribing and product selection

Prescribing information relating to sunscreen products reviewed in the section 'Evidence base for over-the-counter medication' is discussed and summarised in Table 8.40; useful tips relating to patients asking for advice about protection from the sun are given in 'Hints and Tips' in Box 8.12.

Table 8.40
Practical prescribing: Summary of sun protection products

Name of medicine	Use in children	Likely side effects	Drug interactions of note	Patients in which care is exercised	Pregnancy & breastfeeding
Chemical sunscreens	Infant upwards but some manufacturers do have lower age limits	Allergic reactions, but may be linked to the vehicle and not the active ingredients	None	None	OK
Physical sunscreens		None, but may be cosmetically unacceptable			

HINTS AND TIPS BOX 8.12: SUN DAMAGE

Water-resistant sunscreens	These are claimed to be effective after immersion in water. However, studies have shown that sunscreen effectiveness decreases after water exposure. It would be prudent therefore, to re-apply sunscreens after swimming
Eye protection	Prolonged (over years) sun exposure can contribute to age-related macular degeneration. Therefore, wraparound sunglasses and lenses that effectively filter UV light should be worn
Treatment of sunburn?	Mild sunburn can be managed with a combination of topical cooling preparations, such as calamine, moisturisers and systemic analgesia
Medicine-induced photosensitivity	NSAIDs, tetracyclines, chlorpromazine, phenothiazines and amiodarone can cause pruritus and skin rash when the skin is exposed to natural sunlight, primarily due to UVA radiation. Patients on photosensitive drugs should use a broad-spectrum sunscreen, as these filter both UVA and UVB radiation http://www.dermnetnz.org/reactions/drug-photosensitivity.html
Sun protection and vitamin D deficiency	The UK Department of Health issued guidance to healthcare professionals on the danger of vitamin D deficiency. This, in part, has been caused by the use of sunscreens. Guidance is not to stop using sunscreen, but certain patient groups should take supplements https://www.nice.org.uk/guidance/ph56

All products should be applied 20 minutes before exposure to the sun, and reapplied every 2 to 4 hours and after swimming to ensure maximum protection. Standard practice until recently was to match skin type with the level of SPF protection the person required. However, this approach, while preventing sunburn, does not prevent long-term skin damage. Rather than selecting a specific sunscreen for skin type, it is advocated that all Caucasians people should use a sunscreen with an SPF of at least 15 because this level of protection is sufficient as a sun block.

Chemical sunscreens

Chemical sunscreens work by absorbing UV energy and give protection against either UVA or UVB, although they tend to be more effective against UVB radiation. The majority of marketed products contain a combination of agents including benzophenones, cinnamates, dibenzoylmethanes and *para*-aminobenzoic acid. The latter is now infrequently used, as *para*-aminobenzoic acid was frequently associated with contact sensitivity.

Physical sunscreens

Physical sunscreens are opaque reflective agents and offer protection against UVA and UVB radiation. Examples of physical sunscreens include zinc and titanium oxide.

Further reading
Gupta AK, Paquet M, Villanueva E, et al. Interventions for actinic keratoses. Cochrane Database of Systematic Reviews 2012, Issue 12. Art. No.: CD004415. http://dx.doi.org/10.1002/14651858.CD004415.pub2.

Websites
Charities
http://www.skincancer.org/ (The Skin Cancer Foundation)
http://www.cancerresearchuk.org/home/ (Cancer Research UK)
http://www.melanomauk.org.uk

Guidance
British Association of Dermatologists guidelines on 'The prevention, diagnosis, referral and management of melanoma of the skin', 2007: http://www.bad.org.uk/shared/get-file.ashx?id=793&itemtype=document
NICE Guidance on skin cancer protection: http://www.nice.org.uk/ph32

General sites
http://www.sunsmart.com.au/ (Sunsmart website)
http://www.cancer.org.au/ (Cancer Council Australia)
http://www.melanoma.org/ (Melanoma Research Foundation)

8

Self-assessment questions

The following questions are intended to supplement the text. Two levels of questions are provided; multiple choice questions and case studies. The multiple choice questions are designed to test factual recall and the case studies allow knowledge to be applied to a practice setting.

Multiple choice questions

8.1   In which condition is scaling the most prominent?

    a. Allergic dermatitis
    b. Scabies
    c. Fungal infection
    d. Plaque psoriasis
    e. Lichen planus

8.2   Actinic keratosis tends to least affect which part of the body?

    a. Hands
    b. Head
    c. Arms
    d. Neck
    e. Back

8.3   A lesion described as flat and less than 1 cm in diameter is known as a:

    a. Papule
    b. Macule
    c. Patch
    d. Comedone
    e. Nodule

8.4   What lesion symptom/sign is NOT associated with suspected skin malignancy?

    a. Symmetry
    b. Change in sensation
    c. Change in colour
    d. Irregular border
    e. Lesion growth

Questions 8.5 to 8.8 concern the following medicines:

A.   Clotrimazole
B.   Miconazole
c.   Benzoyl peroxide
D.   Salicylic acid
E.   Nicotinamide
F.   Benzyl benzoate
G.   Minoxidil

Select, from A to G, which of the medicines:

8.5   Is associated with the greatest adverse event profile

8.6   Can bleach clothing

8.7   Not used in diabetic patients

8.8   Can produce systemic side effects

Questions 8.9 to 8.17 concern the following conditions:

A.   Chicken pox
B.   Cold Sores
C.   Impetigo
D.   Pityriasis versicolor
E.   Psoriasis
F.   Lichen planus
G.   Tinea corporis
H.   Fifth disease
I.   Molluscum contagiosum
J.   Pityriasis rosea

Select, from A to J, which of the conditions:

8.9   Is associated with a facial rash often resembling a 'slapped cheek'

8.10   Can be mistaken for warts

8.11   Is associated with moderate to severe itching

8.12   Sunlight can trigger symptoms

8.13   Itching, burning or tingling symptoms precede appearance of the lesions

8.14   Reinfection results in shingles

8.15   Is associated with a herald patch

8.16   Central clearing of the rash is often observed

8.17   Is bacterial in origin

Questions 8.18 to 8.20: these questions consist of a statement in the left-hand column, followed by a statement in the right-hand column. You need to:

- decide whether the first statement is true or false
- decide whether the second statement is true or false

Then choose:

A. If both statements are true, and the second statement is a correct explanation of the first statement

B. If both statements are true, but the second statement is NOT a correct explanation of the first statement

C. If the first statement is true, but the second statement is false

D. If the first statement is false, but the second statement is true

E. If both statements are false

Directions summarised

	1st statement	2nd statement	
A	True	True	2nd explanation is a correct explanation of the first
B	True	True	2nd statement is not a correct explanation of the first
C	True	False	
D	False	True	
E	False	False	

	First statement	*Second statement*
8.18	Psoriasis is characterised by rough/scaly rash	Increased cell turnover rate causes skin scaling
8.19	Emollients are the mainstay of treatment in dermatitis	Ointments tend to be less effective than creams
8.20	DLSO discolours and thickens the nail	It can be treated with terbinafine cream

Case study

CASE STUDY 8.1

Mr RJ and his 9-year-old son Jimmy want to buy something for Jimmy's verruca. Mr RJ thinks that Jimmy has had the verruca for about 4 to 6 weeks. He describes it as a circular, discoloured piece of skin that looks like the verrucas he used to get.

a. What course of action are you going to take?

Try and directly question Jimmy. See if Jimmy knows how long the suspected verruca has been there. Ask if the lesion is causing any pain when walking. Instead of asking for further descriptions of what the lesion looks like and where it is positioned, ask if you can look at the lesion.

On further questioning and examination you concur with the self-diagnosis of a verruca. The lesion is small (less than 0.5 cm in diameter) and causes minimal pain when direct pressure is applied.

b. What are you going to recommend?

A salicylic acid-based product is the most suitable product, and you recommend Bazuka after first making sure Jimmy is not a diabetic.

Six weeks later Mrs RJ returns with Jimmy and demands to see the pharmacist. She says the stuff you recommended is rubbish and Jimmy's verruca is bigger than it was before!

c. How are you going to respond?

First, you must stay calm and not be defensive. Ask open-ended questions to find out why Mrs J is unhappy; this approach will generally reveal what the problem is. Second, if the reason is not obvious, then you must find out about compliance. Who has been responsible for applying the product? If the parents have told Jimmy to use it, has he been using the product correctly and at the correct dosage frequency? In addition, many patients have unrealistic expectations on how quickly the verruca will resolve with therapy. Did you tell them how long it would take

before an effect will be seen? This is a vital piece of information to ensure patients realise that treatment is not a quick cure.

You find out that Mrs J has been applying the Bazuka and doing everything the instruction leaflet says. You inspect Jimmy's feet again and from what you can remember, the lesion does look slightly larger.

d. Why might this be the case?

Salicylic acid is destructive in nature and if the product comes in to contact with non-affected skin, then it can damage skin and appear to the patient that the lesion has indeed got bigger.

Mrs J wants to try Bazuka Extra Strength since the normal Bazuka is not helping.

e. What are you going to do?

You must try to stress to Mrs J that she continues with the normal Bazuka because 6 weeks of therapy is not long enough to make a decision to alter therapy.

Reluctantly, Mrs J accepts your advice and leaves the pharmacy promising she will try for a bit longer. One week later she presents a prescription for Cuplex gel for Jimmy.

f. What are you going to do?

It appears that Mrs J was not satisfied or convinced with your advice and has decided to see the GP. You do not know whether Mrs J told the doctor about using an OTC product. You could ring the GP to tell him or her that Mrs J has been using a salicylic acid-based product already; however, this is likely to have little bearing on the outcome of product selection as Jimmy will still need to continue treatment with something for a few more weeks. The prescription should be dispensed and Mrs J counselled appropriately. It would be unprofessional to point out that Cuplex is unlikely to be any better than Bazuka.

CASE STUDY 8.1 (Continued)

When you hand Mrs J the Cuplex, she mentions that the doctor said this was stronger than Bazuka and should do the trick.

g. How do you reply?

Be diplomatic and non-judgemental. It is likely that the doctor knows that Cuplex is no better than Bazuka

but if the parent is convinced that what she is now getting is superior to the previous product, then her motivation to comply with directions might be better and hence eradication of the verruca will occur. It might be worth asking the doctor, next time you have a conversation, what his or her rationale for prescribing Cuplex was.

CASE STUDY 8.2

Ms AH is the mother of an infant son aged 4 months. She asks for your help in treating her son's flaky skin on his scalp. She says he has had the problem on and off for the last 6 weeks. She hasn't yet tried anything except baby shampoo, as recommended by the health visitor. However, she now wants a cream or something to get rid of the problem once and for all.

a. What further information do you require to be in a position to help her?

You need to know more about the severity of the problem, for example whether any other areas of the baby's skin are affected. Does the baby appear to scratch at the rash and what were the previous episodes like? Were they the same as this time or different? Also, is there a family history of atopy or other dermatological conditions in the family.

You decide the child has cradle cap.

b. What treatment are you going to recommend?

The use of a mild tar-based product every other day until the scalp clears would be appropriate. In between using the tar-based product the mother should be instructed to use the baby shampoo.

Ms AH returns to the pharmacy 2 weeks later with another of her children. Impressed that her son's scalp is now clear she now wants some advice for her 7-year-old daughter. She has a sore on the corner of her mouth.

c. What further information do you require to be in a position to help her?

You need to know:

- *How long has the sore been present*
- *How the sore first developed*
- *What symptoms are associated with the sore*
- *The progression of the sore. Has it spread?*
- *Previous history of the rash and any family history*

You find out the sore appeared overnight and is now itchy. On inspection the lesion appears to be weeping a clear exudate.

d. What is the most likely diagnosis?

Based on this information the likely diagnosis is a cold sore.

e. What treatment, if any, are you going to recommend?

No treatment necessary but if the parent insists on therapy, then any product could be given, although antiviral therapy is expensive and the cost is difficult to justify. In addition, advice on minimising transmission could be given such as not sharing towels and trying to avoid kissing (e.g., mum and dad).

CASE STUDY 8.3

Mr RT, an elderly man, asks for some cream to help get rid of a rash he has over part of his chest. The following questions are asked, and responses received.

Information gathering	Data generated
How long had the symptoms	Rash started 3 days ago
What does it look like	Red and angry
Where exactly	Started on his left side below his armpit and now spread under the armpit
Other symptoms	Felt a bit unwell, slight loss of appetite & headache
Any itching or pain?	Some pain – rated as 4 on scale of 1–10
Previous history of presenting complaint	None similar
Past medical history	Slight stroke 1 year ago. Hypertension controlled with medication
	Eczema, contact dermatitis, urticarial reaction to some plants

Information gathering	Data generated
Drugs (OTC, Rx and compliance)	Warfarin, Bendroflumethiazide, Adalat LA
	Double Base cream
	Occasional use of clobetasone (Eumovate) for dermatitis
Allergies	Unknown
Social history Smoking Alcohol Drugs Employment Relationships	Wife died 6 months ago, finding it difficult to cope at times. Does not like to bother children who live locally. Feels very low
Family history	Not asked
On examination	Clusters of papules & vesicles unilaterally along dermatome, affecting left chest and back

Diagnostic pointers with regard to symptom presentation

For skin rash seen on the trunk in the area observed, then herpes zoster seems likely. The expected findings for questions when related to the possible conditions that could be confused with herpes zoster and are seen by community pharmacists are summarised below.

	Vesicles	Unilateral	Recurrent	Pain	Other symptoms
Herpes zoster	Yes	Yes	Unusual	Yes	Tingling/burning before eruption General malaise
Contact dermatitis	Possible	Yes	Yes	Possible	Itch
Herpes simplex	Yes	Yes	Yes	Yes	None of note
Eczema	Possible	Possible	Yes	Possible	Itch
Trauma	No	Possible	No	Yes	Should be an obvious cause

When this information is applied to that gained from our patient (below) we see that his symptoms fit with herpes zoster.

CASE STUDY 8.3 (Continued)

	Vesicles	Unilateral	Recurrent	Pain	Other symptoms
Herpes zoster	✓	✓	✓	✓	✓
Contact dermatitis	✓	✓	✗	✗?	✗
Herpes simplex	✓	✓	✗	✓	✗
Eczema	✓	✓	✗	✗	✗
Trauma	✗	✓	✗	✓	✗

Shingles information

Shingles is an acute infection caused by reactivation of latent varicella zoster virus. Following primary chickenpox infection, the virus lies dormant in the dorsal root ganglia of the spinal cord. When reactivated, it travels along the sensory nerve to affect one or more dermatomes, causing the characteristic shingles rash. Reactivation of the virus probably occurs following a decrease in cell-mediated immunity (e.g., with increasing age, HIV infection, illness). A diagnostic question to ask is previous history of chicken pox. If the patient has never had chicken pox, then they cannot develop shingles.

Course of action

The patient could be given analgesics to help with pain but referred for possible antivirals (e.g., Famciclovir 250 mg tds for 7 days) and warned about postherpetic neuralgia. The patient also seems to be showing signs of depression, which needs further investigation. It would be good practice, in this case, to try and speak with the doctor to arrange an urgent appointment for the patient to treat the rash but also mention your concerns over the patient exhibiting signs of depressive illness.

CASE STUDY 8.4

Mr AC, a man in his late 20s/early 30s, presents with a very itchy rash on his left hand. He asks if you can give him a cream to stop the itching. The following questions are asked, and responses received.

Information gathering	Data generated
How long had the symptoms	Few days
Rash anywhere else	No
Other symptoms/provokes	Not really – just really itchy!
Additional questions	No exposure to chemicals or new tasks involving hand work
Previous history of presenting complaint	No
Past medical history	Epileptic
Drugs (OTC, Rx and compliance)	Na valproate 500 mg bd. Well controlled
Allergies	None
Social history Employment Relationships	Works for the NHS doing patient transports
Family history	Dad has eczema

Information gathering	Data generated
On examination	Left hand and wrist has obvious red papules but look like they have been scratched (this is confirmed by patient)

Marked itching involving the hands is most likely to be scabies. However, other conditions are possible and are noted below:

Probability	Cause
Most likely	Scabies
Likely	Dermatitis, insect bites, pompholyx
Very unlikely	Dermatitis herpetiformis

Using the information gained from questioning and linking this with known epidemiology, it should be possible to make a differential diagnosis.

Diagnostic pointers with regard to symptom presentation

The expected findings for questions when related to the different conditions that can be seen by community pharmacists are summarised below.

	Location other than hands & wrists	Lesion appearance	Itch	Positive family or social history
Scabies	Unusual	Red papules through to vesicles	Intense	Yes
Dermatitis	Often (depends on type of dermatitis)	Red scaling rash that might crust over due to scratching	Moderate to intense	No
Insect bites	Often	Red papules through to vesicles	Moderate to intense	Possible
Pompholyx	Unusual	Vesicles	Intense	No
Dermatitis herpetiformis	Usual	Red papules through to vesicles	Intense	No

When this information is applied to that gained from our patient (below), we see that his symptoms most closely match scabies.

CASE STUDY 8.4 (Continued)

	Location other than hands & wrists	Lesion appearance	Itch	Positive family or social history
Scabies	✓	✓	✓ (intensity points more to scabies than other conditions)	✓ (occupation exposes person to higher risk)
Dermatitis	X?	X	✓	X
Insect bites	X	✓	✓	X?
Pompholyx	✓	X?	✓	X
Dermatitis herpetiformis	X	✓	✓	X

Therapy could be started with permethrin cream, although it is expensive and referral to the GP might be considered. It is also important to try and trace the contact from which he has contracted scabies and also inform work.

CASE STUDY 8.5

A patient asks you for some OTC 1% hydrocortisone cream to treat some eczema on her face. She tells you that she has read on an Internet forum that it is much cheaper to buy this product than to get it on prescription, but that she has also heard that many pharmacists 'make a fuss' about selling this for use on the face. What factors may have contributed to the development of this patient's view?

- Patients believe that they are well-informed, often as a consequence of Internet use
- Patients expect to get what they want at the best price, for medicines as for any other products. Patients often see medicines as commodities and not medicines.

- You need to:
Explain legal/ethical position of pharmacist
Explain risks
Suggest other options
Refuse sale

CASE STUDY 8.6

Atopic eczema, irritant contact dermatitis and allergic contact dermatitis can present in similar ways. For each condition name the features and causative factors that are common to all three.

All present as sore, red itchy skin lesions that appear in different locations. Affected sites help diagnose the condition.

- *Major factor in all three is the impaired barrier function of the epidermis, leading to increased loss of water – dry, cracked skin that allows entrance of irritants and allergens.*
- *Atopic eczema is due to internal factors. Cause thought to involve genetics, environmental triggers, defects in the epidermal skin barrier and the immunological response.*
- *Irritant contact dermatitis – caused by exogenous (external) factors. An irritant must penetrate the outer skin layer to initiate the physiological response, for example, detergents, soaps, solvents, abrasives, oils, etc.*

- *Allergic contact dermatitis – sensitisation must occur. Specific cell-mediated sensitisation by an allergen. Future exposure to the same allergen triggers memory T cells to initiate the inflammatory response. Lesions may appear at sites distant from the sight of exposure, for example, nickel and chromate, cement, cosmetics, rubber, dyes, topical corticosteroids.*

What other dermatological conditions need to be considered when differentiating eczema/dermatitis?

- *Lichen planus: thickened and scaly*
- *Psoriasis: general itch not present, distribution of lesions different*
- *Fungal infections: clearly defined edge, central clearing*
- *Discoid dermatitis: clear edges, circular/oval, symmetrical distribution*
- *Pompholyx: intensely itchy vesicles/blisters on hands/ soles of feet*
- *Urticaria: rash is itchy and red, as seen when stung by nettles. Skin shows signs of oedema, and blanches if pressed*

Answers

1 = d	2 = e	3 = a	4 = a	5 = F	6 = C	7 = D	8 = G	9 = H	10 = I
11 = A	12 = B	13 = B	14 = A	15 = J	16 = G	17 = C	18 = A	19 = C	20 = C

Musculoskeletal conditions

Background

The musculoskeletal system comprises of hard (bone and cartilage) and soft (muscles, tendons, ligaments) tissues. It is responsible for mobility and provides protection to vital structures. Most musculoskeletal problems occur as a result of injury or organic illness. The majority of patients presenting to a community pharmacist will have an acute problem arising from injury, although chronic conditions such as osteoarthritis will be encountered routinely when issuing prescriptions to patients.

The key role of the pharmacist when dealing with patients with a musculoskeletal problem is to establish the cause, its severity and whether it can be self-managed appropriately or requires further investigation.

General overview of musculoskeletal anatomy

The skeletal system of the human body is composed of 206 bones. At the point of contact between two or more bones, an articulation (joint) is formed. This system of bones and joints maximises movement while maintaining stability. There are two basic types of joints:

- synovial joints: allow considerable movement (e.g., shoulder or knee)
- fibrocartilaginous joints: are completely immoveable (e.g., the skull) or permit only limited motion (e.g., spinal vertebrae).

Bones and joints cannot move by themselves. The integrity of the musculoskeletal system depends on the interaction between skeletal muscle and bones, and coordinated movement is only possible because of the way muscle is attached to bone. Tendons attach the end of the muscle to the bone or another structure upon which the muscle acts. To perform such a function, tendons are composed of very dense fibrous tissue.

Joints require additional stability and support. Strong bands of fibrous tissue known as ligaments bind together bones entering a joint to provide this additional support and stability. It is often the integrity of the connecting structures that are damaged in a musculoskeletal injury. The simplified diagram of the medial aspect of the knee joint in Fig. 9.1 illustrates the relationship of the connective structures to the skeleton and musculature.

The knee joint is an example of a synovial joint. The femur, tibia and fibula do not touch each other because they are covered with articular cartilage and separated by the synovial cavity. The knee joint also contains bursae – small fluid sacs – that provide protection at points in the joint where friction or pressure is high. These can become inflamed, leading to bursitis.

History taking

Gaining an accurate history from the patient should provide enough information to determine whether their injury is within the scope of a community pharmacist. By the

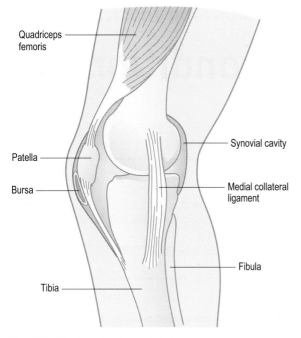

Fig. 9.1 The knee joint: medial view.

very nature of musculoskeletal injuries, if someone manages to come into the pharmacy then the injury is unlikely to be serious. Information gathering should concentrate on when the problem occurred, what precipitated it, the level of discomfort, any restriction in range of motion and whether the symptoms are worsening.

In general any patient who presents with an injury that is causing extreme discomfort or worsening pain or an injury that adversely affects mobility and has been present for more than a week would probably be better managed by a doctor or physiotherapist/sports therapist, and referral should be made.

Acute low back pain

Background

Low back pain is experienced in the lumbosacral area of the back, between the bottom of the ribs and the top of the legs. Acute back pain is classed as episodes lasting 6 weeks or less, and chronic if symptoms persist beyond 6 weeks.

Over 50% of patients will be pain free within 6–12 weeks, although up to two-thirds of patients will have a recurrence within 1 year after initial onset.

Prevalence and epidemiology

Low back pain is extremely common. For example, in the US it is the fifth common reason patients see a medical practitioner and in the UK 7–8% of all adult GP consultations are for low back pain. In 2004–2005, 4.5 million working days were lost through back pain in the UK.

Back pain is most common between the ages of 35 and 55, with prevalence rates similar for men and women, although 50–90% of pregnant women develop low back pain. Studies and statistical data have shown that in developed countries 60–90% of adults will experience an episode of low back pain at some point in their adult lives. Back pain is most common in those with skilled manual, partly skilled and unskilled jobs. Occupational risk factors in developing back pain include those who perform heavy manual labour, frequent bending, twisting and lifting, and people who remain in static positions for long periods of time such as truck and car drivers who drive long distances each year. Sports that involve excessive twisting, such as golf and gymnastics, can also lead to back pain.

Aetiology

In the majority of cases an exact cause cannot be determined for the patient's symptoms and is often referred to as simple, non-specific or uncomplicated low back pain. Pain originates from the lumbosacral region and is often mechanical in origin (Fig. 9.2) and includes problems caused by muscles, tendons, ligaments and discs. Contributory factors in the cause of low back pain are a general lack of fitness, occupational (as above) and psychosocial, for example anxiety and depression. Serious underlying pathology is very rare with infection and malignancy accounting for less than 1% of cases.

Arriving at a differential diagnosis

The vast majority of patients (95%) who present in the pharmacy will have simple back pain that will, in time, resolve with conservative treatment. The remaining cases will have back pain with associated nerve root compression. It is extremely unlikely that a pharmacist will encounter a patient with serious spinal pathology, such as infection or malignancy. However, pharmacists should be mindful that age can affect the diagnosis. Table 9.1 highlights those conditions that can be encountered by community pharmacists and their relative incidence.

Taking a thorough history is of key importance when evaluating a patient with low back pain. Begin questioning the patient with traditional questions regarding the

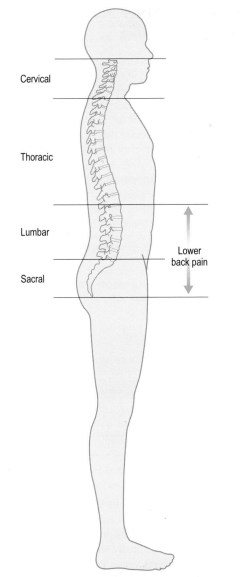

Cervical

Thoracic

Lumbar

Sacral

Lower back pain

Fig. 9.2 Location and distribution of lower back pain: L4–L5, pain radiates down outer calf and onto the top of the foot; L5–S1, pain radiates to the outside and sole of the foot.

pain: location, radiation, evidence of trauma, the effect pain has on mobility and factors which aggravate or relieve the pain (Table 9.2).

Clinical features of acute low back pain

Pain in the lower lumbar or sacral area is usually described as aching or stiffness. Depending on the cause, pain might be localised (e.g., lumbosacral strains after physical activity) or more diffuse (e.g., from postural backache after sit-

Table 9.1 **Causes of back pain and their relative incidence in community pharmacy**	
Incidence	Cause
Most likely	Simple back pain (usually associated with physical activity)
Likely	Sciatica, pregnancy
Unlikely	Osteoarthritis
Very unlikely	Malignancy, osteomyelitis, ankylosing spondylitis

ting incorrectly for a prolonged period). In cases of acute injury the symptoms come on quickly and there will be a reduction in mobility.

Bad posture when seated and poor lifting technique when performing day-to-day tasks, such as cleaning or gardening, are very common predisposing factors.

Conditions to eliminate

Likely causes

Sciatica

Sciatica typically occurs in healthy middle-aged adults. Pain is acute in onset and radiates to the leg. Pain starts in the lower back and as it intensifies radiates into the lower extremity. Disc herniation usually involves those between L4 and L5 and L5–S1 vertebrae (Fig. 9.2), although most occur between L5 and S1. If disc herniation is minimal, pain is dull, deep and aching. Pain spreads from the lumbar spine to the upper part of the leg. If the disc ruptures or herniates under strain, then pain is usually lancinating in quality, shooting down the leg like an electric shock. Valsalva movements, for example, coughing, sneezing or straining at stool, often aggravate pain. Referral is needed for confirmation of the diagnosis. Doctors can perform a straight-leg raising test whereby the pain of sciatica can be induced by elevating the leg of the patient when lying down. Prognosis is good, although improvement and recovery is often slower than in low back pain alone.

Unlikely causes

Osteoarthritis

In the context of low back pain pharmacists should only manage acute problems; however, patients will present with chronic symptoms and seek advice, especially those with degenerative joint disease. It is associated with advancing age, and affects up to one-third of people over

(?) Table 9.2
Specific questions to ask the patient: Back pain

Question	Relevance
Age	Age does influence the relative incidence of conditions seen in the population Under 15 years of age: Although back pain is uncommonly reported in children, children do have higher incidence of identifiable and potentially serious causes, for example, spondylolysis, malignancy and Scheuermann's disease (although pain is experienced in the upper back and neck, rather than the lower back). Also recent studies have linked weight of school bags to back pain. It would seem prudent to refer all children unless backache is associated with recent participation in sport 15–30: prolapsed disc, trauma, fractures, pregnancy and ankylosing spondylitis most likely 30–50: degenerative joint disease (osteoarthritis), prolapsed disc, and malignancy most likely. Older than 50 years of age: the incidence of serious underlying disorders increases, such as osteoporosis, malignancy and metabolic bone disorders (Paget's disease)
Location	Pain that radiates into the buttocks, thighs and legs implies nerve root compression. If pain is felt below the knee, this is highly suggestive of sciatica
Onset	Low back pain that is acute and sudden in onset is likely to be muscle strain in the lumbosacral region and not serious. However, acute low back pain in the elderly should be referred, as even slight trauma can result in compression fractures The patient will normally remember performing some recent exertion (playing sport, gardening, etc.) or say the pain started when they bent forward Low back pain that is insidious in onset should be viewed with caution
Restriction of movement	People with disc herniation usually have difficulty in sitting down for long periods Mechanical causes of pain are exacerbated with physical activity and relieved by rest Systemic causes of backache are usually worse with rest and disturb sleep
Weakness or numbness	Progressive muscle weakness must be referred for further evaluation

65 years of age and is twice as common in women. It can be localised to a single joint or involve multiple joints and most commonly affects the hands, knees, hips, neck and low back. It is thought that an imbalance of synthesis and degradation of cartilage is responsible for the disease, which affects the whole joint. It is characterised by pain of insidious onset that progressively increases over months or years and is exacerbated by exertion and relieved by rest. The affected joints are painful when used and may show a restricted range of motion. Stiffness in the affected joint occurs typically in the morning and after rest, but usually only lasts for 15 to 30 minutes.

Very unlikely causes

Infection (osteomyelitis)

Symptoms of osteomyelitis include bone pain, general malaise and presence of high fever. There may be local swelling, redness and warmth at the site of the infection. Patients also usually exhibit a loss of range of motion to the affected body part.

Ankylosing spondylitis

Spondylitis is characterised by thinning or loss of elasticity of the discs that cushion the vertebrae of the spine. It is three times more common in men and tends to run in families. Symptoms gradually worsen over a period of several months to several years. Patients commonly exhibit fatigue and have marked stiffness on awakening with pain that alternates from side to side of the lumbar spine. Pain may awaken the person at night and worsens at rest, but improves with physical activity. Pain can be made worse by bending, lifting and prolonged sitting in one position (e.g., long car journeys). Up to 40% of patients may also show inflammation of the eye.

Malignancy

Malignancy is very rare; it is more prevalent in patients over 50, although rates are still low – 0.14% in patients under 50 and 0.56% in patients over 50. A history of significant and unexplained weight loss, presence of anaemia, and failure of symptoms to improve over a 4-week period all warrant referral.

Causes of low back pain not related to back pathophysiology

It must be remembered that acute illness, for example, colds and influenza, can give rise to generalised aching or pain. Likewise, pre-rash pain associated with shingles and referred pain from abdominal organs (e.g., pyelonephritis) can present as low back pain. A careful history of the presenting symptoms should enable exclusion of such conditions.

! TRIGGER POINTS indicative of referral

Symptoms/signs	Possible danger/reason for referral
Fever	Infection
Pain that radiates away from lower back area	Sciatica
Young or older people (55 years old) Numbness Persistent and progressively worsening pain Weight loss Feeling unwell	Possible sinister spinal pathology
Bowel or bladder incontinence	Cauda equina syndrome (rare and very unlikely to be seen by a pharmacist)
Back pain from structures above the lumbar region	Outside scope of community pharmacist
Failure of symptoms to improve after 4 weeks	Requires further investigation as pain that becomes subacute/chronic requires medical intervention

---

Evidence base for over-the-counter medication

Pharmacists can appropriately treat patients with uncomplicated acute low back pain. The goal of treatment is to provide relief of symptoms and a return to normal mobility.

Conservative treatment

Bed rest was once widely prescribed for patients with low back pain. However, systematic reviews have now proven that prolonged bed rest is counterproductive (Dahm et al., 2010). The review found two trials ($n = 401$) that showed improvements in pain relief and functional status in patients with acute lower back pain (LBP) who were advised to stay active compared with bed rest. The authors conclude:

Moderate quality evidence shows that patients with acute LBP may experience small benefits in pain relief and functional improvement from advice to stay active compared with advice to rest in bed.

Exercise programmes can help with acute back pain and have been shown to reduce recurrence.

Analgesics (paracetamol, aspirin, ibuprofen)

All systemic analgesics when prescribed as monotherapy have proven efficacy in pain relief at standard doses. However, the use of nonsteroidal anti-inflammatory drugs (NSAIDs) for 7 to 10 days is widely advocated. A systematic review of NSAIDs in acute or chronic low back pain found treatment with an NSAID produced significant short-term improvement compared with placebo (Roelofs et al., 2008). The review identified 65 trials, 28 of which were rated as 'high quality'. The study failed to find any difference among the various NSAIDs. It also found that NSAIDs were no better than paracetamol for LBP. The authors did note that paracetamol had fewer side effects. Based on this observation, paracetamol may be the best first-line choice for most people. Patients must be advised to see their doctor if symptoms fail to improve after 7 days.

Compound analgesics (paracetamol/codeine, aspirin/codeine or paracetamol/dihydrocodeine)

It is recognised that combination analgesics with high doses of opioids are effective in acute and chronic pain. However, in the UK, codeine and dihydrocodeine can only be prescribed over the counter (OTC) provided their respective maximum strengths do not exceed 1.5% and the maximum dose does not exceed 20 or 10 mg, respectively. In practice, this equates to commercially available products with a maximum dose of 12.8 mg of codeine and 7.46 mg of dihydrocodeine. At these doses their painkilling effect has been called into question. In response to the ongoing concerns about codeine-containing products, the MHRA, in 2009, issued new guidance to restrict codeine-containing products for the short-term (3 days) treatment of acute, moderate pain which is not relieved by paracetamol, ibuprofen or aspirin alone. In 2013 the MHRA issued further guidance that codeine should not be given to children under the age of 12.

Caffeine

It has long been claimed that caffeine enhances analgesic efficacy and a number of proprietary products contain caffeine in doses ranging from 15 to 110 mg. A Cochrane review (Derry et al., 2012) identified 19 studies (*n* = 7238), which involved mainly paracetamol or ibuprofen, with 100 to 130 mg caffeine. Findings showed that there was a small, but statistically significant benefit with caffeine used at doses of 100 mg or more, which was not dependent on the pain condition or type of analgesic. The authors concluded that the addition of caffeine (100 mg) to a standard dose of commonly used analgesics provides a small but important increase in the proportion of participants who experience a good level of pain relief. In light of this new data, if recommending caffeine-containing products, only those with 100 mg or more of caffeine should be given.

Topical NSAIDs

A 2015 systematic review identified 61 studies comparing topical NSAIDs to oral NSAIDs and placebo (Derry et al., 2015). The review found that topical NSAIDs are effective in providing pain relief. Furthermore, certain formulations, mainly gel formulations of diclofenac, ibuprofen, and ketoprofen, provide the best results.

Rubefacients

Rubefacients (also known as counter irritants) have been incorporated in topical formulations for decades. They cause vasodilation, producing a sensation of warmth that distracts the patient from experiencing pain. It has also been hypothesised that increased blood flow might help disperse chemical mediators of pain, although this in unsubstantiated. Numerous chemicals are listed as being rubefacients.

Rubefacients containing salicylates have been reviewed (Derry et al., 2014) and shown to be no better than placebo.

Capsaicin

Capsaicin is approved for post-herpetic neuralgia and painful diabetic neuropathy (Axsain, capsaicin 0.075%) and symptomatic relief in osteoarthritis (Zacin, capsaicin 0.025%) in the UK via prescription. Although these are not available OTC, a number of OTC products do contain capsaicin (e.g., Balmosa, 0.035%, Ralgex cream, 0.12% and stick 1.96% capsaicin) at concentrations equivalent or higher than those found in prescription products.

Systematic reviews of the efficacy of capsaicin show mixed results (Mason et al., 2004; Zhang & Po, 1994). It appears its place in therapy is as second line or adjunctive treatment.

Enzymes

Heparinoid and hyaluronidase are included in a number of products. Theoretically they are supposed to disperse fluids in swollen areas, reducing swelling and bruising, but this is unproven.

Complementary therapies

Back pain accounts for more visits to a complementary practitioner than any other pain condition. In one study, 10% of people complaining of back pain had visited a complementary practitioner (osteopath, chiropractor, acupuncturist) (Maniadakis & Gray, 2000).

A limited, but growing body of clinical evidence exists to assess whether complementary therapies are effective. In light of the growing public interest and the expanding volume of literature, four Cochrane reviews have been conducted on heat and cold therapy (French et al., 2006), herbal remedies (Oltean et al., 2014), acupuncture (Furlan et al., 2005) and massage (Furlan et al., 2008) respectively.

Herbal remedies

Several herbal medicines are promoted as treatments for various types of pain, some of which have been tested for the relief of symptoms of low back pain. The Cochrane review reviewed four active constituents: *Harpagophytum procumbens* (Devil's Claw), *Salix alba* (white willow bark), *Capsicum frutescens* (cayenne) and *Solidago chilensis* (Brazilian arnica). Devil's Claw (standardised daily dose of 50 mg or 100 mg harpagoside) reduced pain more than placebo and a standardised daily dose of 60 mg was equally as effective as 12.5 mg of rofecoxib (now withdrawn from the market). Similarly, Willow Bark (standardised daily dose of 120 mg and 240 mg of salicin) was also more effective than placebo, and 240 mg of salicin was as effective as 12.5 mg of rofecoxib. Cayenne (as a cream or plaster) reduced pain more than placebo. One trial of arnica (*n* = 20) found very low quality evidence of reduction in perception of pain and improved flexibility.

Acupuncture

The available evidence for acupuncture in acute low back pain does not support its use, although if used in chronic back pain, acupuncture is more effective for pain relief than no treatment in the short term.

Massage therapy

Thirteen randomised control trials (RCTs) (*n* = 1596) were identified for the review, of which only five were considered of reasonable quality. Overall, the review concluded that massage might be beneficial in non-specific back pain, especially when combined with exercise and education. Acupuncture massage (applying pressure, tension or motion to specific points on the body) may be better than traditional massage. However, more evidence is required to confirm this.

Superficial heat and cold

Applying heat or cold to superficial musculoskeletal injuries, such as non-specific back pain, is a popular lay recommendation. These range from hot water bottles, heat pads and infrared lamps, to ice packs. The Cochrane review identified nine trials that met their inclusion criteria (six trials involved heat and three trials involved cold therapy). The authors concluded that many of the studies were of poor methodological quality, but evidence exists that continuous heat wrap therapy reduces pain and disability in the short-term to a small extent. No conclusions could be drawn on cold therapy due to the limited nature of the three trials reviewed.

Glucosamine

Although glucosamine is not used for acute low back pain, it is widely advertised to the general public as a treatment for osteoarthritis. Glucosamine is naturally found in the body, especially in cartilage, tendons and ligaments, and must be synthesised by the body because significant amounts are not found in the diet. Its active form, D-glucosamine is used in the manufacture of glycosaminoglycan, a precursor to cartilage tissue. Early reviews of glucosamine reported favourable decreases in pain and increase in joint function. However, a review by Towheed et al. (2005), including 20 studies with 2570 patients with osteoarthritis, found mixed results. When studies of sound methodological quality were used, the review failed to find any difference between glucosamine and placebo with regards to pain and changes in the Western Ontario and McMaster Osteoarthritis Index (WOMAC) function score. It still remains uncertain whether the two salts of glucosamine available, sulphate and hydrochloride, are equally active. Also studies so far have been relatively short (2–3 months) and any long-term benefits are still uncertain.

Chondroitin

Early research into the benefit of chondroitin in reducing pain and improving functionality in people with osteoarthritis showed chondroitin to be beneficial. Recent research that involved larger trials has shown no significant benefit. Patients should be advised that if they use chondroitin, then benefits are likely to be modest at best and if they want to use a natural product, that glucosamine would be a better choice (Wandel et al., 2010).

Arnica (Arnica montana)

There are only limited studies with arnica, and they have had mixed results with it having little or no effect on bruising and swelling in soft tissue injuries. Although generally well tolerated, arnica has been reported to produce allergic reactions in some people (Natural Medicines Comprehensive Database 2015).

Summary

Based on evidence, patients with acute low back pain should be encouraged to keep active and be given either paracetamol or a 7-day course of a systemic or topical NSAID unless contraindicated. Evidence for any complementary therapy is poor.

Compound analgesics should be avoided, although patients might perceive that they are getting a stronger pain killer.

Practical prescribing and product selection

Prescribing information relating to systemic analgesics reviewed in the section 'Evidence base for over-the-counter medication' is discussed and systemic proprietary products summarised in Table 9.3; useful tips relating to systemic analgesics are given in Hints and Tips in Box 9.1.

Paracetamol

Paracetamol is the safest analgesic. It can be given to all patient groups, has no significant drug interactions and side effects are very rare. Patients with low back pain will benefit most from taking paracetamol regularly at its maximum dose of 4 g (8 tablets) per day. It is the drug of choice in pregnancy and breastfeeding.

Aspirin

Unlike paracetamol, aspirin is associated with problems in its use. Children under 16 years of age should avoid any products containing aspirin (although children with low back pain should be referred). It can cause gastric irritation and is associated with gastric bleeds, especially in the elderly. For this reason, aspirin should not be given to this patient group or any patient with a history of peptic ulcer. In a small minority of asthmatic patients, aspirin can precipitate shortness of breath, therefore any asthmatic who has previously had a hypersensitivity reaction to aspirin should avoid aspirin. It should be avoided in patients taking warfarin as bleeding time is increased. Aspirin is best avoided in pregnancy because adverse effects to the mother and foetus have been reported. It should also be avoided in breastfeeding.

Nonsteroidal anti-inflammatories

The choice of oral OTC NSAIDs in the UK is limited to ibuprofen (Naproxen is currently only licensed for period

Table 9.3
Systemic proprietary analgesics available OTC (excludes paediatric formulations and products for period pain)

Product	Aspirin	Paracetamol	Ibuprofen	Codeine	Other	Children
Alka-Seltzer Original	324 mg					>16 years
Alka-Seltzer XS	267 mg	133 mg			Caffeine 40 mg	>16 years
Anadin Extra Tabs; Sol. Tabs	300 mg	200 mg			Caffeine 45 mg	>16 years
Anadin Ibuprofen; Anadin Joint Pain; Anadin Liquifast 200 mg Caps; Anadin Period Pain Relief; Anadin Ultra			200 mg			>12 years
Anadin Paracetamol		500 mg				>6 years
Anadin Original	325 mg				Caffeine 15 mg	>16 years
Aspro Clear	300 mg					>16 years
Aspro Clear Maximum Strength	500 mg					>16 years
Care Ibuprofen Tablets			200 mg			>12 years
Care Extra Strength Ibuprofen Tabs 400 mg			400 mg			>12 years
Codis 500	500 mg			8 mg		>16 years
Cuprofen			400 mg			>12 years
Disprin & Disprin Direct	300 mg					>16 years
Feminax Express (ibuprofen lysine 342 mg)			200 mg			>12 years
Hedex		500 mg				>6 years
Hedex Extra		500 mg			Caffeine 65 mg	>12 years
Hedex Ibuprofen			200 mg			>12 years
Ibufem			200 mg			>12 years
Mandanol		500 mg				>6 years
Mandanol Plus		500 mg			Caffeine 65 mg	>12 years
Nurofen Extensive formulation range All deliver 200 or 400 mg of ibuprofen as base. Many products now formulated as lysine salt and marketed to show amount of salt which is higher than the base. For example, Nurofen Maximum Strength Migraine Pain 648 mg Caplets. Formulations include: tablets, caplets, melt-tabs, liquid capsules			200 & 400 mg			>12 years

Table 9.3
Systemic proprietary analgesics available OTC (excludes paediatric formulations and products for period pain) (Continued)

Product	Aspirin	Paracetamol	Ibuprofen	Codeine	Other	Children
Nurofen Back Pain SR Caps			300 mg			>12 years
Nurofen Plus			200 mg	12.8 mg		>12 years
Nuromol		500 mg	200 mg			>18 years
Panadol Original Tabs; Soluble Tabs; Panadol Advance		500 mg				>6 years
Panadol Actifast		500 mg				>12 years
Panadol Actifast Sol		500 mg				>6 years
Panadol Extra Advance Tabs & Extra Sol Tabs		500 mg			Caffeine 65 mg	>12 years
Panadol Night Pain		500 mg			Diphenhydramine 25 mg	>12 years
Panadol Ultra		500 mg		12.8 mg		>12 years
Paracodol Tabs & Caps		500 mg		8 mg		>12 years
Paramol Tabs		500 mg			Dihydrocodeine 7.46 mg	>12 years
Solpadeine Plus Tablets; Capsules & Soluble Tablets		500 mg		8 mg	Caffeine 30 mg	>12 years
Solpadeine Max		500 mg		12.8 mg		>12 years
Solpadeine Max Sol. Tablets		500 mg		12.8 mg	Caffeine 30 mg	>12 years
Solpadeine Migraine			200 mg	12.8 mg		>12 years
Solpadeine Headache Sol. Tabs.		500 mg			Caffeine 65 mg	>12 years
Syndol		500 mg		8 mg	Caffeine 30 mg	>12 years
Ultramol Sol. Tabs.		500 mg		8 mg	Caffeine 30 mg	>12 years
Veganin Tablets		500 mg		8 mg	Caffeine 30 mg	>12 years

HINTS AND TIPS BOX 9.1: ASPIRIN IN CHILDREN

Children and aspirin	Aspirin-taking in children has been linked to Reyes' syndrome; a rare syndrome in which encephalopathy occurs and if not diagnosed early can lead to death
Caffeine-containing analgesics	These might have a mild stimulant effect and should therefore be avoided before going to bed

pain - see page 135 for more information). The recommended dosage of ibuprofen in adults is 200 to 400 mg (one or two tablets) three times a day, although most patients will need the higher dose of 400 mg three times a day.

NSAIDs are best avoided in certain patient groups, such as the elderly, because they are more prone to gastrointestinal (GI) bleeds and have reduced renal function. Patients with a history of peptic ulcers and those asthmatics who are hypersensitive to aspirin should also avoid NSAIDs. NSAIDs can be used in pregnancy but may delay labour; the use of NSAIDs, particularly in the last trimester, should be done under medical advice. They can be used in breastfeeding.

For the majority of patients, NSAIDs are well tolerated, although gastric irritation is a well-recognised side effect. They can interact with many medicines and, although most of these interactions are not significant, NSAIDs can alter lithium levels so that, where possible, an alternative analgesic should be recommended. If an NSAID is given with lithium, then the patient's serum lithium needs to be monitored more closely than normal.

Topical NSAIDs

Topical NSAIDs provide an alternative to those patients who should avoid systemic NSAID therapy. They have fewer side effects than systemic therapy with the most commonly reported adverse events being skin reactions (maculopapular rash or itching) at the site of application. GI side effects have been reported but are rare. Low plasma levels probably explain their low incidence of adverse systemic effects. Most manufacturers recommend avoiding use during pregnancy because of the same potential adverse effects as oral NSAIDs, although the risks should be generally far lower than with oral NSAIDs.

Topical NSAIDs come in a range of formulations, including cream, gel, spray and mousse. Table 9.4 highlights all UK commercially available NSAIDs (as of Sept 2015) and summarises their prescribing information.

Rubefacients (e.g., Deep Heat, Radain B ranges)

Rubefacients should be avoided in young children. Lower age limits vary from manufacturer to manufacturer and from formulation to formulation. Many products are only licensed for people over 12 years of age, although there are a few which can be used from the age of 5 (e.g., Deep Heat range) or 6 years old (e.g., Radian B Muscle Rub). They have no drug interactions, and side effects are localised to excessive irritation at the site of application. The majority of products contain two or more compounds, although most contain nicotinates and/or salicylates. Other compounds in rubefacients include menthol, camphor, capsaicin and turpentine oil. They can be used in all patient groups.

References

Dahm KT, Brurberg KG, Jamtvedt G, et al. Advice to rest in bed versus advice to stay active for acute low-back pain and sciatica. Cochrane Database of Systematic Reviews 2010, Issue 6. Art. No.: CD007612. http://dx.doi.org/10.1002/14651858.CD007612.pub2.

Derry CJ, Derry S, Moore RA. Caffeine as an analgesic adjuvant for acute pain in adults. Cochrane Database of Systematic Reviews 2012, Issue 3. Art. No.: CD009281. http://dx.doi.org/10.1002/14651858.CD009281.pub2.

Derry S, Matthews PRL, Wiffen PJ, et al. Salicylate-containing rubefacients for acute and chronic musculoskeletal pain in adults. Cochrane Database of Systematic Reviews 2014, Issue 11. Art. No.: CD007403. http://dx.doi.org/10.1002/14651858.CD007403.pub3.

Derry S, Moore RA, Gaskell H, et al. Topical NSAIDs for acute musculoskeletal pain in adults. Cochrane Database of Systematic Reviews 2015, Issue 6. Art. No.: CD007402. http://dx.doi.org/10.1002/14651858.CD007402.pub3.

French SD, Cameron M, Walker BF, et al. Superficial heat or cold for low back pain. Cochrane Database of Systematic Reviews 2006, Issue 1. Art. No.: CD004750. http://dx.doi.org/10.1002/14651858.CD004750.pub2.

Furlan AD, van Tulder MW, Cherkin DC, et al. Acupuncture and dryneedling for low back pain. Cochrane Database of Systematic Reviews 2005, Issue 1. Art. No.: CD001351. http://dx.doi.org/10.1002/14651858.CD001351.pub2

Furlan AD, Imamura M, Dryden T, et al. Massage for low-back pain. Cochrane Database of Systematic Reviews 2008, Issue 4. Art. No.: CD001929. http://dx.doi.org/10.1002/14651858.CD001929.pub2.

Maniadakis A, Gray A. The economic burden of back pain in the UK. Pain 2000;84:95–103.

Mason L, Moore, A, Derry S, et al. Systematic review of topical capsaicin for the treatment of chronic pain. BMJ 2004;328(7446):991–996.

Oltean H, Robbins C, van Tulder MW, et al. Herbal medicine for low-back pain. Cochrane Database of Systematic Reviews 2014, Issue 12. Art. No.: CD004504. http://dx.doi.org/10.1002/14651858.CD004504.pub4.

Roelofs PDDM, Deyo RA, Koes BW, et al. Non-steroidal anti-inflammatory drugs for low back pain. Cochrane Database of Systematic Reviews 2008, Issue 1. Art. No.: CD000396. http://dx.doi.org/10.1002/14651858.CD000396.pub3.

Towheed T, Maxwell L, Anastassiades TP, et al. Glucosamine therapy for treating osteoarthritis. Cochrane Database of Systematic Reviews 2005, Issue 2. Art. No.: CD002946. http://dx.doi.org/10.1002/14651858.CD002946.pub2.

Wandel, S, Juni, P, Tendal B, et al. Effects of glucosamine, chondroitin, or placebo in patients with osteoarthritis of hip or knee: network meta-analysis. BMJ 2010;341:c4675. doi:4610.1136/ bmj.c4675.

Zhang W, Po ALW. The effectiveness of topically applied capsaicin. Eur J Clin Pharmacol 1994;46:517–22.

Table 9.4
Proprietary topical NSAID analgesics available OTC

Product	Formulation	Strength	Dosage	Children
Ibuprofen				
Care	Gel	5% & 10%	qds	>14 years
Deep Relief	Gel	5%	tds	>12 years
Fenbid	Gel	5%	Up to qds	>12 years
Fenbid Forte	Gel	10%	Up to qds	>12 years
Ibugel	Gel	5%	No dose stated	>12 years
Ibuleve	Gel	5%	tds	>12 years
Ibuleve Maximum Strength	Gel	10%	tds	>12 years
Ibumousse	Mousse	5%	tds-qds	>12 years
Ibuleve Speed Relief	Gel	5 & 10%	tds	>12 years
Ibuleve Speed Relief	Spray	5%	Up to qds	>12 years
Ibuspray	Spray	5%	tds-qds	>12 years
Mentholatum	Gel	5%	tds	>14 years
Nurofen	Gel	5% & 10%	qds	>14 years
Phorpain & Phorpain Forte	Gel	5% & 10%	qds	>12 years
Radian B Ibuprofen	Gel	5%	qds	>14 years
Other NSAIDs				
Difflam (benzydamine)	Cream	3%	tds but max of six times	No lower age limit stated
Movelat (mucopolysaccharide polysulpahate & salicylic acid)	Cream and Gel	0.2% & 2.0%	qds	>12 years
Traxam Pain Relief (Felbinac)	Gel	3%	bd-qds	>12 years
Voltarol Emulgel P & Voltarol Pain-Eze Emulgel (Diclofenac)	Gel	1.16 %	tds-qds	>14 years
Voltarol 12 hour Emulgel	Gel	2.32%	bd	>14 years

Further reading
Bueff HU, Van Der Reis W. Low back pain. Prim Care 1996;23:345–64.
Deyo RA, Weinstein JN. Low back pain. N Engl J Med 2001;344:363–70.
Henschke N, Maher CG, Refshauge KM. Screening for malignancy in low back pain patients: a systematic review. Eur Spine J 2007;16(10):1673–9.

Koes BW, van Tulder MW, Thomas S. Diagnosis and treatment of low back pain. BMJ 2006;332: 1430–4.
Reichenbach S, Sterchi R, Scherer M, et al. Chondroitin for osteoarthritis of the knee or hip. Ann Intern Med 2007;146:580–90.

Websites
BackCare: the charity for healthier backs: http://www.
backcare.org.uk/
The National Ankylosing Spondylitis Society: http://www.nass.
co.uk/

Activity-related/sports-related soft tissue injuries

This section will discuss common conditions affecting the shoulder, elbow, knee, ankle and foot.

Background

Muscles, tendons, ligaments, fascia and synovial capsules are all soft tissue structures. Damage to any of these structures will result in pain and/or inflammation. The majority of patients will present to a doctor, physiotherapist or casualty department rather than the pharmacy. However, a number of small studies report that when people use the pharmacy, they are satisfied with the advice received.

Prevalence and epidemiology

Most injuries are as a direct result of physical activity or accident. Prevalence is therefore higher in people who actively participate in sports, and injuries involving the lateral ligaments of the ankle account for 25% of all sports injuries.

Aetiology

The aetiology of soft tissue injury depends on the structures affected. Sprains are due to forcing a joint into an abnormal position that overstretches or twists ligaments, and can vary from damage of a few fibres to complete rupture. Strains involve tearing of muscle fibres, which can be partial or complete, and are usually a result of over exertion when the muscle is stretched beyond its usual limits.

Arriving at a differential diagnosis

Patients will often state that they have sprained or strained something. It is important to confirm their self-diagnosis, as these terms are often used wrongly and interchangeably. Although sprains and strains can be graded according to the severity of the injury, it is of little practical value because it has no therapeutic consequence; therefore the major role of the pharmacist is to determine whether the patient can manage the injury or whether referral is needed. This will be primarily based on questions asked (Table 9.5) that can be supported with the aid of a basic physical examination.

Clinical features of soft tissue injury

In general patients will present with pain, swelling and bruising. The extent and nature of symptoms will be determined by the severity of the injury.

Shoulder-specific conditions

The shoulder provides the greatest range of motion of any joint. It is a very mobile and complex interconnected structure (Fig. 9.3); consequently, there are a number of commonly encountered shoulder injuries, such as frozen shoulder, impingement syndromes and rotator cuff syndrome. The prevalence of shoulder-related problems is uncertain, although estimates range from 4% to 20%, with rotator cuff syndrome accounting for up to 70% of shoulder problems.

Within the confines of the community pharmacy, the patient can be asked to perform certain arm movements that will allow the range of motion of the shoulder to be determined (Fig. 9.4). Patients who show marked loss of motion should be referred.

Rotator cuff syndrome
The rotator cuff refers to the combined tendons of the scapula muscles that hold the head of the humerus in place. Rubbing of these tendons causes pain. It is most often seen in patients over the age of 40 and is associated with repetitive overhead activity. Pain tends to be worse at night and might disturb sleep. Reaching behind the back also tends to worsen pain and the patient cannot normally initiate abduction.

Frozen shoulder
Pain is gradual in onset causing aching in the upper arm that can become severe and radiate down the arm to the elbow. As the condition worsens, marked stiffness and restriction in all the major ranges of motion is observed. Pain can interfere with sleep. It is a relatively uncommon cause of shoulder pain accounting for 2% of cases. It often occurs without warning or explanation and can vary in severity from day-to-day. NSAIDs could be offered but if symptoms fail to respond with treatment after 5 days, then referral for alternative treatment and physiotherapy should be considered.

Table 9.5
Specific questions to ask the patient: Soft tissue injuries

Question	Relevance
When did it happen and when did the patient present	The closer these two events are, the more likely the patient will be suffering from a serious problem that is outside the remit of the pharmacist, unless the injury was sustained in close proximity to the pharmacy and the patient has asked for first aid
Presenting symptoms	Marked swelling, bruising and pain occurring straight after injury is suggestive of more serious injury and referral to casualty for x-rays and further tests is needed
Nature of injury	If the injury occurred in which impact forces were great, then fracture becomes more likely Sudden onset, associated with a single traumatic event suggests a mechanical problem such as tendon/ligament tearing If the person has a foot injury and is unable to bear their full weight while walking, then referral is needed
Range of motion	If the affected joint shows marked reduction in normal range of motion, this requires referral for fuller evaluation
Nature of pain	Referred pain suggests nerve root compression, for example, a shoulder injury in which pain is also felt in the hand Pain that is insidious in onset and progressive is more likely to be due to some form of degenerative disease and requires referral
Age of patient	*Children:* Bones are softer in children and therefore more prone to greenstick fractures (fracture of the outer part of the bone) and should be referred to exclude such problems *Elderly:* Risk factors for fracture, such as osteoarthritis and osteoporosis, should be established

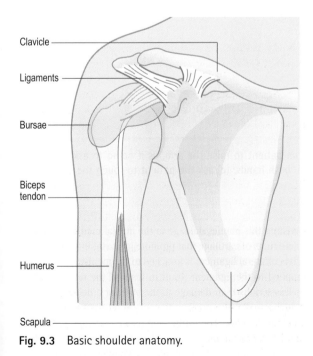

Clavicle

Ligaments

Bursae

Biceps tendon

Humerus

Scapula

Fig. 9.3 Basic shoulder anatomy.

Elbow-specific conditions

Community pharmacists are only likely to see three elbow problems: tennis elbow (lateral epicondylitis), golfer's elbow (medial epicondylitis) and student's elbow (bursitis).

Tennis elbow is characterised by pain and tenderness felt over the outer aspect of the elbow joint that might also spread up the upper arm. The patient should have a history of gradually increasing pain and tenderness. If the patient tries to extend the wrist against resistance, then pain increases. In comparison, the pain of golfer's elbow is noticed on the inner side of the elbow and can radiate down the forearm. Both names are misleading as these conditions are usually related to a repetitive activity, which will often not be associated with sports activity.

Knee-specific conditions

The knee is the largest joint in the body and is subject to extreme forces. Unsurprisingly, it is one of the most common sites of sport injuries, especially among footballers. To help maintain stability, the knee has three main pairs

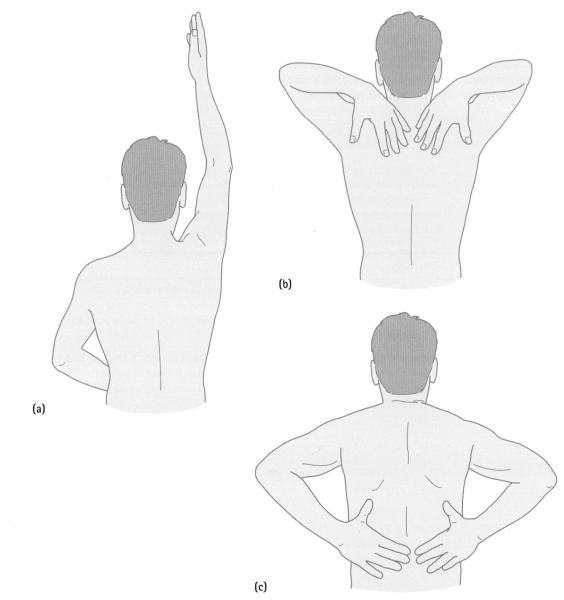

(a)

(b)

(c)

Fig. 9.4 Determining the shoulder's range of motion: (a) ask the patient to raise the arm, as if going to ask a question at school; (b) ask the patient to touch the back of the neck with both hands; (c) ask the patient to touch the back of the scapulae with both hands.

of ligaments: the medial collateral ligament, which connects the femur to the tibia; the lateral collateral ligament, which connects the femur to the fibula and the anterior cruciate ligament, which prevents the tibia from sliding forward on the femur (Fig. 9.5).

Ligament damage

This is most often seen in footballers. Find out from the person how the injury occurred. If the injury occurred when twisting this implies damage to the medial meniscus (incomplete rings of cartilage that promote joint stability) as the medial collateral ligament is attached to the meniscus and forces applied to the ligament result in tears of the meniscus. This is less serious than damage to the anterior cruciate ligament, which usually occurs when the person receives a blow to the back of the knee. The former can usually respond to NSAIDs and physiotherapy, whereas the latter can take months to heal and might stop people from playing competitive sport.

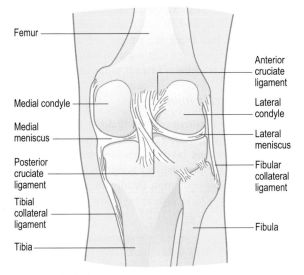

Fig. 9.5 Basic knee anatomy.

Runner's knee (chondromalacia)

This is most commonly noted in recreational joggers who are increasing their mileage, for example, training to run a marathon. It develops insidiously with pain being the predominant symptom. Pain is experienced usually at the front of the knee or behind the kneecap. Pain can be aggravated by prolonged periods of sitting down in the same position or going up and down stairs. Treatment depends on the severity of pain, from NSAIDs if the pain is mild, to total rest and stopping running if severe.

Ankle and foot specific conditions

The majority involve sprained ankles whether through sporting activity or just as a result of accidents.

Ankle sprains

The ankle acts as a hinge joint permitting up and down motion. Three sets of ligaments provide stability to the joint: the deltoid, lateral collateral and syndesmosis. The majority of ankle sprains involve the lateral ligamentous structures due to inversion of the joint leading to injury (Fig. 9.6). Patients usually describe an accident when they 'went over their ankle'. Most patients will walk with a limp because the ankle cannot support their full weight.

Achilles tendon injuries

Injuries to the structures associated with the Achilles tendon are usually seen in runners or athletes involved in jumping sports. Pain is felt behind the heel, just above the calcaneus, and progressively worsens the longer the injury lasts. It often occurs when runners increase their mileage or run over hilly terrain. Depending on the severity of the

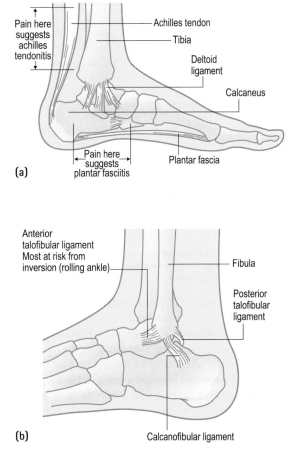

Fig. 9.6 Basic anatomy of the ankle: (a) medial view; (b) lateral view.

injury, treatment could be anything from NSAIDs, complete rest or having a cast fitted. If the injury is recent in onset and pain not too severe, the pharmacist could suggest NSAID therapy and rest. If this fails, then the person should be referred.

Plantar fasciitis

The plantar fascia extends from the calcaneus to the middle phalanges of the toes. Runners are most prone to plantar fasciitis, although it can affect older people. Patients will present with tenderness and pain felt along the plantar surface of the foot and heel. Pain is insidious and progressively worsens, which can limit activity.

Common muscle strains

Thigh strains

Tears of the quadriceps (front of the thigh) and hamstring (back of the thigh) are very common. Patients will not always be able to recall a specific event that has caused the strain. Pain and discomfort is worsened when the patient tries to use the muscle, but daily activities can usually be performed. Rest, ice, compression and elevation (RICE) followed by NSAID treatment will usually resolve the problem; however, referral is needed if daily activities are compromised.

Delayed onset muscle soreness

This is a common problem and follows unaccustomed strenuous activity. For example, the patient might describe playing football for the first time in a long while or having just started going to aerobic classes. Pain is felt in the muscles, which feel stiff and tight. Pain peaks within 72 hours. Patients should be encouraged to properly stretch before exercising to minimise the problem. No treatment is necessary.

Conditions to eliminate

Shin splint syndrome

Recreational runners and people unaccustomed to regular running can experience pain along the front of the lower third of the tibia. Pressing gently on this area will cause considerable pain. It is caused by over stretching the tibial muscle and is usually precipitated by running on hard surfaces. Pain is made worse by continued running or climbing stairs. Treatment involves running less frequently or for shorter distances and NSAID therapy for approximately 1 week.

Bursitis

Bursae can become inflamed, which leads to accumulation of synovial fluid in the joint. Housemaid's knee and student's elbow are such examples. Clinically, joint swelling is the predominant feature, with associated pain and local tenderness.

Stress fractures

These are most commonly associated with the foot. Patients experience a dull ache along the affected metatarsal shaft that changes to a sharp ache behind the metatarsal head. It is often seen in those patients that have a history of increased activity or a change in footwear.

Gout

Acute attacks of gout are exquisitely painful, with patients reporting that even bedclothes cannot be tolerated. Approximately 80% of cases affect the big toe. Gout is more prevalent in men, especially over the age of 50.

Carpal tunnel syndrome

At the base of the palm is a 'tunnel' through which the median nerve passes; this narrow passage between the forearm and hand is called the carpal tunnel. If the median nerve becomes trapped, it can cause numbness and tingling in the hand. Often the patient will awaken in the night with numbness and tingling pain that radiates to the forearm, which sometimes extends to the shoulder.

Repetitive strain injury

This condition, also termed chronic upper limb pain syndrome, often results after prolonged periods of steady hand movement and involves repeated grasping, turning and twisting. The predominant symptom is pain in all or one part of one or both arms. Usually the person's job will involve repetitive tasks such as keyboard operations.

> **❗ TRIGGER POINTS indicative of referral: Soft tissue injury**
>
> | Symptoms/signs | Possible danger/reason for referral |
> |---|---|
> | Acute injuries which show immediate swelling and severe pain | Suggests significant trauma and/or fracture |
> | Marked decrease or excessive range of movement in any joint | May suggest major ligament disruption |
> | Patients unable to bear weight on an injured ankle/foot | Fractures more likely |
> | Children under 12 years of age and elderly patients | |

Evidence base for over-the-counter medication and practical prescribing and product selection

Prescribing information relating to medication for soft tissue injuries is the same as for acute low back pain (see page 287). However, non-drug treatment plays a vital and major role in the treatment of acute soft tissue injuries. Standard advice follows the acronym RICE:

Rest	Rest allows immobilisation, enhancing healing and reducing blood flow
Ice	Ice should be applied while the injury feels warm to the touch. Apply until the skin becomes numb and repeat at hourly intervals. Bags of frozen peas wrapped in a towel are ideal to use on the injury as they conform to body shape and provide even distribution of cold

Compression	A crepe bandage provides a minimum level of compression. Tubular stockings (e.g., Tubigrip) are convenient and easy to apply, but fail to give adequate compression
Elevation	Ideally the injured part should be elevated above the heart to help fluid drain away from the injury

Further reading

Calmbach WL, Hutchens M. Evaluation of patients presenting with knee pain: Part II. Differential diagnosis. Am Fam Physician 2003;68:917–22.

Kayne S, Reeves A. Sports care and the pharmacist-an opportunity not to be missed. Pharm J 1994;253:66–7.

Murrell J. Walton Diagnosis of rotator cuff tears. Lancet 2001;357:769–70.

Polisson RP. Sports medicine for the internist. Med Clin N Am 1986;70:469–89.

Spiegel TM, Crues JV. The painful shoulder: diagnosis and treatment. Prim Care 1988;15:709–24.

West SG, Woodburn J. Pain in the foot. BMJ 1995;310:860–4.

Website

Society of Sports Therapists: http://www.society-of-sports-therapists.org

Self-assessment questions

The following questions are intended to supplement the text. Two levels of questions are provided; multiple choice questions and case studies. The multiple choice questions are designed to test factual recall and the case studies allow knowledge to be applied to a practice setting.

Multiple choice questions

9.1   Which of the following symptoms is commonly associated with sciatica?

   a. Pain that radiates to the thoracic vertebrae
   b. Pain that radiates to the quadriceps
   c. Pain that radiates down the hamstring
   d. Pain that radiates to the groin
   e. Pain that radiates to sacroiliac junction

9.2   A fit young man (early twenties) played football for the first time in over a year, 2 days ago. He telephones the pharmacy for advice because he cannot walk properly as he has stiff legs. Which condition is he most likely to be experiencing from his football activities?

   a. Shin splint syndrome
   b. Thigh strain
   c. Hamstring strain
   d. Delayed onset muscle soreness
   e. Chondromalacia

9.3   Which anatomical structure attaches bone to muscle?

   a. Ligament
   b. Tendon
   c. Bursae
   d. Cartilage
   e. Fibrous tissue

9.4   Mr Smith, a 47-year-old hypertensive and asthmatic patient, asks for a painkiller, as he has 'turned his ankle' while playing golf. Which treatment is most suitable?

   a. Aspirin
   b. Ibuprofen
   c. Heat rub
   d. Paracetamol
   e. Arnica

Questions 9.5 to 9.10 concern the following conditions/symptoms:

A.   Lateral epicondylitis
B.   Medial epicondylitis
C.   Rotator cuff syndrome
D.   Bursitis
E.   Plantar fasciitis
F.   Chondromalacia
G.   Stress fracture
H.   Sciatica

Select, from A to H, which condition/symptom is most associated with:

9.5   Radiating pain

9.6   Increased pain when sedentary

9.7   Worsening pain at night

9.8   Joint swelling

9.9   Pain over the outer elbow

9.10 Repetitive activity

Questions 9.11 to 9.14 concern the following medicines:

A.   Paracetamol
B.   Aspirin
C.   Naproxen
D.   Ibuprofen
E.   Diclofenac
F.   Caffeine
G.   Glucosamine
H.   Codeine
I.   White willow bark

Select, from A to I, which of the above medicines:

9.11 Is only available topically

9.12 Is safest for pregnant women

9.13 Has a stimulant effect

9.14 Analgesic effect has been called in to question

Questions 9.15 to 9.17: for each of these questions *one or more* of the responses is (are) correct. Decide which of the responses is (are) correct. Then choose:

A. If a, b and c are correct
B. If a and b only are correct
C. If b and c only are correct
D. If a only is correct
E. If c only is correct

Directions summarised

A	B	C	D	E
a, b and c	a and b only	b and c only	a only	c only

9.15 Caffeine is incorporated into analgesics. The effect caffeine has is:

   a. To enhance the analgesic effect
   b. To speed up absorption of analgesics
   c. To stimulate peristalsis

9.16 In which scenario should the patient be referred when presenting with low back pain?

   a. Radiating pain
   b. Numbness
   c. General malaise

9.17 Carpal tunnel syndrome causes:

   a. Pain that radiates into the hand
   b. Tingling sensation in the hand
   c. Numbness in the hand

Questions 9.18 to 9.20: these questions consist of a statement in the left-hand column, followed by a statement in the right-hand column. You need to:

- decide whether the first statement is true or false
- decide whether the second statement is true or false

Then choose:

A. If both statements are true, and the second statement is a correct explanation of the first statement
B. If both statements are true, but the second statement is NOT a correct explanation of the first statement
C. If the first statement is true, but the second statement is false
D. If the first statement is false, but the second statement is true
E. If both statements are false

Directions summarised

	1st statement	2nd statement	
A	True	True	2nd explanation is a correct explanation of the first
B	True	True	2nd statement is not a correct explanation of the first
C	True	False	
D	False	True	
E	False	False	

	First statement	*Second statement*
9.18	Elevation of the limb is advocated in soft tissue injuries	Elevation allows the fluid to drain away from the injury
9.19	Gout is usually observed in the body extremities	Uric acid crystals precipitate out giving rise to symptoms
9.20	Stress fractures are almost exclusively seen in children	Fractures are mostly seen in the foot

Case study

Mrs BB, a 69-year-old woman, hobbles into your pharmacy, supported by her husband. She has just slipped off the pavement edge and believes she has sprained her ankle.

a. To ascertain if referral is necessary, describe the questions you would ask Mrs BB.

Find out the exact nature of the pain and its location. It is likely that the anterior talofibular ligament has been damaged. Symptoms that would warrant referral are severe pain in any bone prominence, if Mrs BB is unable to walk unsupported for at least four steps and marked swelling and bruising occurred straight after the fall. Mrs BB should be told to go to casualty if these symptoms are present. You decide that Mrs BB has indeed sprained her ankle, but referral is unnecessary. Mrs BB asks to purchase some OTC analgesia to alleviate her pain. Her regular medication is as follows:

- *Bendroflumethiazide 2.5 mg od: used to treat hypertension; taken for 5 years*
- *Fybogel sachets, 1 bd: taken for 4 years for constipation*
- *Lansoprazole 15 mg od: maintenance therapy in treatment of gastro-oesophageal reflux disease (GORD) associated with hiatus hernia.*

b. Which OTC systemic analgesics would be most suitable for Mrs BB? Explain how you arrived at your choice and why you eliminated others.

- *Aspirin: can cause GI disturbance; Mrs BB has GORD; therefore, aspirin is contraindicated.*
- *Ibuprofen: NSAIDs can cause fluid retention and Mrs BB has hypertension. However, this is unlikely*

to be clinically significant, especially if only NSAIDs are recommended for only a few days. Like aspirin, ibuprofen can cause GI disturbances.
- *Paracetamol and/or products with codeine: combinations with aspirin/ibuprofen need to be avoided. Paracetamol and codeine combinations could be offered but the analgesic effect of codeine is questionable, and the codeine content is likely to worsen her already existing constipation. This leaves paracetamol as the medicine of choice for Mrs BB.*

Mrs BB asks if she should also use a cream on her ankle.

c. Describe which would be suitable to recommend to Mrs BB. Give the reasons for your decision(s).

Rubefacients contain essential oils, salicylates, nicotinates, capsicum, camphor, turpentine and menthol. Evidence is lacking with regard to their efficacy in decreasing pain but they help in masking pain symptoms. These could be recommended to Mrs BB but ideally recommend a product with no salicylate present as there is a low risk of systemic absorption and gastric irritation.

Topical NSAIDs: relatively low doses reach the bloodstream, and there is therefore less risk of GI problems than with systemic NSAIDs. Use of topical NSAIDs are unlikely to cause side effects if used for short periods of time (5–10 days) and could be given to Mrs BB even though she has GORD. However, she should be told that if she experiences any indigestion-type symptoms to stop using the product.

9

CASE STUDY 9.2

Mr JD, a 47-year-old male, asks you for something for low back pain. On questioning you find out the following:

Information gathering	Data generated
Describe the pain	Pain described as aching and dull and spreads to bottom on the right hand side
How long have you had the symptoms?	Came on about 2 days ago. Woke up with the pain
Where is the pain?	Pain is diffuse over low back
Any other symptoms?	No other symptoms
When do you get the symptoms?	Constant
Does the pain move anywhere?	Top of the bum (as above)
Does anything make the symptoms better/worse?	Pain is made worse if sitting over a long period of time
Additional questions asked	Cannot remember doing anything to precipitate it. Severity – 5/6 out of 10

Information gathering	Data generated
Previous history of presenting complaint	No
Past medical history (PMH)	No PMH
Drugs (OTC, Rx and compliance)	Esomeprazole 1 od for last year to help with indigestion
Social history	Works in an office No lifestyle changes
Family history	Not asked
On examination	Not performed

Diagnostic pointers with regard to symptom presentation

The next table summarises the expected findings for questions when related to the different conditions that can be seen by community pharmacists.

	Age	Radiation of pain	Onset	Absence of systemic or neurological signs	Precipitating factors
Simple back pain	All adults	No	Acute	Yes	Yes
Sciatica	>30 years	Yes (buttocks and leg)	Acute	Yes	Yes
Osteoarthritis	>30 years but more common with increased age	No	Chronic	Yes	No
Osteomyelitis	All ages	No	Acute	No	No
Ankylosing spondylitis	>50 years	Yes (side-to-side of back)	Chronic	Yes	No
Malignancy	>50 years	No	Chronic	No	No

When this information is applied to that gained from our patient (in next table), we see that his symptoms most closely match sciatica. Acute onset and radiation are very suggestive of this condition despite their being no obvious cause.

CASE STUDY 9.2 (Continued)

	Age	Radiation of pain	Onset	Absence of systemic or neurological signs	Precipitating factors
Simple back pain	✓	✗	✓	✓	✗
Sciatica	✓	✓	✓	✓	✗
Osteoarthritis	✓	✗	✗	✓	✓
Osteomyelitis	✓	✗	✓	✗	✓
Ankylosing spondylitis	✗?	✓	✗	✓	✓
Malignancy	✗?	✗	✗	✗	✓

Outcome

Referred pain is usually an indication to refer the patient. However, analgesia could be given while the patient waits to see a doctor, but since he takes a proton pump inhibitor, it would be best to recommend paracetamol.

Answers

1 = c	2 = d	3 = b	4 = d	5 = H	6 = F	7 = C	8 = D	9 = A	10 = C
11 = E	12 = A	13 = F	14 = H	15 = D	16 = A	17 = C	18 = B	19 = B	20 = D

Paediatrics

Background

A number of conditions are encountered much more frequently in children than the rest of the population. It is these conditions that this chapter focuses on. A small number of conditions that affect all age groups but are often associated with children are not included, for example, middle ear infection. Such conditions are covered in other chapters and where appropriate will be cross-referenced to the relevant sections within the text.

History taking

In the majority of cases pharmacists will be heavily dependent on getting details about the child's problem from their parents or an adult responsible for the child's welfare. This presents both benefits and problems to the pharmacist. Parents will know when their child is not well and asking the parent about the child's general health will help determine how poorly the child actually is. For example, a child who is running around and lively is unlikely to be acutely ill and referral to a doctor is less likely. The major problem faced by all healthcare professionals is the difficulty in gaining an accurate history of the presenting complaint. This poses difficulties in assessing the quality and accuracy of the information as children find it hard to articulate their symptoms. If the child can be asked questions, these often have to be posed in either closed or leading formats to elicit information.

As a rule of thumb, any child who appears visibly ill should always be seen by the pharmacist and referral might well be needed, whereas children who are acting normally and appear generally well will often not need to see the GP and can be managed by the pharmacist.

Head lice

Background

Humans act as hosts to three species of louse: *Pediculus capitis* (head lice), *Pediculus corporis* (body lice) and *Pediculus pubis* (pubic lice). Only head lice are discussed in this section.

Prevalence and epidemiology

Head lice affect all ages, although they are much more prevalent in children aged 4 to 11 years, especially girls. Studies conducted in schools show wide variation of current lice infestation ranging from 4% to 20% of pupils. Head lice can occur at any time and do not show any seasonal variation. Most parents will have experienced a child who has head lice, or received letters from school alerting parents to head lice infestation within the school.

Aetiology

Head lice can only be transmitted by head-to-head contact. Fleeting contact will be insufficient for lice to be transferred between heads. Once transmitted lice begin to reproduce. The adult louse lives for approximately 1 month. Throughout this time the female louse lays several eggs at the base of a hair shaft each night. Eggs hatch after 7 to 10 days, leaving the egg case attached to the hair shaft (known as a 'nit'). In the course of maturing to adulthood, the young louse (the nymph) undergoes three moults. Shortly after maturing, the female louse is sexually mature and able to mate.

Arriving at a differential diagnosis

Most parents will diagnose head lice themselves or be concerned that their child has head lice because of a recent local outbreak at school. Occasionally parents will also want to buy products to prevent their child contracting head lice. It is the role of the pharmacist to confirm a self-diagnosis and stop inappropriate sales of products. It should also be remembered that an itching scalp in children is not always due to head lice. Asking a number of symptom-specific questions should enable a diagnosis of head lice to be easily made (Table 10.1).

Clinical features of head lice

Observation of live lice is diagnostic. They are commonly found in the occipital and post-auricular areas. Scalp itching is also seen in approximately a third of patients. Itching is caused due an allergic response of the scalp to the saliva of the lice and can take weeks to develop.

Conditions to eliminate

Dandruff

Dandruff can cause irritation and itching of the scalp. However, the scalp should be dry and flaky. Skin debris might also be present on clothing.

Seborrhoeic dermatitis

Typically, seborrhoeic dermatitis will affect areas other than the scalp, most notably the face. If only scalp involvement is present, then the child might complain of severe and persistent dandruff. In infants the child will have large yellow scales and crusts of the scalp (cradle cap).

	Table 10.1
	Specific questions to ask the patient: Head lice

Question	Relevance
Have live lice been seen?	The presence of live lice is diagnostic
	Pharmacists can advise patients on how best to check for infection. Currently, both wet and dry combing are advocated
	Dry combing
	Straighten and untangle the dry hair using an ordinary comb
	Once the hair moves freely, switch to a detection comb. Starting from the back of the head, comb the from the scalp down to the end of the hair
	After each stroke examine the comb for live lice
	Continue to comb all the hair in sections until the whole head has been combed
	This process can take 5 or more minutes in people with shoulder length hair
	Wet combing
	Wash the hair with a normal shampoo
	Apply hair conditioner
	Repeat steps 1–4 as for dry combing
	Rinse out the conditioner
	Wet combing is more time consuming than dry methods and both should be performed on all family members
Empty egg shells (nits)	This does not constitute evidence of current infestation. This is a common misconception held by the general public and the pharmacist must ensure that parents seeking treatment have observed live lice
	Egg shells are not removed by using insecticides. Patients need to be reassured that the presence of egg shells does not mean treatment failure
Presence of itching	Itching is not always present in head lice. Inspection of the scalp should be made to check for signs of dandruff, psoriasis or seborrhoeic dermatitis

> **! TRIGGER POINTS indicative of referral: Head lice**
>
> • Parents who find cost of treatment prohibitive

Evidence base for over-the-counter medication

Treatment options include insecticides, wet combing and physical agents. All treatments available in the UK have shown varying degrees of clinical effectiveness, but it is difficult to assess which is most effective as very few comparative trials have been performed, and insecticidal resistance varies from region to region. No treatment is 100% effective and failure has been linked with poor adherence to each treatment regimen.

Insecticides

Of the treatment approaches, insecticides have been most studied but only malathion should be now be used as all other insecticides show very poor cure rates.

Wet combing

Wet combing is an alternative treatment option, however, cure rates are reported to be only 40–60% with the low cure rates attributed to poor adherence (Roberts et al., 2000; Hill et al., 2005).

Physical agents

Dimeticone is a relatively recent introduction to the market and is thought to work by coating the lice both internally and externally, which leads to disruption in water excretion, causing the gut of the lice to rupture from osmotic stress (Burgess, 2009). Its inclusion in treatment options seems to stem from one robust trial conducted by Burgess et al. (2005). Dimeticone was compared against phenothrin with cure rates determined at days 9 and 14. Dimeticone was shown to have comparable cure rates to phenothrin (69% compared with 78%). The study has been criticised for using dry detection methods and using different detection days (days 5 and 12 as recommended by the department of health); however, a further trial in 2007 supports the 2005 trial results. In the latter study, 4% dimeticone lotion, applied for 8 hours or overnight was compared with 0.5% malathion liquid applied for 12 hours or overnight. The results found dimeticone was significantly more effective than malathion, with 30/43 (70%) participants cured using dimeticone compared with 10/30 (33%) using malathion.

Dimeticone is also available in a much higher concentration (92%) marketed as NYDA. A randomised controlled trial compared the efficacy of a product containing dimeticone 92% to a permethrin 1% lotion. Both products were applied twice, 7 days apart, and the results showed that cure rates on day 9 were 97% with dimeticone and 68% with permethrin, but cure rates were not given for day 14 (Heukelbach et al., 2008).

Isopropyl myristate is another physical insecticide product and works by blocking the tracheal breathing system and coating the surface of lice with a thin film of fluid (Drugs and Therapeutics Bulletin, 2009). Evidence of efficacy comes from two trials that compared isopropyl myristate against permethrin. Results found isopropyl myristate was significantly more effective than permethrin (82% vs 19%). Although these results seem impressive, the comparator drug was permethrin – a product not recommended due to its poor efficacy.

Coconut, anise and ylang ylang spray (CAY; Lyclear Spray Away) acts by coating lice in an oily film, obstructing the respiratory system. CAY spray has been evaluated and was shown to have a good success rate (Mumcuoglu et al., 2002).

In summary, treatment used will be driven by individual preference, the patient's medical history and previous exposure to treatment regimens. Wet combing (available as bug-busting kits) is time consuming and requires patient motivation but is helpful in areas of high insecticidal resistance. Insecticides, dimeticone and isopropyl myristate are simpler to use than bug-busting kits and appear to have higher cure rates. **Based on current evidence it seems dimeticone is the treatment of choice.**

Practical prescribing and product selection

Prescribing information relating to medicines for head lice reviewed in the section 'Evidence base for over-the-counter medication' is discussed and summarised in Table 10.2; useful tips relating to patients presenting with head lice are given in 'Hints and Tips' in Box 10.1. All products have to be used more than once; insecticides have to be repeated 7 days after first application (this is based on expert opinion, as the second application is intended to kill nymphs emerging from eggs that have survived the first application); wet combing every 4 days for at least 2 weeks.

All products, except isopropyl myristate, can be used on children older than 6 months. Dimeticone or wet combing is recommended for pregnant and breastfeeding women. When applying all products, pay particular attention to the areas behind the ears and at the nape of the neck, as these areas are where lice are most often found.

Table 10.2
Practical prescribing: Summary of head lice medicines

Name of medicine	Use in children	Likely side effects	Drug interactions of note	Patients in which care is exercised	Pregnancy & breastfeeding
Malathion	>6 months (NYDA Spray >2 years)		None	None	OK
Dimeticone					
Isopropyl myristate	>2 years	None reported			OK

HINTS AND TIPS BOX 10.1: HEAD LICE

Who to treat?	Only those individuals with an active head lice infestation should be treated
Products for prevention	No credible evidence exists for any product marketed for prevention. The patient/parent should be counselled on when treatment is required
Treatment failure?	It is recommended that detection combing is performed after any treatment to confirm head lice eradication
	For wet combing
	Wet combing should be continued if necessary until no full-grown lice have been seen for 3 consecutive sessions
	For insecticides, dimeticone and isopropyl myristate
	Perform detection combing (wet or dry) 2–3 days after completing treatment. If no adult or nymph lice are found, repeat detection, combing 8–10 days after treatment. Treatment is successful if no lice are found in both detection combing sessions after treatment
Myths	Public misconceptions about head lice need to be dispelled
	Head lice are not only associated with dirty hair
	Head lice do not only affect children
	Children should not be kept from attending school

Malathion (Derbac–M liquid)

Derbac-M should be applied to dry hair and left for 12 hours before washing off.

Dimeticone 4% Lotion & Spray (Hedrin)

The lotion is applied to dry hair ensuring that it is spread evenly from the hair root to the tips. The spray should be applied approximately 10 cm from the hair making sure it is evenly distributed over dry hair. Both need to be left on for a minimum of 8 hours (overnight is preferable) before being washed out with shampoo.

Dimeticone 4% Gel (Hedrin Once Liquid gel)
The gel is applied in the same way as the lotion but only needs to be left on the hair for 15 minutes.

Dimeticone 92% Spray (NYDA)
The hair should be combed with a fine-toothed comb before applying the spray over the entire head. Once applied, leave on the hair for 30 minutes before re-combing the hair. The dimeticone should be left on the hair and scalp for 8 hours or overnight, and then washed out using shampoo.

Isopropyl myristate in cyclomethicone (Full Marks Solution and Spray)
This is applied in the same manner as dimeticone, but the contact time is only 10 minutes. It is only recommended for adults and children over the age of 2 years.

References
Burgess IF. The mode of action of dimeticone 4% lotion against head lice, *Pediculus capitis*. BMC Pharmacol 2009;9(1):3.
Burgess IF, Brown CM, Lee PN. Treatment of head louse infestation with 4% dimeticone lotion: randomised controlled equivalence trial. Br Med J 2005;330:1423–5.
Heukelbach J, Pilger D, Oliveira FA, et al. A highly efficacious pediculicide based on dimeticone: Randomized observer

blinded comparative trial. BMC Infectious Diseases 2008;8:115.

Hill N, Moor G, Cameron MM, et al. Single blind, randomised, comparative study of the Bug Buster kit and over the counter pediculicide treatments against head lice in the United Kingdom. Br Med J 2005;331:384–7.

Mumcuoglu KY, Miller J, Zamir C et al. The in vivo pediculicidal efficacy of a natural remedy. Isr Med Assoc J 2002;4:790–3.

Roberts RJ, Casey D, Morgan DA, et al. Comparison of wet combing with malathion for treatment of head lice in the UK: a pragmatic randomised controlled trial. Lancet 2000;356:540–4.

Further reading

Burgess IF, Brown CM, Peock S, et al. Head lice resistant to pyrethroid insecticides in Britain. Br Med J 1995;311:752.

Burgess IF, Lee PN, Matlock G. Randomised, controlled, assessor blind trial comparing 4% dimeticone lotion with 0.5% malathion liquid for head louse infestation. PLoS ONE 2007;2(11):e1127. doi:10.1371/journal.pone.0001127

Connolly M. Recommended management of headlice and scabies. The Prescriber 2013;June:17-29.

Websites

Community Hygiene Concern: http://www.chc.org/bugbusting/
Pediculosis.com: http://www.pediculosis.com/
Once a week – take a peek: http://www.onceaweektakeapeek.com/

Threadworm (*Enterobius vermicularis*)

Background

Worm infections are extremely common in both the developed and developing world. In Western countries the most common worm infection is threadworm (known in some countries as pinworm), which is a condition that causes inconvenience and embarrassment. Social stigma surrounds the diagnosis of threadworm, with many patients believing that infection implies a lack of hygiene. This belief is unfounded as infection occurs in all social strata. The patient might benefit from reassurance, explaining that the condition is very common and is nothing to be ashamed or embarrassed about.

Prevalence and epidemiology

Threadworm is the most common helminth infection throughout temperate and developed countries. Threadworm prevalence is difficult to establish due to the high number of people who self medicate or are asymptomatic. However, UK prevalence rates have been estimated at 20% in the community, rising to 65% in institutionalised settings. Threadworms are much more common in school or pre-school children than adults, because of their inattention to good personal hygiene.

Aetiology

Eggs are transmitted to the human host primarily by the faecal–oral route (autoinfection) but also by retroinfection and inhalation. Faecal–oral transmission involves eggs lodging under fingernails, which are then ingested by finger sucking after anal contact. Retroinfection occurs when larvae hatch on the anal mucosa and migrate back into the sigmoid colon. Finally, threadworm eggs are highly resistant to environmental factors and can easily be transferred to clothing, bed linen and inanimate objects (e.g., toys), resulting in dust-borne infections. Once eggs are ingested, duodenal fluid breaks them down and releases larvae, which migrate into the small and large intestines. After mating, the female migrates to the anus, usually at night, where eggs are laid on the perianal skin folds, after which the female dies. Once laid, eggs are infective almost immediately. Transmission back into the gut can then take place again via one of three mechanisms outlined, and so the cycle is perpetuated.

Arriving at a differential diagnosis

Threadworm diagnosis should be one of the more simple conditions to diagnose as patients present with very specific symptoms.

Clinical features of threadworm

Night-time perianal itching is the classic presentation (caused from the mucous produced by females when laying eggs). However, patients might experience symptoms ranging from a local 'tickling' sensation to acute pain. Any child with night-time perianal itching is almost certain to have threadworm. Itching can lead to sleep disturbances, resulting in irritability and tiredness the next day. Diagnosis can be confirmed by observing threadworm on the stool, although they are not always visible.

Complicating factors such as excoriation and secondary bacterial infection of the perianal skin can occur due to persistent scratching. The parent should be asked if the perianal skin is broken or weeping.

Conditions to eliminate

Other worm infections

Roundworm and tapeworm infections are encountered occasionally. However, these infections are usually contracted abroad when visiting poor and developing countries.

Contact irritant dermatitis

Occasionally, dermatitis can cause perianal itching (especially in adults). If there is no recent family history of threadworm or there is no visible sign of threadworm on the faeces, then dermatitis is possible.

> ❗ **TRIGGER POINTS indicative of referral: Threadworm**
>
> | Symptoms/signs | Possible danger/reason for referral |
> | --- | --- |
> | Medication failure | Possible misdiagnosis |
> | Secondary infection of perianal skin due to scratching | Need for assessment and possible systemic antibiotics |

Evidence base for over-the-counter medication

Mebendazole is available OTC for the treatment of threadworm. There is a large body of evidence to support the effectiveness of mebendazole in roundworm infections but for other worm infections, including threadworm, cure rates are lower. For threadworm, cure rates between 60% and 82% for single-dose treatment of mebendazole have been reported (Rafi et al., 1997; Sorensen et al., 1996).

Practical prescribing and product selection

Prescribing information relating to mebendazole is reviewed in the section 'Evidence base for over-the-counter medication' and summarised in Table 10.3; useful tips relating to patients presenting with threadworm are given in 'Hints and Tips' in Box 10.2.

Treatment should ideally be given to all family members and not only the patient with symptoms, as it is likely that other family members will have been infected even though they might not show signs of clinical infection. A repeated dose 14 days later is often recommended to ensure worms maturing from ova at the time of the first dose are also eradicated.

Mebendazole should be avoided in pregnancy because foetal malformations have been reported; however, it appears as safe in breastfeeding women. Pregnant women should be advised to practise hygiene measures for 6 weeks to break the cycle of infection.

Mebendazole (e.g., Ovex)

The dose for adults and children over 2 is 100 mg (either a single tablet or 5 mL of suspension). Young children might prefer to chew the tablet, and it has been formulated to taste of orange. Side effects include abdominal pain/discomfort (most commonly reported side effect), diarrhoea and rash. It does interact with cimetidine, increasing mebendazole plasma levels, but this is of little clinical

Table 10.3 Practical prescribing: Summary of medicines for threadworm

Name of medicine	Use in children	Likely side effects	Drug interactions of note	Patients in which care is exercised	Pregnancy & breastfeeding
Mebendazole	>2 years	Abdominal pain, rash	Phenytoin and carbamazepine	None	Avoid in pregnancy; OK in breastfeeding

HINTS AND TIPS BOX 10.2: THREADWORM

Hygiene measures	Complementary to drug treatment is the need for strict personal hygiene Nails should be kept short and clean. Careful washing and nail scrubbing before meals and after each visit to the toilet is essential to prevent autoinfection Bed linen, towels and sleepwear should be washed on the first day of treatment Underwear should be worn underneath night clothes to prevent scratching Shower daily, immediately on rising, washing around the anus Damp dusting and daily vacuuming are recommended to remove eggs

consequence. Phenytoin and carbamazepine decrease mebendazole plasma levels, and the dose of mebendazole may need to be increased.

References

Rafi S, Memon A, Billo AG. Efficacy and safety of mebendazole in children with worm infestation. J Pak Med Assoc 1997;47:140–1.

Sorensen E, Ismail M, Amarasinghe DK, et al. The efficacy of three anthelmintic drugs given in a single dose. Ceylon Med J 1996;41:42–5.

Further reading

Abbas A. Diagnosis and treatment of helminth infections. The Prescriber 2014; 19 May: 19–25.

Albonico M, Smith PG, Hall A, et al. A randomized controlled trial comparing mebendazole and albendazole against Ascaris, Trichuris and hookworm infections. Trans R Soc Trop Med Hyg 1994;88:585–9.

Anon. Management of threadworms in primary care. Merec Bulletin 1998;18:11–13.

Zaman V. Other gut nematodes. In: Weatherall DJ, Ledingham JGG, Warrell DA (eds). Oxford textbook of medicine. Oxford: Oxford University Press; 1987.

Colic

Background

There is no universally agreed definition of colic. A widely used definition of colic is that proposed by Wessel et al. (1954) and has come to be known as the 'rule of threes'. Wessel proposed that an infant could be considered to have colic if he or she cries for more than 3 hours a day for more than 3 days a week for more than 3 weeks. However, the definition by Wessel is arbitrary and few parents are willing to wait 3 weeks to see if the infant meets the criteria for colic. As a result in the clinical setting colic is usually defined as repeated episodes of excessive and inconsolable crying in an infant that otherwise appears to be healthy.

Prevalence and epidemiology

Due to no universally accepted definition of colic its prevalence is difficult to determine, and estimates vary widely from 3% to 40%, dependent on which definition is used. Studies reporting lower figures strictly applied Wessel's criteria, whereas higher figures used wider definitions. It is likely that prevalence falls between the two extremes and affects 10–20% of infants.

Colic starts in the first few weeks of life and usually resolves by the age of 3 to 5 months old.

Aetiology

The cause of colic is poorly understood but seems to be multifactorial. It has been linked to a disorder of the GI tract, where spasmodic contraction of smooth muscle causes pain and discomfort, which might be caused by allergy to cow's milk or lactose intolerance. It has also been suggested that it might stem from emotional, behavioural and social problems that include underdeveloped parenting skills, inadequate social network, postpartum depression, and parental anxiety and stress.

Arriving at a differential diagnosis

It can be difficult to determine whether the baby has colic or is just excessively crying, as the diagnosis of the condition is dependent on qualitative descriptions. However, the term 'colic' is often wrongly applied to any infant who cries more than usual. Asking a number of symptom-specific questions should enable a diagnosis of colic to be made (Table 10.4).

Clinical features of colic

Excessive crying and inconsolable crying are obvious clinical features accompanied by facial flushing and drawing up of the legs. Pain may be mild, merely causing the child to be restless in the evenings or severe, resulting in rhythmical screaming attacks lasting a few minutes at a time, alternating with equally long quiet periods in which the

Table 10.4
Specific questions to ask the patient: Colic

Question	Relevance
History of crying	Excessive crying is not isolated and will have been present for some time. Acute infections are normally sudden in onset, and the baby will not exhibit a long-standing history of excessive crying
Aggravating factors	Infants may excessively cry for reasons other than a medical cause, for example, hunger, thirst, being too hot or cold and trapped wind. These should be explored as part of your questioning strategy before diagnosing colic

child almost goes to sleep before another attack starts. Attacks appear to be more common in the early evening, giving rise to the name '6:00 pm colic'.

Conditions to eliminate

Acute infection

Colic and acute infections of the ear or urinary tract can present with almost identical symptoms. However, in acute infection the child should have no previous history of excessive crying and have signs of systemic infection such as fever.

Intolerance to cows' milk protein

Colicky pain in infants is sometimes due to intolerance to cows' milk protein. This is far less common than generally believed but should be considered if the infant is failing to thrive.

Gastro-oesophageal reflux disease (GORD)

Infants frequently have regurgitation that is accompanied with excessive crying. A diagnosis of GORD is usually made if regurgitation happens more than five times a day and is associated with failure to gain weight and refusal to feed.

> **! TRIGGER POINTS indicative of referral: Colic**
>
> | Symptoms/signs | Possible danger/reason for referral |
> |---|---|
> | Infants that are failing to put on weight | This may indicate GORD or intolerance to cow's milk |
> | Overanxious parents | Parents might need further medical opinion reassurance |

Evidence base for over-the-counter medication

Parents should be reassured that the child's symptoms will subside over time, that their baby is well and they are not doing something wrong. Most parents will want some form of treatment. Treatments include simeticone, lactase enzymes, low-lactose milk formulas and gripe mixtures. None have a credible evidence base.

Simeticone is reported to have antifoaming properties, reducing surface tension and allowing easier elimination of gas from the gut by passing flatus or belching. It is widely used yet has very limited evidence of efficacy. Of three trials reported, only one found a small improvement in the number of crying attacks. This trial was small ($n = 26$) and suffered from methodological flaws, so results should be viewed with caution.

Lactase breaks down lactose present in milk to glucose and galactose. This reduction in lactose concentration is reported to improve colic symptoms, but four small trials investigating its effect were inconclusive.

Low-lactose formulas should not be recommended as studies conducted to date have been of poor methodological quality. No trial data exists for gripe mixtures and therefore should be avoided.

Summary

Although evidence for simeticone and lactase enzymes is not strong, it would seem unreasonable not to let parents try either for a trial period of a week if they are finding it difficult to cope. If no response is seen, then referral to the doctor for an alternative formula feed would be advisable.

Practical prescribing and product selection

Prescribing information relating to dimethicone is discussed and summarised in Table 10.5; useful tips relating to colic are given in 'Hints and Tips' in Box 10.3.

Simeticone (e.g., Infacol and Dentinox)

Simeticone is pharmacologically inert; it has no side effects, drug interactions or precautions in its use and can therefore be safely prescribed to all infants. The dose for both products is 2.5 mL (21 mg) after each feed.

Lactase enzyme (Colief)

The dose of Colief differs depending if the baby is formula or breastfed: if breastfeeding, four drops should be

Table 10.5
Practical prescribing: Summary of medicines for colic

Name of medicine	Use in children	Likely side effects	Drug interactions of note	Patients in which care is exercised	Pregnancy & breastfeeding
Simeticone	Infant upwards	None	None	None	Not applicable
Lactase					

HINTS AND TIPS BOX 10.3: COLIC

| Review feeding technique | Before recommending a product, it is worth checking the feeding technique. Underfeeding the baby can result in excessive sucking and in air being swallowed, leading to colic-like symptoms. Additionally the teat size of the bottle should be checked. When the bottle is turned upside down the milk should drop slowly from the bottle |

added to a small amount of expressed milk and the baby breastfed as normal; if using an infant formula, then the feed should be made up as usual and four drops added to warm, but not hot, formula. If making up the formula in advance, then add two drops of Colief and store in the fridge for 4 hours.

Reference

Wessel MA, Cobb JC, Jackson EB, et al. Paroxysmal fussing in infancy, sometimes called 'colic'. Paediatrics 1954;14:421–4.

Further reading

Barr RG, Lessard J. Excessive crying. In: Bergman AB (ed). 20 Common Problems in Paediatrics. USA: McGraw-Hill; 2001.

Garrison MM, Christakis DA. A systematic review of treatments for infant colic. Pediatrics 2000;106:184–90.

Lucassen PL, Assendelft WJ, Gubbels JW, et al. Effectiveness of treatments for infantile colic: systematic review. Br Med J 1998;316:1563–9.

Kanabar D. Current treatment options in the management of infantile colic. The Prescriber 2008;5 April:24–9.

Websites

CRY-SIS: www.cry-sis.org.uk

The Breastfeeding Network: https://www.breastfeedingnetwork.org.uk

General sites on colic: http://www.colichelp.com/, http://www.infacol.co.uk/home and http://www.colief.co.uk/

Atopic dermatitis

Background

Atopic dermatitis is a chronic non-infective inflammatory skin condition characterised by an itchy red rash. It usually starts within the first 6 months of life and predominantly affects young children. The majority (60–70%) of patients will 'grow out' of the condition by their early teens. However, in a small number of patients atopic dermatitis persists into adulthood where the condition becomes chronic. Atopic dermatitis can impair the quality of life of patients and their families. Typical distribution of atopic dermatitis is illustrated in Fig. 10.1.

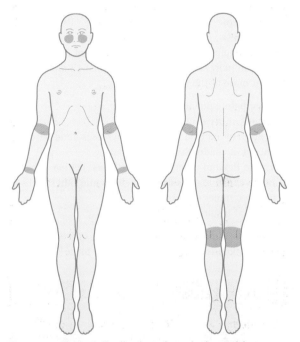

Fig. 10.1 Typical distribution of atopic dermatitis.

Prevalence and epidemiology

The prevalence of atopic dermatitis is unclear. Rates vary from country-to-country. In the UK prevalence rates have been rising, and it now affects 15–20% of children, although over 80% are reported to have mild disease. The condition usually presents in infants aged between 2 and 6 months, but it can occur in older children. Upward of 60% of children will have onset within the first year, rising to 80% within the first 5 years. Atopic dermatitis is much less common in adults, affecting only 1–3% of people.

Aetiology

Atopic dermatitis has a strong genetic component, although the precise genetic cause is unknown. Two-thirds of people with the disease have a family history of atopic dermatitis, asthma or hay fever. Atopic dermatitis is present in approximately 80% of children where both parents are affected and in 60% if one parent is affected.

In addition a number of environmental factors have been implicated in the development or worsening of the condition and include certain foods (e.g., dairy products), stress, extremes of heat and humidity, and irritants such as detergents and chemicals.

Arriving at a differential diagnosis

An itchy rash with very early childhood onset is indicative of atopic dermatitis (Fig. 10.2 & Fig. 10.3). To help with diagnosis, criteria-based protocols are available. For example atopic dermatitis can be diagnosed if the person has had an itchy skin condition in the past 12 months plus three or more of the following:

- onset before the age of 2 years
- history of dry skin
- history of eczema in the skin creases (and also the cheeks in children under 10 years)
- visible flexural eczema (inside elbows, behind knees or involvement of the cheeks/forehead and outer limbs in children under 4 years)
- personal history of other atopic disease

Asking a number of symptom-specific questions should enable a diagnosis of atopic dermatitis to be made (Table 10.6).

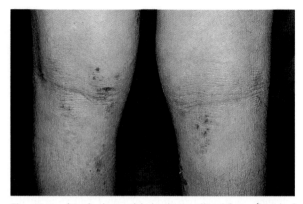

Fig. 10.3 Atopic dermatitis in the popliteal fossa (bend of knee). Reproduced from DJ Gawkrodger, 2007, Dermatology: An Illustrated Colour Text, 4th edition, Churchill Livingstone, with permission.

Clinical features of atopic dermatitis

A typical presentation of a child with atopic dermatitis is an irritable, scratching child with dermatitis of varying severity. Itching is the predominant symptom which can induce a vicious cycle of scratching, leading to skin damage, which in turn leads to more itching – the so called 'itch scratch itch' cycle. The child might have had the symptoms for some time and the parent has often already tried some form of cream to help control the itch and rash. Scratching can lead to broken skin, which can become infected. There is a tendency to have dry, sensitive skin, even in those who have 'outgrown' of the disease.

Once a diagnosis has been established and before treatment is considered, it is important to make an assessment on the severity and social impact of the condition (Table 10.7).

Conditions to eliminate

Seborrhoeic dermatitis

Seborrhoeic dermatitis in infants typically occurs in the first 6 months. Itching is generally not present and the condition usually spontaneously resolves after a few weeks and seldom recurs. It usually affects the scalp, face and napkin area. Large yellow scales and crusts often appear on the scalp and are often referred to as cradle cap (Fig. 8.10).

Psoriasis

Psoriasis can be mistaken for atopic dermatitis because the rash is erythematous and can occur on parts of the body such as the scalp, elbows and knees, which is a common location for atopic dermatitis in older children. However, the rash is raised and has well defined boundaries with a

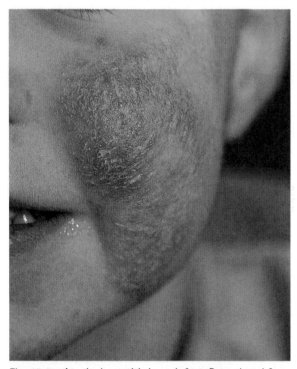

Fig. 10.2 Atopic dermatitis in an infant. Reproduced from B J Zitelli, H W Davis, 1997, Atlas of Pediatric Physical Diagnosis, 3rd edition, Mosby, with permission.

Table 10.6
Specific questions to ask the patient: Atopic dermatitis

Question	Relevance
Is itching present?	Atopic dermatitis is classically associated with intense itching Psoriasis and seborrhoeic dermatitis are not usually associated with itching
Distribution of rash	Varies according to age (Fig. 10.1) but in infants the nappy area is not involved and is a useful distinction between atopic dermatitis and seborrhoeic dermatitis
Age of child	Presentation varies with age Babies: facial involvement (the cheeks) is common along with patchy red scaly lesions on the wrists and hands (Fig. 10.2) Toddlers and older children: the antecubital (in front or at the bend of the elbow), popliteal fossae (behind the knee), and ankles are more commonly involved (Fig. 10.3)
Family history of atopy	If a parent has eczema, hay fever or asthma, then the likelihood of atopic dermatitis rises

Table 10.7
Severity and social impact of atopic dermatitis

Severity*	Psychological impact*
Clear: normal skin, no evidence of active eczema.	None: no impact on quality of life.
Mild: areas of dry skin, infrequent itching (with or without small areas of redness).	Mild: little impact on everyday activities, sleep and psychosocial well-being.
Moderate: areas of dry skin, frequent itching, redness (with or without excoriation and localised skin thickening).	Moderate: moderate impact on everyday activities and psychosocial well-being, and frequently disturbed sleep.
Severe: widespread areas of dry skin, incessant itching, redness (with or without excoriation, extensive skin thickening, bleeding, oozing, cracking and alteration of pigmentation).	Severe: severe limitation of everyday activities and psychosocial functioning, and loss of sleep every night.

*Adapted from NICE guidelines 2007.

silvery-white, scaly appearance that are typically symmetrical. Itch, if present, is mild (Fig. 8.3).

Contact dermatitis

Seen as a red itchy skin rash seen at any site related to exposure border (Fig. 8.27).

Fungal infection

The rash is a pink or red, itchy, slightly raised annular patch with a well-defined inflamed border (Fig. 8.14). It can occur on all body surfaces.

Chapter 8 – dermatology has more information on the skin conditions discussed in this section.

TRIGGER POINTS indicative of referral: Atopic dermatitis

Symptoms/signs	Possible danger/reason for referral
Children with moderate or severe atopic dermatitis Medication failure – patient suffers two or more flare-ups per month	Outside scope of community pharmacist; patient probably needs corticosteroid therapy
Presence of secondary infection (weeping and crusting lesions)	Potentially needs systemic antibiotics

Evidence base for over-the-counter medication

The mainstay of treatment for atopic dermatitis consists of avoiding potential irritants, managing dry skin, controlling itching and using topical corticosteroids to treat flare-ups. Unfortunately, the latter option is not available to children under the age of 10 due to OTC license restrictions.

Avoiding irritants

Where practical, factors that worsen dermatitis should be avoided. The use of highly perfumed soaps and detergents should be discouraged and replaced with soap substitutes (e.g., Alpha Keri, Neutrogena, Dove). Patients should be told to have lukewarm, not hot, baths because in some patients hot water can aggravate the problem. In addition a bath additive should be used to help skin hydration.

Emollients

It is believed emollients add moisture to the skin and repair the lipid barrier function while also helping to prevent penetration by irritants and decrease the need for steroids. Despite a lack of high quality randomised controlled trials, emollients are well established as first-line treatment for atopic dermatitis. No trials appear to have addressed whether one emollient is superior to another. Patients might have to try several emollients before finding one that is most effective for their skin.

Antihistamines

There appears to be no clinical trial data on the use of sedative antihistamine for reducing pruritus in atopic dermatitis; however, they are often prescribed to children to help with itching. The American Academy of Dermatology guidelines on the treatment of atopic dermatitis report there is little evidence for the use of antihistamines; however, they suggest that sedating antihistamines may be useful where there is significant sleep disruption due to itching (Hanifin et al., 2004).

Corticosteroids

A substantial body of evidence exists for corticosteroids in controlling all types of dermatitis, including atopic dermatitis. If the symptoms warrant corticosteroid therapy, then children need to be referred to the doctor. Usually mild steroids, such as hydrocortisone (1–2.5%), preferably in an ointment base, should be prescribed twice daily.

Practical prescribing and product selection

Prescribing information relating to medicines for atopic dermatitis reviewed in the section 'Evidence base for over-the-counter medication' is discussed and summarised in Table 10.8; useful information regarding emollients containing lanolin is given in Hints and Tips in Box 10.4.

Emollients

There are a plethora of emollient products marketed and which one a patient uses will be dictated by patient response and acceptability. All emollients should be regularly and liberally applied with no upper limit on how often they can be used. All are chemically inert and therefore can be safely used from birth upwards. For a summary of emollient products, see Table 8.32.

Table 10.8
Practical prescribing: Summary of medicines for atopic dermatitis

Name of medicine	Use in children	Likely side effects	Drug interactions of note	Patients in which care is exercised	Pregnancy & breastfeeding
Emollients	Birth onwards	None	None	None	Not Applicable
Sedating antihistamines					
Chlorphenamine	>1 year	Sedation	Increased sedation with opioid analgesics, anxiolytics, hypnotics and antidepressants. However, it is unlikely a child will be taking such medicines	None	Not Applicable
Clemastine	>1 year				
Cyproheptadine	>2 years				
Promethazine	>2 years				

HINTS AND TIPS BOX 10.4: ATOPIC DERMATITIS

General self-help	If possible, avoid scratching. Keep nails short and rub with fingers to alleviate itch to minimise skin trauma
Lanolin-containing emollients	Emollients that contain lanolin (e.g., Keri Lotion and E45) should be avoided as they are known to cause sensitisation
Applying emollients	They are best applied when the skin is moist, for example, during bath times Apply as frequently as possible The more oily the emollient, the more effective they tend to be

Sedating antihistamines

Chlorphenamine (Piriton)

Chlorphenamine can be given from the age of 1 year. Children up to the age of 2 years should take 2.5 mL of syrup (1 mg) twice a day. For children aged between 2 and 5 years, the dose is 2.5 mL (1 mg) three or four times a day and those over the age of 6 years should take 5 mL (2 mg) three or four times a day.

Clemastine (Tavegil)

Clemastine is taken twice a day by children over the age of 1 year. Those aged between 1 and 3 years should take 250 to 500 μg (1/4 to 1/2 a tablet), children aged between 3 and 6 years should take 500 μg (1/2 a tablet) and for those over the age of 6 years, the dose is 500 μg to 1 mg (1/2 to 1 tablet).

Cyproheptadine (Periactin)

Children between the ages of 2 and 6 years should take 2 mg (half a tablet) and for children over the age of 7 years, the dose is 4 mg (1 tablet) two or three times a day.

Promethazine (Phenergan Elixer 5 mg/5 mL and 10 mg and 25 mg tablets)

Children between the ages of 2 and 5 years should take 5–15 mg (5–15 mL) daily in one to two divided doses and for those over the age of 5 years, the dose is 10 –25 mg daily in one to two divided doses.

Reference
Hanifin JM, Cooper KD, Ho VC, et al. Guidelines of care for atopic dermatitis, developed in accordance with the American Academy of Dermatology (AAD)/American Academy of Dermatology Association 'Administrative Regulations for Evidence-Based Clinical Practice Guidelines'. J Am Acad Dermatol 2004;50(3):391–404.

Further reading
Brown S, Reynolds NJ. Atopic and non-atopic eczema. Br Med J 2006;332:584–8.
Clark C, Hoare C. Making the most of emollients. Pharm J 2001;266:227–9.
CG57 Atopic eczema in children: NICE guideline 2007. http://www.nice.org.uk/guidance/cg57
Management of atopic eczema in primary care. Guideline 125. SIGN, March 2011. http://sign.ac.uk/guidelines/fulltext/125/index.html
MacKenzie A, Schofield O. Recommended diagnosis and management of atopic eczema. Prescriber 2013;19th November:18-28.

Websites
National Eczema Society: http://www.eczema.org/
General dermatology site: http://www.dermatologist.co.uk/index.html

Fever

Background

Fever is simply a rise in body temperature above normal. Normal oral temperature is 37 °C (98.6 °F), plus or minus 1 °C, although rectal temperature is about 0.5 °C higher and under arm temperature 0.5 °C lower than oral temperature. During the course of 24 hours minor fluctuations in temperature are observed. Fever is often classified as being either mild (low-grade) (up to 39 °C) or high (above 39 °C).

In a practice setting, for those under 5 years of age, the best temperature to take is under the arm, using an electronic or chemical dot thermometer. Infrared tympanic thermometers are also advocated (NICE guidance No. 160, May 2013). Forehead strip thermometers are popular because they are easy to use, but should be avoided as they are unreliable.

Prevalence and epidemiology

Fever is a common symptom of many conditions; in children viral and to a lesser extent bacterial causes are most commonly implicated. It has been reported that fever is probably the most common reason for a child to be taken to a doctor.

Aetiology

Body temperature is regulated closely because temperature changes can significantly alter cellular functions and, in extreme cases, lead to death. Thermoregulation is a balance between heat production and heat loss. Cellular metabolism produces heat and this means that energy – in the form of heat – is produced continually by the body. This heat production is lost through the skin by radiation, evaporation, conduction and convection. The thermoregulation centre located in the hypothalamus controls the whole process. When body temperature reaches its 'set point' (approximately 37 °C), mechanisms to lose or conserve heat are activated. When a person suffers from a fever, this suggests that there is some defect in the temperature-regulating control system. In fact the system is functioning normally but with an adjusted higher 'set point'. This process is complex but involves the production of pyrogens (fever-causing substances) that alter the set point.

Arriving at a differential diagnosis

Establishing fever is usually a subjective perception by the parent that the child feels warm or is off colour. The importance of the parent's perception should not be underestimated or dismissed if the child's temperature has not been taken. Many healthcare professionals often place too much value on an empirical figure when in many instances the look of the child is more important than the height of the fever. Asking a number of symptom-specific questions should enable the pharmacist to treat or refer the child with fever (Table 10.9).

NICE recommend using a 'traffic light' system to assess the seriousness of fever (Table 10.10). In a pharmacy setting any child that shows symptoms or signs of intermediate (amber) or high (red) risk should be referred to the doctor.

Clinical features of fever

A child with fever will generally be irritable, off his or her food and seek greater parental attention. Other signs that might be seen include facial flushing and shivering.

Conditions to eliminate

Likely causes

Urinary tract infection
One of the most common causes of fever in children is urinary tract infection. Often the child will present only with fever. Other symptoms can be present and include irritability, poor feeding, vomiting or abdominal pain. Referral is needed.

Roseola infantum (sixth disease)
Roseola infantum is probably caused by a neurodermotropic virus and is most prevalent in children under 1 year of age. Onset is with a sudden high fever (40 °C)

> **Table 10.9**
> **Specific questions to ask the patient: Fever**

Question	Relevance
How old is the child?	Children under 3 months should be referred automatically because diagnosis can be very difficult and serious complications can arise
How poorly is the child?	The parent will know how poorly the child is relative to normal behaviour. A child might have a high temperature but appear relatively normal whereas a child with a mild temperature might be quite poorly
Associated symptoms	Viral upper respiratory tract infections are usually accompanied with one or more symptoms including cough, cold or sore throat
	Glandular fever is usually accompanied with fatigue and lymph node enlargement (usually seen in teenagers)
	If no other symptoms are present it suggests a bacterial infection, often a urinary tract infection

Table 10.10
Assessment of the seriousness of fever in children under 5 years of age

	Green–low risk	Amber–intermediate risk	Red–high risk
Colour	Normal colour of skin, lips and tongue	Pallor reported by parent/carer	Pale/mottled/ashen/blue
Activity	Responds normally to social cues Content/smiles Stays awake or awakens quickly Strong normal cry/not crying	Not responding normally to social cues Awakens only with prolonged stimulation Decreased activity No smile	No response to social clues Appears ill to the pharmacist Unable to rouse or if roused does not stay awake Weak, high-pitched or continuous cry
Respiratory		Nasal flaring 6–12 months, RR >50 breaths/min >12 months, RR 40 breaths/min	Grunting RR >60 breaths/minute
Hydration	Normal skin and eyes Moist mucous membranes	Dry mucous membrane Poor feeding in infants CRT ≥3 seconds Reduced urine output	Reduced skin turgor
Other	NONE of the amber or red signs or symptoms	Fever ≥ 5 days Swelling of a limb/joint	0–3 months ≥38 °C 3–6 months ≥39 °C Non-blanching rash Neck stiffness Bulging fontanelle Seizures

CRT, capillary refill time; RR, respiration rate.
Table adapted from NICE. CG 160 Feverish illness in children: assessment and initial management in children younger than 5 years. London: National Institute for Health and Clinical Excellence, 2013. Reproduced with permission. Guidelines are accurate at time of going to press. Latest guidelines are available at http://www.nice.org.uk/guidance/cg160

that usually subsides by the third or fourth day once the rash, which blanches when pressed, appears on the trunk and limbs. The condition is self-limiting.

Unlikely causes

Upper respiratory tract infections
It is rare for upper respiratory tract infections to present with fever alone. Cough, cold or sore throat is usually present. Treatment can be offered and referral is generally not needed unless secondary bacterial infection is suspected; earache symptoms might suggest this.

Medicine-induced fever
A number of medicines can elevate body temperature and should be considered if no other cause can be determined. Penicillins, cephalosporins, macrolides, tricyclic antidepressants, anticonvulsants and anti-inflammatory medicines,

when associated with hypersensitivity, have all been associated with increasing temperature.

Very unlikely causes

Meningitis
Meningitis should be considered in any feverish child who is obviously systemically unwell and exhibits symptoms such as severe headache, photophobia, lethargy, drowsiness and neck stiffness. The classic textbook sign of a non-blanching rash is often seen late in symptom presentation and should not be routinely expected to be seen in children. Further information can be found on page 323.

Pneumonia
Children who exhibit increased respiration rates and fever need referral for further evaluation as pneumonia is a possibility.

Glandular fever

Glandular fever is most commonly seen in young adults rather than children but any patient who has a long-standing history of fatigue and a low-grade fever should be referred for further evaluation.

! TRIGGER POINTS indicative of referral: Fever

Symptoms/signs	Possible danger/reason for referral
Any feverish child under 3 months old	Outside scope of community pharmacist and person requires further assessment
Fever accompanied with no other symptoms	
Fever of 5 days or longer	
Febrile convulsion/seizures	
Stiff neck	Suggests meningitis
Obviously ill child or child who fails to respond to stimuli	
Signs of dehydration that fall in 'amber' or 'red' categories (see Table 10.10)	Oral rehydration may be inadequate and intravenous fluids may be needed

---

Evidence base for over-the-counter medication

Paracetamol and ibuprofen are effective in reducing fever, but UK guidelines recommended they should only be used in children who are unwell or distressed. Either could be used as monotherapy and if the first is not helping, then switch to the other. If both appear to be ineffective, then consider alternating between the two (Wong et al., 2013).

Non-pharmacologically intervention – tepid sponging

Two reviews by Meremikwu & Oye-Ita (2002, 2003) looked at the effect of paracetamol and tepid sponging in reducing fever. Conclusions from both reviews were guarded in stating they were effective, due to the small number of trials reviewed that met their inclusion criteria. This of course does not mean to say that these approaches are ineffective but that better, larger trials are required.

Practical prescribing and product selection

Prescribing information relating to medicines for fever reviewed in the section 'Evidence base for over-the-counter medication' is discussed and summarised in Table 10.11; useful tips relating to patients presenting with fever are given in Hints and Tips in Box 10.5.

Paracetamol (e.g., Calpol)

Paracetamol is available in a number of dosage forms – liquid, soluble tablets, sachets and melt tabs. Dosing of paracetamol in children falls in to a number of age bands (Table 10.12).

For all age bands the maximum number of doses per day is four. Paracetamol has no commonly occurring side effects, does not interact with any medicines and so can be safely taken by all children.

Ibuprofen (e.g., Nurofen, Calprofen)

Ibuprofen can be given to children over 3 months old. Doses for ibuprofen, like paracetamol, are age dependent. The dosing schedule that follows is taken from the British National Formulary (Note some OTC products' dosing schedules are different to this):

- Age 3 months to 5 months: 50 mg three times a day.
- Age 6 months to 1 year: 50 mg three to four times a day.
- Age 1 year to 4 years: 100 mg three times a day.
- Age 4 years to 7 years: 150 mg three times a day.
- Age 7 years to 10 years: 200 mg three times a day.
- Age 10 years to 12 years: 300 mg three times a day.

Ibuprofen can cause gastrointestinal side effects, such as nausea and diarrhoea, and also interacts with many

---

Table 10.11
Practical prescribing: Summary of medicines for fever

Name of medicine	Use in children	Likely side effects	Drug interactions of note	Patients in which care is exercised	Pregnancy & breastfeeding
Paracetamol	>3 months	None	None	None	Not applicable
Ibuprofen	Note: Paracetamol from 2 months for post-immunisation pyrexia	GI disturbances		Children with known hypersensitivity to NSAIDs	

HINTS AND TIPS BOX 10.5 FEVER

Drinking fluids	Children should be told to drink additional fluid to prevent dehydration, as a fever will make them sweat more than usual

Table 10.12
Dosing schedule for paracetamol

3–6 months	2.5 mL	120 mg/mL	
6–24 months	5.0 mL		
2–4 years	7.5 mL		
4–6 years	10 mL		
6–8 years		5 mL	250 mg/mL
8–10 years		7.5 mL	
10–12 years		10 mL	

other medicines, although those medicines that interact with ibuprofen are very unlikely to be taken by children. Any child who has previously taken an NSAID and had an allergic reaction to it should avoid ibuprofen.

References

Meremikwu MM, Oyo-Ita A. Paracetamol versus placebo or physical methods for treating fever in children. Cochrane Database of Systematic Reviews 2002, Issue 2. Art. No.: CD003676. http://dx.doi.org/10.1002/14651858.CD003676.

Meremikwu M, Oyo-Ita A. Paracetamol for treating fever in children. Cochrane Database of Systematic Reviews 2003. Issue 2.

Wong T, Stang AS, Ganshorn H, et al. Combined and alternating paracetamol and ibuprofen therapy for febrile children. Cochrane Database of Systematic Reviews 2013, Issue 10. Art. No.: CD009572. http://dx.doi.org/10.1002/14651858. CD009572.pub2.

Further reading

Dodd SR, Lancaster GA, Craig JV, et al. Sensitivity and specificity of aural compared with rectal thermometers: a meta-analysis. J Clin Epidemiol 2006;59(4):354–7.

Infectious childhood conditions

Background

A number of infectious diseases are more prevalent in children than the rest of the population. Many of these diseases are now vaccine preventable and the provision of immunisation programmes has almost eradicated them from developed countries. However, some conditions have no vaccine or incomplete vaccine cover is provided, which means contraction of the disease is still possible. This usually results in the child suffering from mild symptoms from which a full and speedy recovery is made but in some circumstances, for example meningitis, infection can result in death.

Most likely conditions to be encountered

Chicken pox

Chicken pox is very common and is probably the most likely infectious childhood rash seen in community pharmacy. It is the primary infection observed when the patient contracts the varicella zoster virus, which is transmitted either by droplet infection or with contact with vesicular exudates. The incubation period ranges from 10 to 20 days and before the rash develops, the patient might experience up to 3 days of prodromal symptoms that could include fever, headache and sore throat. The rash typically begins on the face, stomach and back before spreading to other parts of the body. Initially, they appear as small red lumps that rapidly develop into vesicles, which crust over after 3 to 5 days. New lesions tend to occur in crops of 3 to 5 for the first 4 days so that at its height of infectivity lesions appear in all stages of development (Fig. 10.4). The vesicles are often extremely itchy and secondary bacterial infection due to the vesicles being scratched is not unusual. Chicken pox is highly contagious, from a few days before the onset of rash until all lesions have crusted over (in the UK >80% of people have been infected by the age of 10 years). Reinfection results in people suffering from shingles (Fig. 10.5). A vaccination has been available since the mid 1990s and has shown to be 70–90% effective. It is part of standard vaccination schedules in countries such as the USA and Australia but currently not the UK.

Molluscum contagiosum

Caused by a pox virus, molluscum contagiosum is usually transmitted by indirect contact, for example sharing towels, although it is not very contagious. The face and axillae are common sites of infection. They generally appear in crops and appear as pink pearl-like spots usually less than 0.5 cm in diameter. All lesions have a central punctum that is a diagnostic feature (Fig. 10.6). Confusion should not arise with other conditions other than viral warts (for further information on warts, see page 245). The condition will spontaneously resolve (usually within 12 months) but if the parent or child is anxious, then referral to the GP should be made because liquid nitrogen can be used to remove the lesions.

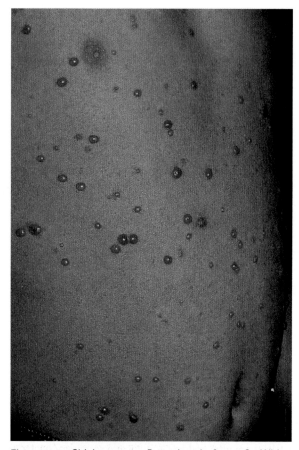

Fig. 10.4 Chicken pox. Reproduced from G White, 2004, Color Atlas of Dermatology, 3rd edition, Churchill Livingstone, with permission.

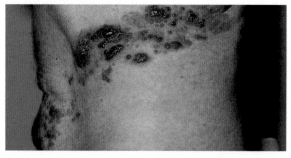

Fig. 10.5 Typical dermatomal distribution of herpes zoster. Reproduced from J Wilkinson et al., 2004, Dermatology in Focus, Churchill Livingstone, with permission.

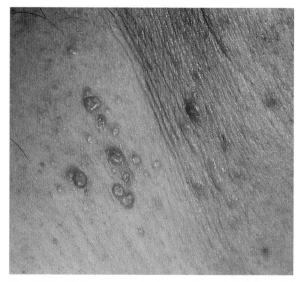

Fig. 10.6 Molluscum contagiosum. Reproduced from DJ Gawkrodger, 2007, Dermatology: An Illustrated Colour Text, 4th edition, Churchill Livingstone, with permission.

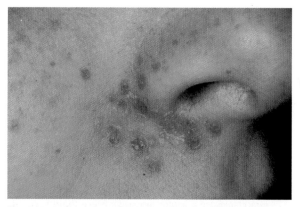

Fig. 10.7 Impetigo. Reproduced from TB Habif, 2010, Clinical Dermatology: A Color Guide To Diagnosis And Therapy, Mosby, with permission.

Impetigo

Impetigo is caused by a bacterial infection, most notably *Staphylococcus aureus* or *Streptococcus pyogenes*. It presents mainly on the face, around the nose and mouth. It usually starts as a small red itchy patch of inflamed skin that quickly develops into vesicles that rupture and weep. The exudate dries to a brown, yellow sticky crust (Fig. 10.7). It is contagious and children should be kept off school until the rash clears. General hygiene measures should include not sharing towels, which will help stop household contacts contracting the infection. The child's nails should be kept short to stop him or her from scratching the lesions. Treatment involves topical or systemic antibiotics (e.g., fusidic acid or flucloxacillin), which currently are not available OTC in most Western countries.

10

Unlikely conditions to be encountered

Erythema infectiosum

Erythema infectiosum is also called 'slapped cheek disease' or 'fifth disease'. It is caused by parvovirus B19 and predominantly affects children between the ages of 3 and 15. Cold-like symptoms appear a couple of days before the rash appears. Typically the rash appears on the cheeks and presents as red and inflamed marks (like the person has been slapped). Itch is often present, and the rash can spread to the arms and legs.

Glandular fever (infectious mononucleosis)

Glandular fever is caused by the Epstein–Barr virus and is most commonly seen in patients aged between ages 15 and 24. In Western countries it is rare in children under 5 years and less frequent in those aged between 5 and 14.

It is transmitted from close salivary contact, is also known as the 'kissing disease' and has an incubation period of 4 to 7 weeks. Symptoms are vague but characterised by fatigue, headache, sore throat and swollen and tender lymph glands. A macular rash can also occur in a small proportion of patients. The symptoms tend to be mild but can linger for many months.

Very unlikely conditions to be encountered

Meningitis

The peak incidence of contracting meningitis is between 6 and 12 months. Signs and symptoms are non-specific in the early stages of the disease and are similar to flu. Symptoms range from fever, nausea, vomiting, headache and irritability. Symptoms can develop quickly – in a matter of hours – and be unpredictable, especially in infants and young children. Symptoms of fever, lethargy, vomiting and irritability are common in children aged between 3 months and 2 years. In infants, floppiness and the dislike of being handled are also common features. Symptoms more common in older children include severe headache, stiff neck and photophobia. Any child who experiences neck pain when asked to place their chin on their chest must be immediately referred.

In the latter stages of the disease a petechial or purpuric non-blanching rash characteristically develops in meningococcal infection.

The number of cases in the UK is now at an all-time low. On average 3000 cases are seen each year; the fall in cases is down because of the introduction of the Hib (active against *Haemophilus influenzae*) and meningococcal C conjugate (active against serogroup C *Meningococcus*) vaccines in to the UK vaccination programme. Further falls

in cases are expected as from September 2015; a meningococcal group B vaccine was introduced into the UK vaccination programme. This strain currently accounts for 50% of cases each year.

Measles

It is caused by an RNA virus and spread by droplet inhalation. Approximately 7% of patients develop respiratory complications such as otitis media and pneumonia, but encephalitis is seen in about one in every 600 to 1000 cases of measles.

Measles has an incubation period of between 7 to 14 days, which is then followed by 3 or 4 days of prodromal symptoms where the child will have a fever, head cold, cough and conjunctivitis. On the inner cheek and gums small white spots are visible, like grains of salt and are known as Koplik's spots; these are diagnostic for measles. A blotchy red rash appears around the ears before moving to the trunk and limbs. Immediate referral to the GP is needed.

Mumps

Mumps is caused by a paramyxovirus and is transmitted by airborne droplets from the nose and throat. It is the least contagious of the childhood diseases and requires close personal contact before infection can occur. There is an incubation period of 16 to 21 days, then fever, followed by swelling of one or both parotid glands. The child will experience pain when the mouth is opened.

Mumps is much more unpleasant if contracted as an adult, and in 20% to 30% of men the disease affects the testicles, with a serious infection that can possibly cause sterility. The most serious complication from mumps is meningitis (seen in approximately 10% of people).

German measles (rubella)

Rubella is caused by an RNA virus and spread by either close personal contact or airborne droplets. It is less contagious than measles and if contracted, many people suffer from mild symptoms and the infection passes undiagnosed. After the incubation period of 14 to 21 days the child experiences up to 5 days of prodromal symptoms, which include cold-like symptoms and swollen glands in the neck before a rash appears on the face that quickly moves to the trunk and extremities. The rash tends to be pinpoint and macular. The biggest threat posed by rubella is to women in early pregnancy, as foetal damage is possible.

To aid the differential diagnosis of childhood conditions, see Table 10.13.

Table 10.13
Differential diagnosis of childhood conditions

	Measles	German measles	Meningitis	Glandular fever	Chicken pox	Molluscum contagiosum	Mumps	Impetigo	Erythema infectiosum
Prodromal stage									
Fever	Yes	No	Yes	Yes	Yes, in older individuals	No	Yes	No	No
Swollen glands	No	Yes	No	Yes	No	No	Yes	No	No
Cold-like symptoms	Yes	Yes	No	No	No	No	No	No	Yes
Other signs	Koplik's spots	Malaise	Lethargy, stiff neck, vomiting, photophobia	Malaise & headache	Malaise & headache	None	None	None	No
Rash									
Location	Ears & face, progressing to trunk & limbs	Face moving quickly to trunk	Trunk and limbs	Trunk	On trunk & face; rarely on extremities	Face and axillae	Not applicable	Facial area, especially around nose & mouth	Face before moving to arms and legs
Character	Maculopapular	Macules, often pinpoint by 2nd day	Purplish blotches. Do not blanch	Maculopapular; about 10% have rash	Lesions discrete and appear in crops	Pink pearl-like spots with central punctum*		Vesicles that exude forming yellow crusts	'Slapped' skin
Epidemiology									
Age group most affected	Children & adolescents	Children under 12 years old	90% before age of 5	15–24 year old most at risk	Very common in children	Young children	Children under 12 years old	School-aged children	Children & adolescents

*Diagnostic.

Websites
Charities: www.meningitis.org and https://www.
    meningitisnow.org

Nappy rash

Background

Nappy rash (also known as nappy dermatitis or diaper rash) is a non-specific term used to describe inflammatory eruptions in the nappy area.

Prevalence and epidemiology

The incidence and prevalence of nappy rash is difficult to determine because of variability between studies. Nappy rash is most commonly seen between 6 and 12 months of age and in one UK study, 25% of infants under 1 month of age had an episode of nappy rash.

Aetiology

Friction and maceration of the skin are key to its cause. This is compounded by excessive heat and moisture combined with the effect of faecal and urinary enzymes when in prolonged contact with the skin (faeces breakdown produces ammonia, and is considered a contributory cause, as ammonia is only irritant when in contact with damaged skin). Greater exposure of skin surfaces to moisture impairs the skin's barrier function and makes the skin more susceptible to secondary infection.

Arriving at a differential diagnosis

The diagnosis is straightforward, although identifying the cause can be more difficult. There are four forms of nappy rash, with irritant nappy rash being the most common. Table 10.14 highlights the key differences in symptom presentation between the four forms.

Clinical features of irritant nappy rash

The rash affects primarily the buttocks (i.e., the area in contact with the irritant) but can involve the lower abdomen and upper thighs. The flexures, which are protected from exposure, are usually spared.

Conditions to eliminate

Secondary infection

An environment that is wet and warm creates an ideal breeding ground for opportunistic infections. Most commonly secondary infections are caused by *Candida albicans* (but other pathogens such as *Staphylococcus aureus* can be involved). Candidiasis is associated with satellite lesions (i.e., away from the main skin involvement). The lesions tend to be papular or pustular.

Seborrhoeic dermatitis

Seborrhoeic dermatitis presents as a rash, which is bright red and confluent. The flexures are not spared, and the rash can take on a diffuse, red shiny or greasy look. It is common for other sites to be involved, such as the scalp and face.

Psoriasiform nappy eruptions

Infants usually develop this form of nappy rash within the first 4 months of life. It presents as well demarcated erythematous plaques. It can show scaling that resembles psoriasis, although this is uncommon. Involvement away from the nappy area is common and affects the limbs, face and scalp.

Table 10.14
Differences in symptom presentation between the four causes of nappy rash

	Irritant	Candidal	Seborrhoeic	Psoriasiform
Flexure involvement	No	Yes	Yes	Yes
Satellite lesions	No	Yes	No	No
Other sites involved	No	Yes	Yes	Yes *limbs, face, scalp*
Rash description	Red, raw	Bright red and well demarcated *pustular*	Shiny/greasy *scalp face*	Atypical for psoriasis as usually no scaling is present *erythematous plaques limb*

HINTS AND TIPS BOX 10.6: NAPPY RASH

Preventative measures	Leave the nappy off for as long as possible each day
	Avoiding using soaps for cleaning
	Washed nappies should be thoroughly rinsed to ensure that they do not contain residues of soap and detergent
	Change nappies as soon as they have been soiled

TRIGGER POINTS indicative of referral: Nappy rash

Symptoms/signs	Possible danger/reason for referral
Involvement of rash away from nappy area	Suggests other causes such as psoriasis
OTC treatment failure	Requires prescription-only treatments
Severe rash	

Evidence base for over-the-counter medication

Management centres on reducing skin irritation (Hints and Tip in Box 10.6), applying a protective layer of barrier cream and reducing any inflammation and/or eliminating infection.

Barrier creams are designed to rehydrate and soothe the skin. A number of chemical constituents are formulated into barrier creams and include silicone, antiseptics and protectorants. Many proprietary products are available and often consist of a combination of ingredients. Secondary infection with *Candida* can be treated with imidazole products.

Practical prescribing and product selection

Barrier creams/protectorants should be applied to all skin surfaces, including the skin folds after each nappy change. They have no side effects, although some products do contain potential sensitising agents; it is best to patch test an area of skin before application. Commonly prescribed products include Drapolene, Metanium and Sudocrem.

For cases causing discomfort (in general those that are secondarily infected with *Candida*) the use of an imidazole twice a day is recommended. Parents should be told not to use a barrier cream until the infection has settled.

Further reading

Baer EL, Davies MW, Easterbrook KJ. Disposable nappies for preventing napkin dermatitis in infants. Cochrane Database of Systematic Reviews 2006, Issue 3. Art. No.: CD004262. http://dx.doi.org/10.1002/14651858.CD004262.pub2.

Self-assessment questions

The following questions are intended to supplement the text. Two levels of questions are provided; multiple choice questions and case studies. The multiple choice questions are designed to test factual recall and the case studies allow knowledge to be applied to a practice setting.

Multiple choice questions

10.1 A 12-week-old baby is brought to the pharmacy by his mother. He has a sore mouth. What is the most likely diagnosis?

a. Teething
b. Mouth ulcer
c. Thrush
d. Leukoplakia
e. None of the above

10.2 Which measurement of fever do NICE (National Institute of Health and Clinical Excellence) recommend for children under 5 years of age?

a. Under arm
b. Forehead
c. Oral
d. Anal
e. Either oral or under arm

10.3 Mrs Ng tells you that while combing her daughter's hair, she saw a head louse. You decide to advise a dimeticone lotion, and Mrs Ng asks how to use it. Which one of the following is the most appropriate way to apply the lotion?

a. Apply once only
b. Apply today, then reapply every 7 days for the next 2 weeks
c. Apply today, then reapply in 7 days' time
d. Apply today, then reapply at 3- to 4-day intervals for the next 2 weeks
e. Apply today, then reapply twice more at 14-day intervals

10.4 What confirms the presence of a head louse infection?

a. Presence of egg cases (nits) in the hair
b. An itchy scalp
c. A live louse
d. Louse faeces on the pillow
e. Dead lice on a pillow

10.5 Which statement concerning threadworm management is incorrect?

a. All family members should be treated
b. Mebendazole can be given from 6 months upwards
c. A repeated dose after 14 days is recommended
d. Mebendazole can cause GI upset
e. Bed linen should be washed at start of treatment

10.6 Nappy rash that becomes secondarily infected with *Candida* is most commonly associated with:

a. Itch and pain
b. Shiny, bright red lesions
c. Satellite lesions
d. Flexure involvement
e. Scaling lesions

10.7 Which sign/symptom represents high risk of infant dehydration?

a. Decreased activity
b. Respiration rate of less than 50
c. Reduced urine output
d. Pallor
e. Reduced skin turgor

10.8 At what age does colic usually resolve?

a. Within the first few weeks of birth
b. Before 6 months old
c. Between 6 and 12 months
d. Between 12 and 18 months
e. Before the age of 2 years old

Questions 10.9 to 10.14 concern the following:

A. Chicken pox
B. Molluscum contagiosum
C. Fifth disease (Erythema infectiosum)
D. Impetigo
E. Psoriasis
F. Atopic dermatitis
G. Roseola infantum

Select, from A to G, which of the conditions:

10.9 Is associated with a facial rash, often resembling a 'slapped cheek'

10.10 Can be mistaken for warts

10.11 Can lead to shingles in later life

10.12 Commonly affects cheeks and behind the knee

10.13 Is associated with high grade fever

10.14 Is caused by bacterial infection

Questions 10.15 to 10.17: for each of these questions *one or more* of the responses is (are) correct. Decide which of the responses is (are) correct. Then choose:

A. If a, b and c are correct
B. If a and b only are correct
C. If b and c only are correct
D. If a only is correct
E. If c only is correct

Directions summarised

A	B	C	D	E
a, b and c	a and b only	b and c only	a only	c only

10.15 Atopic dermatitis is characterised by:

 a. History of dry skin
 b. Flexural eczema
 c. Onset before 2 years old

10.16 Which of the listed symptoms about headache in a young child would raise sufficient concern to refer to a doctor?

 a. Irritability
 b. Fever
 c. Photophobia

10.17 Which statements about treating fever with analgesia are true?

 a. Paracetamol is effective in reducing fever
 b. Alternating between paracetamol and ibuprofen is not recommended
 c. Evidence for tepid sponging is inconclusive

Questions 10.18 to 10.20: these questions consist of a statement in the left-hand column, followed by a statement in the right-hand column. You need to:

● decide whether the first statement is true or false
● decide whether the second statement is true or false

Then choose:

A. If both statements are true, and the second statement is a correct explanation of the first statement
B. If both statements are true, but the second statement is NOT a correct explanation of the first statement
C. If the first statement is true, but the second statement is false
D. If the first statement is false, but the second statement is true
E. If both statements are false

Directions summarised

	1st statement	2nd statement	
A	True	True	2nd explanation is a correct explanation of the first
B	True	True	2nd statement is not a correct explanation of the first
C	True	False	
D	False	True	
E	False	False	

	First Statement	*Second statement*
10.18	Chicken pox is contagious until all lesions have crusted over	Children should be kept away from school until no longer contagious
10.19	Impetigo is commonly seen on the trunk	Children should be kept away from school until no longer contagious
10.20	Roseola infantum is characterised with a blanching rash	Children should be kept away from school until no longer contagious

Case study

CASE STUDY 10.1

Ms JP, a young mother of two children, comes into the pharmacy one afternoon, clutching a letter from the children's primary school. The letter says that there is a head lice outbreak and instructs parents to treat their children for head lice.

a. How do you respond?

You need to find out if her children actually have head lice or she is trying to buy a product to stop them from getting head lice. She should be told that products cannot be bought to prevent her children contracting head lice, and that she should inspect their heads regularly and that only when live lice are found, should a product be bought. Ms JP should be told how to inspect her children's hair for signs of head lice.

Ms JP returns to the pharmacy 4 days later and says her youngest daughter does now have head lice. She is 5 and suffers from no medical problems.

b. What product are you going to recommend?

Insecticides or a physical agent would be acceptable treatment options. Due to insecticidal resistance and high cure rates seen with dimeticone, it would seem reasonable to use this as treatment of choice.

Ms JP says she has heard that you can use conditioner and that will get rid of the problem.

c. How do you respond?

Ms JP is probably referring to the 'bug busting' technique. She should be told that the effectiveness of bug busting is lower than using dimeticone or insecticides but can be tried. You should stress that it is very important to adhere to the regimen, as poor compliance with the bug-busting method is probably why it has been shown to be less effective.

Ms JP then asks you whether her older daughter, Samantha, should also be treated even though she has not got head lice.

d. What do you say?

Only those with a live lice infestation should be treated. Ms JP should be asked to keep checking Samantha's hair on a regular basis.

CASE STUDY 10.2

Mr PB is looking after his 4-year-old grandson for the weekend. He asks for some advice because he has noticed a rash on his grandson's body and wants something to help get rid of it.

a. What do you need to know?

You need to know:

- *The location of rash*
- *What the rash looks like*
- *When the rash appeared*
- *Associated symptoms such as itch*
- *General health of the child*
- *What, if any, symptoms the child had before the rash appeared*

All Mr PB is able to tell you is that his grandson has been with him for the past day and only noticed the rash this morning when he was dressing him. The rash is on his chest and back; Mr PB describes them as spots. He thinks it is probably itchy because he saw his grandson scratching this morning.

b. What do you think could be the problem?

Without seeing the child and the rash, it is always difficult to make a differential diagnosis from information from a third party, but it appears the child might have chicken pox, given his age, location of rash and that the spots itch.

c. Are there any further questions you could ask the man to confirm your diagnosis?

Further questions you could ask are:

- *Are the spots coming out in groups?*
- *Have any of the spots turned into little blisters?*
- *Has he been exposed to other children with chicken pox?*

Knowing about the grouping and look of the spots is helpful as the chicken pox rash often appears in clusters. Knowing about prior exposure is very useful as this should help confirm your differential diagnosis.

Mr PB is unsure and concerned that his grandson is OK.

d. What could you do?

It appears that his grandson is not poorly ill and unless his condition deteriorates, there is probably no need to call out the doctor. You could recommend an antihistamine to help with the itching and reassure him that his grandson will be OK, but if his symptoms become worse, the doctor should be contacted. You also tell him that the rash fits the description of chicken pox but without seeing the rash, you cannot be sure. It would therefore be useful if you could see the child or if the child could be seen by someone over the next couple of days to confirm your suspicions.

CASE STUDY 10.3

A mother of a 2-month-old girl asks for help with her baby – she seems to be crying all the time.

Information gathering	Data generated
Presenting complaint (possible questions)	
Describe symptoms	Baby cries and will not be consoled, even after feeding, burping and nappy changes. Brings knees to her chest as she cries
How long has she had the symptoms?	About a month but just not getting better. Usually worse in the evening
Severity of pain/ distress of child	Difficult to say, but she is obviously worse than other babies she knows about
Other symptoms/ provokes?	As already stated
Any previous symptoms previous?	Has always had times where she has cried a lot but is just far worse in the last month

Information gathering	Data generated
Additional questions	Baby is bottle-fed Baby is gaining weight satisfactorily. No stomach distension and baby is passing stool adequately
Past medical history	Bought a gripe mixture last week on advice of a relative. This seems to have had no effect
Social history	Mother has changed formula milk twice in the last month. Mother is frustrated and appears tired
Family history	None for presenting complaint

This case obviously relates to whether the baby has colic.

Diagnostic pointers with regard to symptom presentation

The next table summarises the expected findings for questions when related to the different conditions that can be seen by community pharmacists.

	History	Weight gain	Systemic symptoms	Inconsolability
Colic	Weeks	OK	No	Yes
Infection	Days/hours	OK	Yes	Yes?
GORD	Weeks	OK	No	No
Intolerance to cows' milk protein	Weeks	Poor	No	No

When this information is applied to that gained from our patient (provided in next table), we see that everything points to a diagnosis of colic. To further eliminate GORD, questions about regurgitation could be asked and also the duration of the crying.

CASE STUDY 10.3 (Continued)

	History	Weight gain	Systemic symptoms	Inconsolability
Colic	✓	✓	✓	✓
Infection	✗	✓	✗	✓?
GORD	✓	✓	✓	✗
Intolerance to cows' milk protein	✓	✗	✓	✗

Reassure the parent that symptoms are transient. Although something has already been tried, it is probably worth starting with a dimeticone or Colief for 1 week. If that fails to help, then referral to the GP is appropriate.

Answers

1 = c	2 = a	3 = c	4 = c	5 = b	6 = c	7 = e	8 = b	9 = C	10 = B
11 = A	12 = F	13 = G	14 = D	15 = A	16 = E	17 = D	18 = B	19 = D	20 = C

Specific product requests

Background

Many patients will present in the pharmacy requesting a specific product rather than wanting advice on symptoms. Regardless of the reason why they are asking for the product, it is the responsibility of the pharmacist to ensure that the patient receives the most appropriate therapy. This chapter therefore deals with situations where patients ask for a particular product but where more information from the patient is needed before complying with their request.

Motion sickness

Background

Motion sickness is a symptom complex that is characterised by nausea, pallor, vague abdominal discomfort and occasionally, vomiting. Symptoms of fatigue, weakness and an inability to concentrate can also be experienced. Symptoms tend to resolve over prolonged exposure to motion. For example, sea sickness disappears over time – a characteristic called adaptation or habituation. Motion sickness can affect any individual and involve any form of movement, from moving vehicles to fairground rides.

Prevalence and epidemiology

The exact prevalence of motion sickness is unknown. Children between the ages of 2 and 12 are most commonly affected and it tends to affect women more than men. However, certain sectors of the population understandably show higher prevalence rates, for example naval crew and pilots.

Aetiology

It is widely believed that motion sickness results from the inability of the brain to process conflicting information received from sensory nerve terminals concerning movement and position, the sensory conflict hypothesis. Motion sickness occurs when motion is expected but not experienced, or the pattern of motion differs from that previously experienced.

Evidence base for over-the-counter medication

First-generation antihistamines (cyclizine, cinnarizine and promethazine) and anticholinergics (hyoscine and scopolamine) are routinely recommended to prevent motion sickness. All have shown various degrees of effectiveness. A Cochrane review (14 studies, $n = 1025$) found scopolamine to be superior to placebo and metoclopramide, and as good as antihistamines (Spinks et al., 2011).

Ginger has long been advocated for use as an anti-emetic. A review by Chrubasik et al. (2005) identified four studies with ginger in the prevention of motion sickness. The results suggested ginger was better than placebo, and similar in efficacy to other pharmacological agents. However, studies involved small numbers of patients and were of uncertain quality; the authors of the review concluded that further studies are required to confirm the effectiveness of ginger.

Non-pharmacological approaches to prevent motion sickness are also available OTC. Bruce et al. (1990) investigated the use of Sea Band acupressure bands versus hyoscine and placebo. Eighteen healthy volunteers were subjected to simulated conditions to induce motion sickness. The findings showed hyoscine exerted a preventative effect, although Sea Bands were no more effective than placebo. Further trials have confirmed these findings, although one small trial by Stern et al. (2001) reported positive findings. Accurate placement of the pressure bands seems to be important, and further trials are needed as acupressure has shown positive effects for nausea and vomiting associated with pregnancy.

Summary

Current evidence indicates that hyoscine and first-generation antihistamines are effective. Choice between the various agents will be driven by patient acceptability.

Practical prescribing and product selection

Prescribing information relating to medicines for motion sickness reviewed in the section 'Evidence base for over-the-counter medication' is discussed and summarised in Table 11.1. They are most effective when given before experiencing motion sickness and products should be selected based on matching the length of the journey with the duration of action of each medicine (see 'Hints and Tips' in Box 11.1).

Antihistamines

Antihistamines promoted for use in motion sickness are first-generation H_1 antagonists and are associated with sedation. They have the same side effects, interactions and precautions in use as other first-generation antihistamines used in cough and cold remedies. For further information see page 17.

Cyclizine

Cyclizine is now rarely used as it is subject to abuse and consequently many pharmacies do not stock it. If taken, adults and children over the age of 12 should take one tablet (50 mg) three times a day. The dose for children over the age of 6 is half the adult dose.

Table 11.1
Practical prescribing: Summary of medicines for travel sickness

Name of medicine	Use in children	Likely side effects	Drug interactions of note	Patients in which care is exercised	Pregnancy & breastfeeding
Cyclizine	>6 years	Dry mouth, sedation	Increased sedation with alcohol, opioid analgesics, analgesics, anxiolytics, hypnotics and antidepressants	Angle-closure glaucoma, prostate enlargement	Standard references state OK, although some manufacturers advise avoidance
Cinnarizine (Stugeron 15)	>5 years				
Promethazine (Avomine)	>5 years				
Hyoscine Joy-Rides	>3 years	Dry mouth, sedation	Increased anticholinergic side effects with TCAs and neuroleptics	Angle-closure glaucoma, prostate enlargement	Avoid if possible in pregnancy In breastfeeding, may cause drowsiness, which would lead to poor feeding in long-term use but OK for short journeys
Kwells	>10 years				
Kwells Kids	>4 years				

HINTS AND TIPS BOX 11.1: TRAVEL SICKNESS

How to minimise effects of motion	Planes – sit over the wing Ships – sit in the middle, close to the water line Cars – sit in the front Avoid rear-facing seats in any form of transport Focus on stationary objects Avoid alcohol or overeating before journeys Avoid reading or focusing on games Ensure good ventilation, for example, open a window
Dry mouth problems	Many people will complain of a dry mouth with travel sickness medicines. This is easily overcome by sucking on a sweet, which will stimulate saliva production
Matching up length of journey with product	Hyoscine should be recommended for journeys up to 4 hours; cinnarizine for journeys over 4 hours but less than 8 hours and promethazine for journeys longer than 8 hours

Cinnarizine (Stugeron 15)

Adults and children over the age of 12 should take two tablets (30 mg) 2 hours before travel. The dose can be repeated every 8 hours (1 tablet) if needed. For children aged between 5 and 12 the dose is half (15 mg) the adult dose.

Promethazine (Avomine)

Avomine can be given for both prevention and treatment of travel sickness. For prevention, adults and children over the age of 10 should take one tablet (25 mg) at least 1 or 2 hours before travel. For treatment, 1 tablet should be taken as soon as sickness is felt, followed by a second tablet 6 to 8 hours later. For children over the age of 5 the dose should be half that of the adult dose in both prevention and treatment.

Hyoscine

Hyoscine can be swallowed or chewed (e.g., Joy-Rides and Kwells). Products should be taken 20 to 30 minutes before the time of travel; because they have a short half-life, they have a short duration of action, and the dose might therefore have to be repeated on journeys longer than 4 hours. Anticholinergic side effects are more obvious than with antihistamines, and it does interact with other medicines that have anticholinergic side effects. Because hyoscine hydrobromide crosses the blood–brain barrier, it can cause sedation. It appears to be safe in pregnancy, although the manufacturers state it should be avoided.

Joy-Rides

Joy-Rides can be given from age 3 upwards. Children aged between 3 and 4 years should take half a tablet (75 µg) and no more than 1 tablet (150 µg) in 24 hours. Children between the age of 4 and 7 should take one tablet (150 µg) with a maximum of 2 tablets (300 µg) in 24 hours, and children aged between 7 and 12 should take one to two tablets.

Kwells

Kwells can only be given to children aged 10 and over. Children over the age of 10 should take half to one tablet. For adults the dose is one tablet.

Kwells Kids

Kwells Kids contain half the amount of hyoscine (150 µg) than Kwells and are marketed at children under the age of 10, although older children can take them. Children aged between 4 and 10 should take ½–1 tablet.

References

Bruce DG, Golding JF, Hockenhull N, et al. Acupressure and motion sickness. Aviat Space Environ Med 1990;61:361–5.

Chrubasik S, Pittler M, Roufogalis B. Zingiberis rhizoma: a comprehensive review on the ginger effect and efficacy profiles. Phytomedicine 2005;12:684–701.

Spinks A, Wasiak J. Scopolamine (hyoscine) for preventing and treating motion sickness. Cochrane Database of Systematic Reviews 2011, Issue 6. Art. No.: CD002851. http://dx.doi.org/10.1002/14651858.CD002851.pub4.

Stern RM, Jokerst MD, Muth ER, et al. Acupressure relieves the symptoms of motion sickness and reduces abnormal gastric activity. Altern Ther Health Med 2001;7:91–4.

Further reading
Dahl E, Offer-Ohlsen D, Lillevold PE, et al. Transdermal scopolamine, oral meclizine and placebo in motion sickness. Clin Pharmacol Ther 1984;36:116–20.
Klocker N, Hanschke W, Toussaint S, et al. Scopolamine nasal spray in motion sickness: a randomised, controlled and crossover study for the comparison of two scopolamine nasal sprays with oral dimenhydrinate and placebo. Eur J Pharm Sci 2001;13:227–32.
Pingree BJ, Pethybridge RJ. A comparison of the efficacy of cinnarizine with scopolamine in the treatment of seasickness. Aviat Space Environ Med 1994;65:597–605.

Emergency hormonal contraception

Background

Emergency hormonal contraception (EHC) is one of only a handful of deregulated products, which targets preventative health care and fits with UK government public health policy. Like other Western countries, the UK has high teenage pregnancy rates and associated high abortion rates.

The intention of UK government policy on making EHC available through pharmacies was to improve access for patients requiring EHC at times when other providers might be closed, for example at weekends and evenings. This policy appears to have been effective. Since EHC availability (2001) the percentage of EHC provided through community pharmacies has steadily increased. Community pharmacists are now the main provider of EHC, and studies have consistently demonstrated that women obtain EHC more quickly from community pharmacies than from other providers. This is relevant as EHC is more effective the sooner it is taken after unprotected sex.

Two products are now available OTC in the UK for emergency contraception; levonorgestrel (deregulated in 2001) and ulipristal (deregulated in 2015).

Aetiology

The exact mechanism of action for levonorgestrel is not clear. It appears to have more than one mode of action at more than one site. It is thought to work mainly by preventing ovulation and fertilisation if intercourse has taken place in the pre-ovulatory phase. It is also suggested that it causes endometrial changes that discourage egg implantation. Ulipristal works by inhibiting or delaying ovulation via suppression of the luteinising hormone surge.

Evidence base for over-the-counter medication

Trial data for levonorgestrel have found it to prevent 86% of expected pregnancies when treatment was initiated within 72 hours. Levonorgestrel is more effective the earlier it is taken after unprotected sex; it prevents 95% of pregnancies if taken within 24 hours, 85% between 24 and 48 hours, and 58% if used within 48 to 72 hours. Data from two trials for ulipristal show it to have similar efficacy to levonorgestrel between 0 and 72 hours after unprotected intercourse or contraceptive failure. When these data are pooled ulipristal shows superior efficacy over levonorgestrel at 24, 72 and 120 hours.

Practical prescribing and product selection

Prescribing information relating to EHC is discussed and summarised in Table 11.2.

Table 11.2
Practical prescribing: Summary of medicines for EHC

Name of medicine	Use in children	Likely side effects	Drug interactions of note	Patients in which care is exercised	Pregnancy & breastfeeding
Levonelle One-Step	>16 years	Nausea, headache, disturbed menstrual cycle	Anticonvulsants, rifampicin, griseofulvin, St. John's Wort and ciclosporin	Conditions in which absorption may be impaired, for example, Crohn's disease	Pregnancy – not applicable; Breastfeeding – safe to use
EllaOne	>16 years	Nausea, headache, dizziness and disturbed menstrual cycle	Anticonvulsants, rifampicin, St. John's Wort and ritonavir	None	Pregnancy – not applicable; Breastfeeding – avoid for 1 week

Assessing patient suitability

Before any sale or supply of EHC the pharmacist has to be in a position to determine whether the patient is suitable to take the medicine. To do this an assessment has to be made on the likelihood that the patient is pregnant:

- First, has the patient had unprotected sex, contraceptive failure or missed taking contraceptive pills in the last 72 to 120 hours? If more than 120 hours have elapsed the patient needs to be referred to her doctor for further assessment.
- Is the patient already pregnant? Details about the patient's last period should be sought. Is the period late, and if so, how many days late? Was the nature of the period different or unusual? If pregnancy is suspected a pregnancy test could be offered.
- What method of contraception is normally used? Patients who take combined oral contraceptives might not need EHC. Guidelines from the Faculty of Sexual and Reproductive Healthcare (2011) state:

For one missed pill (a missed pill is defined as one that is more than 24 hours late) or starting a new pack 1 day late:

No additional or emergency contraception is usually necessary. The patient should take the missed pill and continue to take the rest of the pack as usual.

For two or more missed pills or starting new pack 2 or more days late:

The patient should take the last pill missed immediately and continue to take the rest of the pack as usual and use an extra method of contraception for the next 7 days.

If pills are missed in the first week (Pills 1–7): EHC should be considered if unprotected sex occurred in the pill-free interval or in the first week of pill-taking.

If pills are missed in the second week (Pills 8–14): No indication for EHC if the pills in the preceding 7 days have been taken consistently and correctly (assuming the pills thereafter are taken correctly and additional contraceptive precautions are used).

If pills are missed in the third week (Pills 15–21): Omit the pill-free interval by finishing the pills in the current pack (or discarding any placebo tablets) and starting a new pack the next day.

If the patient uses a progestogen-only form of contraception: After a missed or late pill a woman should be advised to abstain or use additional contraception, such as condoms, for the next 2 days (48 hours after the pill has been taken). Emergency contraception may be indicated if unprotected sex occurs during this 48-hour period.

A number of useful checklists have been produced and are used in practice. Many pharmacists ask patients to complete one of these forms, instead of asking potentially embarrassing questions in the pharmacy.

Levonelle One Step

Levonelle should be taken as soon as possible and within 72 hours after unprotected sex or contraceptive failure. The dose consists of a single tablet (levonorgestrel 1500 µg). About one in five patients experience nausea but only 1 in 20 go on to vomit. If the patient vomits within 3 hours of taking the dose she should be advised that a further supply of EHC would be needed. A number of medicines do, theoretically, interact with Levonelle, most notably those that are enzyme inducers and include anticonvulsants, rifampicin, griseofulvin and St. John's Wort, although the clinical significance of the interactions appear low as only a handful of drug interaction reports have been received by the manufacturers. It seems prudent, until such time that more substantial evidence is available, that patients taking these medicines are best referred to the doctor. In such circumstances, increasing the dose of Levonelle is commonly practised (although not licensed).

Advanced sale of levonorgestrel is also permitted. However, pharmacists must consider the clinical appropriateness of a supply, and should consider declining repeated requests for advance supply and advise patients to use more reliable methods of contraception. See 'Hints and Tips' in Box 11.2.

Ulipristal acetate (EllaOne)

The treatment consists of one tablet to be taken as soon as possible but no later than 120 hours (5 days) after unprotected sex or contraceptive failure. If vomiting occurs within 3 hours another tablet should be taken. Common side effects that affect up to 10% of women are mood disorders, headache, dizziness, nausea, pain (abdominal, back or period), breast tenderness and fatigue. Like levonorgestrel it can interact with a number of medicines including antiepileptics (carbamazepine, fosphenytoin, oxcarbazepine, phenobarbital, phenytoin, primidone), rifampicin, ritonavir and St. John's wort. Ulipristal passes into breast milk and women should not breastfeed for 1 week after use.

Further reading

Anderson C, Blenkinsopp A. Community pharmacy supply of emergency hormonal contraception: a structured literature review of international evidence. Hum Reprod 2006;21(1):272–84.

Piaggio G, von Hertzen H, Grimes DA, et al. Timing of emergency contraception with levonorgestrel or the Yuzpe regimen. Task Force on Postovulatory Methods of Fertility Regulation. Lancet 1999;353:721.

11

HINTS AND TIPS BOX 11.2: EMERGENCY HORMONAL CONTRACEPTION

Consumer awareness	Studies have shown that most women have heard of EHC (>90%), although their knowledge on when it can be taken and its effectiveness is lower; for example, less than half of women are aware of how long EHC remains effective and less than two thirds are aware it was most effective the sooner it was taken after intercourse. It is highly likely that lower levels of awareness surround ulipristal and that it is effective for up to 5 days after unprotected sex compared with 72 hours for levonorgestrel.
Potential for misuse?	Some concerns have been raised about women misusing EHC because of its greater accessibility. However, a review of international experience with pharmacy supply of EHC found only a small proportion of women use EHC repeatedly (6.8% using it twice in 6 months, and 4.1% using it three times) (Anderson & Blenkinsopp, 2006).
EHC failure?	Taking EHC can affect the timing of the next menstrual period and patients should be told that their period might be earlier or later than usual. However, if the period is different than normal or more than 5 days late, then she should be advised to have a pregnancy test.
Awareness of effectiveness	Studies have shown that most women have heard of EHC (>90%), although their knowledge on when it can be taken and its effectiveness is lower; for example, less than half of women are aware of how long EHC remains effective and less than two thirds are aware it was most effective the sooner it was taken after intercourse.
Do you have to supply EHC?	The supply of EHC is at the discretion of each pharmacist and some, for religious beliefs, might choose not to supply EHC. However, the patient should be advised on other local sources of supply.

Websites

British Pregnancy Advisory Service: http://www.bpas.org
Brook Advisory Centres: http://www.brook.org.uk/
Contraceptive services with a focus on young people up to the age of 25. NICE public health guidance 51: https://www.nice.org.uk/guidance/ph51
Family Planning Association: http://www.fpa.org.uk
Marie Stopes International: http://mariestopes.org

Nicotine replacement therapy

Background

Smoking represents the single greatest cause of preventable illness and premature death worldwide. In 2010 over 100 000 people in the UK died as a result of smoking; putting this in context, smoking caused about 20% of all cancer deaths, 14% of all circulatory deaths and over 35% of all respiratory disease deaths.

Prevalence and epidemiology

The number of smokers over the age of 16 in the UK is falling – from a high of 45% in 1974 to 19% in 2013, although over recent years the smoking rate has remained at around 1 in 5 adults. Unemployed people (39%) are around twice as likely to smoke as those in employment (21%). Smoking is most common in those under the age of 35; 29% in people between 20 and 24 years of age, and 27% in those aged 25 to 34. It is least common (13%) in people over 60.

Aetiology

Hundreds of compounds have been identified in tobacco smoke; however, only three compounds are of real clinical importance:

- tar-based products, which have carcinogenic properties
- carbon monoxide, which reduces the oxygen-carrying capacity of the red blood cells
- nicotine, which produces dependence by activation of dopaminergic systems

Tolerance to the effects of nicotine is rapid. Once plasma nicotine levels fall below a threshold, patients begin to suffer nicotine withdrawal symptoms and will crave another cigarette. Treatment is therefore based on maintaining plasma nicotine just above this threshold.

Evidence base for over-the-counter medication

Nicotine replacement therapy (NRT) has established itself as an effective treatment option. A 2008 Cochrane review (Stead et al., 2008) found 111 trials (n >40 000) comparing NRT to placebo or non-NRT treatments, and the results indicated that

NRT increases rates of quitting smoking by 50–70%. It is not possible to say if one delivery system is better than another because comparative trials between delivery systems have not been conducted. Personal choice will therefore be the determining factor in which is chosen as being most suitable. In addition, the effectiveness of NRT is also affected by the level of additional support provided to the smoker, and many smoking cessation services are offered through pharmacy as part of their contractual arrangements with local commissioners.

Numerous intervention strategies have been used involving NRT. These include nurse-led services, workplace interventions, and doctor and pharmacy-based services. A 2012 review reported good levels of evidence that community pharmacists can deliver effective smoking cessation campaigns, and that structured interventions and counselling were better than opportunistic intervention (Brown et al., 2012).

It should be noted that relapse is a normal part of the quitting process and occurs on average three to four times. If a smoker has made repeated attempts to stop and has failed, experienced severe withdrawal or has requested more intensive help, then referral to a specialist smoking cessation service should be considered. Electronic cigarettes are becoming increasingly popular and in 2015 Public Health England concluded that e-cigarettes are 95% safer than smoking tobacco. In 2016, the MHRA issued a licence for an e-cigarette, paving the way for it to be prescribed by doctors. Additionally, the MHRA is introducing new rules for nicotine-containing e-cigarettes and refill containers that come into force in 2017 that will ensure minimum standards for the safety and quality of all e-cigarettes and refill containers.

Practical prescribing and product selection

Prescribing information relating to medicines for NRT reviewed in the section 'Evidence base for over-the-counter medication' is discussed and summarised in Table 11.3.

Before instigation of any treatment it is important that the patient does want to stop smoking. Work has shown that

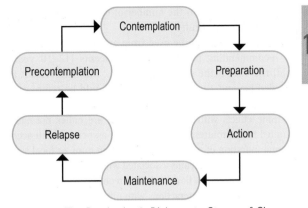

Fig. 11.1   The Prochaska & Diclemente Stages of Change Model.

motivation is a major determinant for successful smoking cessation, and interventions based on the transtheoretical model of change put forward by Prochaska and colleagues have proved effective (Fig. 11.1). The model identifies six stages, progress through which is cyclical, and patients need varying types of support and advice at each stage.

Most patients who ask directly for NRT will be at the preparation stage of the model and ready to enter the action stage. However, a small number of patients may well be buying NRT to please others and are actually in the precontemplation stage and do not want to stop smoking.

NRT is formulated as gum, lozenges, patches, nasal spray, inhalator, mouth spray, sublingual and orodispersible tablets; therefore there should be a treatment option to suit all patients.

A number of approaches to NRT regimens are advocated. In general, the strength of the formulation is tailored to the number of cigarettes smoked, and one form of NRT is tried at a time. However, it is possible for patients to use more than one form of NRT together, and there is evidence that this produces better results in patients with a high level of dependence. Additionally, patients can use

Table 11.3 Practical prescribing: Summary of medicines used as nicotine replacement therapy					
Name of medicine	**Use in children**	**Likely side effects**	**Drug interactions of note**	**Patients in which care is exercised**	**Pregnancy & breastfeeding**
Nicorette	>12 years	GI disturbances, headache, dizziness	None	Patients with heart disease and diabetes	OK
Nicotinell					OK but manufacturers of Nicotinell liquorice gum advise it not to be used in pregnancy
NiQuitin					

NRT to 'cut down' on the number of cigarettes smoked or as a nicotine substitute.

Most products can be used from age 12 years onwards. If recommending products for adolescents (12–18 years old) the dose is the same as for adults, but if treatment is needed beyond 12 weeks the person should be referred to a more formal structured programme run.

Side effects with NRT are rare and are either normally limited to gastrointestinal (GI) problems associated with accidental ingestion of nicotine when chewing gum, or local skin irritation and vivid dreams associated with patches. Headache, nausea and diarrhoea have also been reported. NRT appears to have no significant interactions with other medicines.

Nicorette

Nicorette is available as a gum (2 and 4 mg), inhalation cartridge (15 mg), microtab (2 mg), nasal spray (10 mg/mL) patches (10, 15 and 25 mg), mouth spray (1 mg/spray) and lozenge (2 mg).

Gum

Nicorette gum is available as either fruit or mint flavours (unflavoured gum leaves a bitter taste in the mouth). The strength of gum used will depend on how many cigarettes are smoked each day. In general, if the patient smokes less than 20 cigarettes a day, then the 2-mg gum should be used. If more than 20 cigarettes a day, then the 4-mg strength may be needed. A maximum of 15 pieces of gum can be chewed in any 24-hour period.

Inhalation cartridge

The inhalator can be particularly helpful to those smokers who still feel they need to continue the hand-to-mouth movement. Each cartridge is inserted into the inhalator and air is drawn into the mouth through the mouthpiece. A maximum of six cartridges can be used in 24 hours. Each cartridge can be used for approximately eight 5-minute sessions, with each cartridge lasting approximately 40 minutes of intense use.

The amount of nicotine from a puff is less than that from a cigarette. To compensate for this, it is necessary to inhale more often than when smoking a cigarette.

Microtabs (2 mg)

Microtabs are licensed for either smoking cessation or smoking reduction. For smoking cessation, the standard dosage is one tablet per hour in patients who smoke less than 20 cigarettes a day (doubled for heavy smokers). This can be increased to two tablets per hour if the patient fails to stop smoking with the one tablet per hour regimen, or for those whose nicotine withdrawal symptoms remain so strong they believe they will relapse. Most patients require

between 8 and 24 tablets a day, although the maximum is 40 tablets in 24 hours. Treatment should be stopped when daily consumption is down to 1 or 2 tablets a day.

For those reducing the number of cigarettes smoked, the tablets should be used between cigarettes to try and prolong the smoke-free period.

Nasal spray (each spray delivers 0.5 mg nicotine)

At the start of treatment one spray should be put into each nostril twice an hour to treat cravings. The maximum daily limit is 64 sprays, equivalent to two sprays in each nostril every hour for 16 hours.

Patches

The patches are usually applied in the morning and removed at bedtime (a 16-hour patch). Patients who want to stop smoking should start on the highest strength patch (25 mg – known as Step One) for 8 weeks before stepping down to the middle strength (15 mg – Step Two) for a further 2 weeks. The lowest strength patch (10 mg – Step Three) should be finally worn for another 2 weeks.

Mouth spray (each spray delivers 1 mg nicotine)

The mouth spray can be used for either smoking cessation or smoking reduction. Smokers wanting to reduce the number of cigarettes smoked should use the mouth spray, as needed, between smoking episodes to prolong smoke-free intervals. For smoking cessation, one spray should be used when cravings emerge. If this first spray fails to control cravings a second spray can be used. Most smokers will require one to two sprays every 30 minutes to 1 hour. The maximum number of sprays in a 24-hour period is 64.

Lozenge (2 and 4 mg)

Lozenges, like other dose forms, can be used for either smoking cessation or smoking reduction. The 2-mg lozenge is used for those who smoke 20 cigarettes or less a day. Most smokers require 8 to 12 lozenges per day (maximum 15 lozenges per day). Reduction strategies are the same as other dose forms in that the lozenges are used when needed between smoking cigarettes to prolong smoke-free intervals and with the intention to reduce smoking as much as possible.

Nicotinell

Nicotinell is available as gum (2 or 4 mg), patches (7, 14 and 21 mg) and lozenges (1 and 2 mg).

Nicotinell gum

Nicotinell gum is flavoured and available as fruit, mint or liquorice. The dosage and administration of Nicotinell gum is the same as that for Nicorette gum.

Patches

The patches are worn continuously and changed every 24 hours, thus Nicotinell patches are suitable for those smokers who must have a cigarette as soon as they wake up, as nicotine levels will be above the threshold of nicotine withdrawal. Treatment, like Nicorette, is based on a stepwise reduction over a maximum period of 3 months. People who smoke more than 20 cigarettes a day should use the highest strength patch (TTS 30 patch, 21 mg) for 3 to 4 weeks, after which the strength of the patch should be reduced to the middle strength (TTS 20 patch, 14 mg) for a further 3 to 4 weeks before finally using the lowest patch (TTS 10 patch, 7 mg). If the patient smokes less than 20 cigarettes a day, then he or she should start on the middle-strength patch.

Lozenge

The strength of lozenge used will depend on the number of cigarettes smoked. For those smoking less than 20 cigarettes a day the 1-mg lozenge should be used and for those smoking 30 or more cigarettes a day, the 2-mg strength is recommended. For those smoking between 20 to 30 cigarettes a day, then 1- or 2-mg lozenges can be used depending on patient response. Patients should be instructed to suck one lozenge every 1–2 hours when they have the urge to smoke. The usual dosage is 8 to 12 lozenges per day, with a maximum of 30 lozenges in 24 hours. Patients should be advised to gradually reduce the number of lozenges needed until they are only using one to two lozenges per day. At this point they should stop treatment.

Lozenges are mint flavoured and should be sucked until the taste becomes strong and then placed between gum and cheek (similar to the gum) until the taste fades, when sucking can recommence. Each lozenge takes approximately 30 minutes to dissolve completely.

NiQuitin

NiQuitin is available as gum (2 or 4 mg), patches (7, 14 and 21 mg), lozenge (2 and 4 mg, or NiQuitin minis: 1.5 and 4 mg) and orodispersible tablets (NiQuitin Strips 2.5 mg).

Patches

Like Nicotinell, patches are designed to be worn continuously (24-hour patch) and dosing is based on a sequential reduction of nicotine over time. Patients who smoke more than 10 cigarettes a day should use the 21-mg patch (Step 1) for 6 weeks, followed by the 14-mg patch (Step 2) for 2 weeks and finally the 7-mg patch (Step 3) for the last 2 weeks. If the person smokes less than 10 cigarettes each day the patient should start on Step 2 for 6 weeks, followed by Step 3 for a final 2 weeks.

NiQuitin lozenge

The low-strength lozenge (2 mg) is aimed at smokers who have their first cigarette of the day more than 30 minutes after waking up and the higher strength (4 mg) for those who smoke within 30 minutes of awakening. Like patches the dose of lozenges are marketed as Steps. For smoking cessation the dosing schedule is:

Step 1 × 6 weeks	1 lozenge every 1–2 hours
Step 2 × 3 weeks	1 lozenge every 2–4 hours
Step 3 × 3 weeks	1 lozenge every 4–8 hours

After this programme patients can use one to two lozenges a day over the next 12 weeks when strongly tempted to smoke.

For smoking reduction, as with other products, the lozenges should be used in between cigarettes to try and prolong the smoke-free period.

Niquitin Minis lozenge

Dosing of this version of the lozenge does vary from NiQuitin lozenges. The low strength (1.5 mg) is marketed for people who smoke less than 20 cigarettes a day and the high strength (4 mg) for those who smoke more than 20 cigarettes a day. For smoking cessation, it is recommended in either strength that the person should use between 8 and 12 lozenges per day (up to a maximum of 15 per day) and stop altogether when only using one or two lozenges per day.

For smoking reduction, as with NiQuitin lozenges, the lozenges should be used in between cigarettes to try and prolong the smoke-free period.

Gum

Gum can be used for smoking cessation or smoking reduction. Like lozenges, the lower strength (2 mg) is aimed at smokers who have their first cigarette of the day more than 30 minutes after waking up and the higher strength (4 mg) for those who smoke within 30 minutes of awakening. The 'chew and rest' technique, as with Nicorette and Nicotinell, is used. For smoking cessation, it is recommended in either strength that the person should use between 8 and 12 pieces of gum per day (up to a maximum of 15 per day) and stop altogether when only using one or two pieces of gum per day.

For smoking reduction, as with NiQuitin lozenges, the gum should be used in between cigarettes to try and prolong the smoke-free period.

Orodispersible Tablets (NiQuitin Strips)

A stepwise approach is again used for smoking cessation. Step 1 (6 weeks): one tablet should be used every 1 to 2 hours. Step 2 (3 weeks): one tablet should be used every

2 to 4 hours and Step 3 (3 weeks): one tablet should be used every 4 to 8 hours. After 12 weeks if the person has the urge to smoke, then 1 or 2 tablets can be taken per day.

See 'Hints and Tips' in Box 11.3 for tips on nicotine replacement therapy.

References

Brown D, Portlock J, Rutter P. Services to support the Healthy Living Pharmacy – a literature review. Int J Clin Pharm 2012;34(3):399–409.

Stead LF, Perera R, Bullen C, et al. Nicotine replacement therapy for smoking cessation. Cochrane Database of Systematic Reviews 2008, Issue 1. Art. No.: CD000146. http://dx.doi.org/10.1002/14651858.CD000146.pub3.

Further reading

Chaplin S, Hajek P. Nicotine replacement therapy options for smoking cessation. The Prescriber 2010;5th October:62–5.

Sinclair HK, Bond CM, Stead LF. Community pharmacy personnel interventions for smoking cessation. Cochrane Database of Systematic Reviews 2004, Issue 1. Art. No.: CD003698. http://dx.doi.org/10.1002/14651858.CD003698.pub2.

Websites

Action on Smoking and Health (ASH): http://www.ash.org/
QUIT (UK charity): http://www.quit.org.uk/

Malaria prophylaxis

Background

Malaria is a parasitic disease spread by the female *Anopheles* mosquito. Four species of the protozoan *Plasmodium* produce malaria in humans: *P. vivax*, *P. ovale*, *P. malariae* and *P. falciparum*. *P. falciparum* is the most virulent form of malaria and is attributable for the majority of deaths associated with malaria infection.

Prevalence and epidemiology

Malaria is a leading cause of death in areas of the world where the infection is endemic, with almost 600 000 deaths in 2013 – mostly among African children.

However, malaria is not only confined to endemic malarial areas, and the number of cases reported in Western countries, for example the UK, is on the increase as more and more people travel to countries where malaria is common. There are between 1500 and 2000 cases reported in the UK each year. In 2014 there were 1586 cases. Figures for that year show that *P. falciparum* accounted for 74% of cases (1169), *P. vivax* 14% (225), *P. ovale* 8% (130) and just 3% (41) for *P. malariae*.

For people travelling to countries where malaria is present, the risk of contracting malaria varies greatly. It depends on the area visited, the time of year, altitude (parasite maturation cannot take place above 2000 metres) and how many infectious bites are received. In general, risk tends to increase in more remote areas than in urban/tourist areas, after rainy or monsoon seasons, and at low altitude. It is therefore possible to have a different risk of contracting malaria within the same country, for example, visiting the southern lowlands of Ethiopia after the rainy season would pose a very high risk, whereas trekking in the Simien mountains in the north of the country during the dry season would pose minimal risk.

HINTS AND TIPS BOX 11.3: NICOTINE REPLACEMENT THERAPY

Application of patches	Patches should be applied to non-hairy skin on the hip, chest or upper arm. The next patch should be placed on a different site to avoid skin irritation
16- or 24-hour patches?	A 16-hour patch will be suitable for most patients; however, if a patient requires a cigarette within the first 20–30 minutes after waking, then a 24-hour patch should be given If sleep disturbances are experienced with the 24-hour patches, the patient can switch to a 16-hour patch or alternatively remove the 24-hour patch when they go to bed
Diabetics	Should monitor their blood sugar levels more closely than usual when NRT is started as carbohydrate metabolism can be affected
Gum chewing technique – 'chew and rest' technique	The gum should be chewed slowly until the taste becomes strong, it should then be rested between the cheek and gum until the taste fades. The gum can then be re-chewed. Each piece of gum lasts approximately 30 minutes.

Aetiology

Malarial parasites are transmitted to humans when an infected female anopheles mosquito bites its host. Once in the human host, the parasites (which at this stage of their life cycle are known as sporozoites) are transported via the bloodstream to the liver. In the liver they divide and multiply (they are now known as merozoites). After 5 to 16 days the liver cells rupture to release up to 400 000 merozoites, which invade the human host's erythrocytes. The merozoites reproduce asexually in the erythrocytes before causing them to rupture and release yet more merozoites into the bloodstream to invade yet more erythrocytes. Any mosquito that bites an infected person at this stage will ingest the parasites and the cycle will begin again. It is worth noting that *P. vivax* and *P. ovale* parasites can remain dormant in the liver, which explains why malarial symptoms can manifest months after return from an infected region.

Clinical symptoms

The most common symptom is fever, although it may initially present with chills, general malaise, nausea, vomiting and headache. Malaria should be considered as a differential diagnosis in anyone who presents with a febrile illness while in or recently leaving a malarious area. *P. falciparum* is unlikely to present more than 3 months after exposure but symptoms associated with *P. vivax* malaria can take up to a year to manifest.

Evidence base for over-the-counter medication

Effective bite prevention should be the first line of defence against malarial infection. Total avoidance of being bitten is not practical and patients must ensure that protective measures from being bitten are always taken.

Insect repellents containing *N,N*-diethyl-*m*-toluamide (DEET) in high concentrations are recommended (see 'Hints and Tips' in Box 11.4). In controlled laboratory studies DEET provides the longest protection compared with other products. Evidence for other insect repellents suggest they have comparable efficacy to low concentrations of DEET but have shorter duration of protection than DEET (Fradin & Day, 2002).

Besides applying DEET, other preventative measures to reduce the chance of being bitten include wearing long, loose-fitting, sleeved shirts and trousers, especially at dawn and dusk. Protection of ankles appears to be particularly important. Hotel windows should be checked to make sure they have adequate screening, windows and doors should remain closed, and ideally the bed should have a mosquito net. Mosquito nets do reduce the incidence of being bitten. Ideally they should be impregnated with insecticide as they are more effective than non-impregnated nets (Lengeler, 2004). If the person is travelling to more remote areas they should purchase their own mosquito net that has been impregnated with an insecticide. There are a number of travel centres and specialty outdoor shops where such products, including insecticidal impregnated clothes, can be bought.

HINTS AND TIPS BOX 11.4: MALARIA

Application of DEET	The concentration of DEET in commercial products varies widely. Products with concentrations in excess of 50% can cause skin irritation and occasionally skin blistering. It is advisable that these are patch tested first before widespread application
	The higher the concentration of DEET, the greater the length of protection:
	• 50% DEET provides protection for up to 12 hours
	• 30% DEET provides protection for up to 6 hours
	• 20% DEET provides protection for 1–3 hours
	Note: reapplication is necessary after swimming or sweating
	DEET can damage certain plastics, for example, sunglasses. It is important to emphasise to the patient that they wash their hands after applying DEET
	Make sure exposed areas, such as feet and ankles, are adequately protected
	DEET reduces the effectiveness of sunblock but sunblock does not affect the effectiveness of DEET
Electronic mosquito repellents	These products are designed to repel female mosquitoes by emitting high-pitched sounds almost inaudible to the human ear. There is no evidence in field studies to support any repelling effects
Alternative remedies	There is currently insufficient evidence supporting the use of vitamin B$_1$, garlic, tea tree oil, herbal remedies, Marmite or repellents containing lemon eucalyptus (e.g., Mosi-guard), or picaridin
	They should not be routinely recommended

Chemoprophylaxis

In addition to taking precautions to avoid being bitten, travellers should also take antimalarial medication. Chloroquine and proguanil are available OTC in the UK. Unfortunately, resistance to these two medicines (e.g., chloroquine-resistant *P. falciparum*) is now widespread, and limits their usefulness.

It is important to check current guidelines for the destination the person is travelling to or through. Two easily available UK reference sources in which recommendations can be found are the *British National Formulary* and *MIMS*. In addition, a number of organisations produce reference material (e.g., the National Pharmacy Association's vaccination updates). In most instances the *MIMS* would be a first-line reference source as the guidelines are updated monthly (compared with the *British National Formulary's* biannual publication) and are more likely to be still up to date. For people who are travelling to very high risk areas (usually sub-Saharan Africa or south-east Asia) or for long periods of time, it might be better to refer the person to a specialist centre.

Practical prescribing and product selection

Prescribing information relating to medicines for malaria reviewed in the section 'Evidence base for over-the-counter medication' is discussed and summarised in Table 11.4; useful tips relating to patients travelling to regions where malaria is endemic are given in 'Hints and Tips' in Box 11.4.

Medicine regimens

Antimalarials need to be taken at least 1 week before departure, during the stay in the malaria endemic region and for 4 weeks on leaving the area. Taking the medication before departure allows the patient to know whether they are going to experience side effects and, if they do, still have enough time to obtain a different antimalarial before departure. It also helps establish a medicine-taking routine

that will, hopefully, help with compliance. Medicine taking for a further 4 weeks after leaving the region is to ensure that any possible infection that could have been contracted during the final days of the stay does not develop into malaria.

Chloroquine (e.g., Avloclor, Nivaquine)

Chloroquine, as a single agent, is now almost obsolete against *P. falciparum* but still remains effective against the other forms of malaria.

Adults and children over 13 should take 300 mg of chloroquine base each week; this is equivalent to two tablets. Chloroquine can be given to children of all ages and is based on a milligram per kilogram basis. Nivaquine is formulated as a syrup (50 mg of base/5 mL) and should be recommended for children because accurate dosing can be achieved.

Chloroquine is associated with a number of side effects including nausea, vomiting, headaches and visual disturbances. Most patient groups, including pregnant women, can take chloroquine, although it is contraindicated in epilepsy because it might lower the seizure threshold and tonic-clonic seizures have been reported with prophylactic doses. Patients with psoriasis might notice a worsening of their condition. Chloroquine should be avoided in patients taking amiodarone because there is a risk of QT prolongation and ventricular arrhythmia. It should also be avoided with ciclosporin (increased ciclosporin levels), cimetidine (increased chloroquine levels) and possibly digoxin (increased digoxin levels).

Proguanil (Paludrine)

Proguanil is always used in combination with chloroquine unless the patient is contraindicated from taking chloroquine. Adults and children over the age of 13 should take 200 mg (two tablets) daily. Like chloroquine, it can be given to children of all ages and the dose ideally should be on a milligram per kilogram basis. Side effects associated with

Table 11.4
Practical prescribing: Summary of medicines for malaria prophylaxis

Name of medicine	Use in children	Likely side effects	Drug interactions of note	Patients in which care is exercised	Pregnancy & breastfeeding
Chloroquine	All ages	GI disturbances and visual problems	Amiodarone, ciclosporin, cimetidine, digoxin	Avoid in epilepsy	OK
Proguanil		Diarrhoea	None	Renal impairment	

proguanil are usually mild and include diarrhoea. Patients with known mild renal impairment should take 100 mg daily, and the dose should be further reduced if renal impairment is moderate or severe. To aid compliance a travel pack suitable for adults on a 2-week holiday is available and combines 14 chloroquine tablets with 98 proguanil tablets.

References
Fradin MS, Day JF. Comparative efficacy of insect repellents against mosquito bites. N Engl J Med 2002;347:13–18.
Lengeler C. Insecticide-treated bed nets and curtains for preventing malaria. Cochrane Database of Systematic Reviews 2004, Issue 2. Art. No.: CD000363. http://dx.doi.org/10.1002/14651858.CD000363.pub2.

Further reading
Enayati AA, Hemingway J, Garner P. Electronic mosquito repellents for preventing mosquito bites and malaria infection. Cochrane Database of Systematic Reviews 2007, Issue 2. Art. No.: CD005434. http://dx.doi.org/10.1002/14651858.CD005434.pub2.

Websites
Fit for travel http://www.fitfortravel.nhs.uk/home.aspx
Liverpool School of Tropical Medicine: http://www.liv.ac.uk/lstm
Malaria Reference Laboratory: http://www.malaria-reference.co.uk
The National Travel Health Network and Centre: http://www.nathnac.org/travel/index.htm

Bites and stings

Background

A whole host of animals (and plants) have the capacity to cause injury to the skin, and depending on the severity, this can result in systemic symptoms. The majority of cases in the UK are caused by insects and are of nuisance value.

Prevalence and epidemiology

The prevalence of bites and stings is largely unknown. Most people self-treat and never seek advice. Biting and stinging insects are generally more common in warmer climates and during warmer months.

Aetiology

Stinging insects are broadly defined as those that use some sort of venom as a defence mechanism or to immobilise their prey. Examples include bees, wasps and ants. The venom is usually 'injected' using a stinger and includes proteins and substances that help break down cells and increase the penetration of the venom, e.g., phospholipase A and hyaluronidase. People can develop allergic reactions to these substances and, unlike with most biting insects, can occasionally suffer significant reactions, including anaphylaxis, to stings. The severity of the reaction depends on the quantity of the venom injected and the person's predisposition to hypersensitivity.

Biting insects are those that feed off the blood supply of humans and other creatures. They include mosquitoes, ticks, and fleas. Apart from having some sort of apparatus to draw the blood, these insects usually secrete anticoagulant-like substances to facilitate feeding. It is these anticoagulant substances that people will react to. However, it is only after repeated bites that sensitivity occurs. Some insects (e.g., horseflies, midges) do not have specialised mouthparts and take blood by biting a hole through the skin. These are typically more painful.

In the UK the most common plant that causes skin reactions is the stinging nettle. An urticarial-type reaction occurs as hairs on the leaf pierce the skin, releasing histamine, acetylcholine and serotonin.

Clinical features of bites and stings

Itching papules, which can be intense, is the hallmark symptom of insect bites. Weals, bullae and pain can occur, especially in sensitised individuals. Lesions are often localised and grouped together, and occur on exposed areas, e.g., hands, ankles and face. Scratching can cause excoriation, which might lead to secondary infection. In contrast, stings are associated with intense burning pain. Erythema and oedema follow but usually subside within a few hours. If systemic symptoms are experienced, they occur within minutes of the sting.

Ticks and Lyme disease

Ticks can be picked up when walking in open grassy areas and feed on the human host. A small proportion of ticks carry a spirochete bacterium that can lead to the person developing Lyme disease. A person with a history of a tick bite (even months previously) who develops an erythematous spreading rash or fever needs to be referred. If a tick is found on the body it will need removal. Ticks should be removed with fine tweezers by gripping the insect close to the skin and pulling straight up. Twisting movements should be avoided as these increase the chance that mouthparts will be left in the skin.

11

Evidence base for over-the-counter medication

Avoiding bites and stings in the first place is obviously important. This means using an effective insect repellent and avoiding times and places when insects are about. DEET is the most effective insect repellent and found in most commercial preparations. For avoidance measures and more information on DEET see page 343.

Topical OTC treatments for bites and stings include local anaesthetics, corticosteroids and antihistamines. However, there is a lack of evidence for the efficacy of these treatments and, in general, recommendations for treatment are based on expert opinion and clinical experience.

Antihistamines (both topical and systemic) have been used for their antipruritic properties. There are limited studies in the treatment of insect bites and stings. Some studies, with systemic antihistamines, have shown efficacy of the less sedating antihistamines for mosquito bites

(Foëx & Lee, 2006). They are probably most useful for their sedating properties when itching is disturbing sleep.

Practical prescribing and product selection

Prescribing information relating to products for bites and stings is reviewed in the section 'Evidence base for over-the-counter medication' and summarised in Table 11.5.

Before OTC treatment is offered, the severity of symptoms should be assessed because small local reactions can be managed primarily with topical products, whereas large local reactions will generally require systemic treatment. Patients with systemic symptoms should be referred.

If the person has been stung and the stinger is still in situ, then this should be removed. The best way of removal is to scrape the stinger away with a sharp edge (e.g., card or knife blade) or alternatively a fingernail.

Table 11.5
Practical prescribing: Summary of medicines used for insect bites and stings

Name of medicine	Use in children	Likely side effects	Drug interactions of note	Patients in which care is exercised	Pregnancy & breastfeeding
Benzocaine Lanacane	>12 years	Can cause sensitisation reactions	None	None	OK
Lidocaine Dermidex	>4 years	Can cause sensitisation reactions	None	None	OK
Savlon Bites and Stings Pain Relief Gel	>12 years				
Hydrocortisone	>10 years	None	None	None	OK
Crotamiton	>3 years	None	None	None	OK
Chlorphenamine	>1 year	Dry mouth, sedation and constipation	Increased sedation with alcohol, opioid analgesics, anxiolytics, hypnotics and antidepressants	Glaucoma, prostate enlargement	Pregnancy OK. Standard references state OK, although some manufacturers advise avoidance. This is presumably because it has the potential to cause drowsiness and may lead to poor feeding

Small local reactions

Local pain and swelling is best treated with cold compresses/ice and, if needed, oral pain killers (ibuprofen or paracetamol). Local itching can be treated with topical crotamiton or low-potency corticosteroids (hydrocortisone 1%). If itching interferes with sleep, then an oral sedating antihistamine might be helpful at night.

Large local reactions

Occasionally, severe pain and swelling can extend beyond the immediate surroundings of the lesion. They should be managed with oral pain killers and antihistamines.

Local anaesthetics (e.g., benzocaine [Lanacane], lidocaine [Dermidex & Savlon Bites and Stings Pain Relief Gel])

Local anaesthetics can be used in adults and children over the age of 4 years and are in general applied three times a day. They are safe to use in pregnancy and are generally well tolerated. Local anaesthetics are known to be skin sensitisers and can produce contact dermatitis.

Local anaesthetic/antihistamine combination (Wasp-Eze Spray)

This product contains benzocaine 1% and mepyramine 0.5%. It can be used on people over the age of 2 years. The dosage is one spray onto the affected area of skin for 2 to 3 seconds. This dose can be repeated after 15 minutes if required.

Hydrocortisone (e.g., Dermacort)

Hydrocortisone is applied once or twice a day to the affected areas. It can be used in adults and children over 10 years of age. It can be used for a maximum of 7 days.

Sedating antihistamines (e.g., chlorphenamine)

Chlorphenamine is associated with sedation, as are all antihistamines. They interact with other sedating medication, resulting in potentiation of the sedative properties of the interacting medicines. They also possess antimuscarinic side effects, which commonly result in dry mouth and possibly constipation. It is these antimuscarinic properties that mean patients with glaucoma and prostate enlargement should ideally avoid their use because it could lead to increased intraocular pressure and precipitation of urinary retention.

Chlorphenamine (e.g., Piriton)

Chlorphenamine can be given from the age of 1 year. Children up to the age 2 should take 2.5 mL of syrup (1 mg) twice a day. For children aged between 2 and 5, the dosage is 2.5 mL (1 mg) three or four times a day, and for those over the age of 6, the dosage is 5 mL (2 mg) three or four times a day. Adults should take 4 mg (one tablet) three or four times a day.

Crotamiton (Eurax)

Adults and children over 3 years of age should apply crotamiton two or three times a day. A combination product containing hydrocortisone is available (Eurax HC) but is best avoided if possible. This is to decrease the exposure of patients to unnecessary corticosteroids and their potential adverse effects.

References
Foëx BA, Lee C. Oral antihistamines for insect bites. Emerg Med J 2006;23:721–2.

Further reading
Anon. Management of simple insect bites: where's the evidence? DTB 2012;50:45–8.
Henderson D, Easton RG. Stingose: a new and effective treatment for bites and stings. Med J Aust 1980;2:143–50.
Kennedy J. Self-care of insect bites and stings. SelfCare 2011; 2(4):111–14.

Websites
http://www.lymediseaseaction.org.uk

Weight loss

Background

Obesity is a growing epidemic, particularly in Western countries. As a consequence the risk of diseases such as diabetes and cardiovascular disease are also increasing, resulting in a situation where the current and future generations could have a shorter life span than their parents. Although a number of measures of obesity have been proposed, the internationally accepted measure is the body mass index (BMI). This is calculated as weight (kg) divided by height squared (m^2). A BMI of over 25 is classified as overweight and for obesity the value is 30.

Prevalence and epidemiology

In 2013, a quarter of adults in England were classified as obese and this is almost double the values seen in 1993. Figures are even higher for those classed as overweight – 42% of men and 32% of women. This equates to 63% of adults being overweight or obese. Figures for Wales and Scotland are similar. Only the US (36%), Mexico (30%), Hungary (29%) and New Zealand (28%) have higher rates of obesity.

Aetiology

Although a number of causes of obesity have been proposed, and genetics may play an important role, for a significant proportion of the population it results from an imbalance between energy intake (food and beverages) and energy expenditure (exercise). Other factors associated with obesity include cultural norms, socioeconomic status, gender and ethnicity. See 'Hints and Tips' in Box 11.5 for guidance on weight loss.

Evidence base for over-the-counter medication

Diet and exercise are the first-line treatment for obesity. Orlistat inhibits pancreatic and gastric lipase, which reduces the absorption of fat from the gut. Clinical trials have shown that orlistat produces a modest weight loss of approximately 5–10% of body weight (Hill et al., 1999). The best results with orlistat are seen in the short term (6–12 months); long-term results rely heavily on lifestyle changes.

Practical prescribing and product selection

Orlistat (Alli)

Orlistat is indicated for weight loss in adults (18 or over) who are overweight (body mass index $\geq 28\,kg/m^2$) and should be taken in conjunction with a mildly hypocaloric, lower-fat diet.

The recommended dose of orlistat is one 60-mg capsule three times daily. The capsule should be taken immediately before, during or up to 1 hour after each main meal. If a meal is missed or contains no fat, the dose of orlistat should not be taken. If weight loss has not been achieved after 12 weeks, then the patient should stop taking orlistat.

Side effects include GI disturbances/GI upsets such as faecal urgency and incontinence, oily evacuation and spotting, flatus and abdominal pain. These can be minimised by restricting fat intake to less than 20 g per meal. Supplementation with fat-soluble vitamins (A, D, E and K) is recommended and can be achieved by taking a multivitamin. Because of the effect on vitamin K levels, patients on warfarin should avoid using orlistat. Orlistat may decrease ciclosporin levels and requires close monitoring. There are limited data of orlistat being used in pregnant and breastfeeding women, and it is therefore not recommended.

Reference
Hill J, Hauptman J, Anderson J. Orlistat, a lipase inhibitor, for weight maintenance after conventional dieting: a 1-y study. Am J Clin Nutr 1999;69:1108–16.

Further reading
Lindgarde F. The effect of orlistat on body weight and coronary heart disease risk profile in obese patients: the Swedish Multimorbidity Study. J Intern Med 2000;248:245–54.
Managing overweight and obesity in adults – lifestyle weight management services: NICE public health guidance 53: https://www.nice.org.uk/guidance/ph53

Benign prostatic hyperplasia (symptoms of)

Background

Tamsulosin was reclassified from POM to P in the UK in 2010. This represents the first medicine deregulated in the UK to treat a chronic, progressive symptomatic condition. This deregulation is also notable for the fact that it may encourage men to take more of an interest in their welfare through community pharmacies, especially as the majority of men with benign prostatic hyperplasia (BPH) do not consult their doctor when experiencing symptoms.

HINTS AND TIPS BOX 11.5: WEIGHT LOSS

Realistic weight loss goals	Recommended goals are 1–4 kg per month in the short term, and 10–20% of body weight in the medium to long term.
Exercise	People should be encouraged to start with regular, moderate exercise (e.g., brisk walking) three times a week, with the aim of increasing exercise to a minimum of 80 minutes per day to maintain weight loss

Prevalence and epidemiology

Men over the age of 50 commonly experience lower urinary tract symptoms (LUTS). It is estimated that 10–30% of men over 70 years of age suffer from symptoms, with the most common cause being benign prostatic enlargement.

Aetiology

LUTS in men can be caused by structural or functional abnormalities in one or more parts of the lower urinary tract. Often the prostate gland is enlarged, which places pressure on the bladder and urethra. Symptoms can also be caused via peripheral or central nervous system abnormalities that affect control of the bladder and sphincter.

Lower urinary tract symptoms

Patients will present with a range of symptoms, typically symptoms such as hesitancy, weak stream and urgency. Symptoms are often classified as being either 'obstructive' or 'irritative'. Obstructive symptoms are related to bladder emptying and are experienced by the patient as incomplete emptying, intermittency and straining. Patients may use terms such as 'stopping and starting' or 'dribbling'. Irritative symptoms are related to bladder filling and involve increased frequency, urgency and nocturia.

Evidence base for over-the-counter medication

Studies show that tamsulosin is significantly better than placebo in improving urinary flow and reducing symptoms.

Tamsulosin is an alpha$_1$-adrenoceptor antagonist blocker that binds selectively and competitively to post-synaptic alpha$_1$-receptors, in particular to the subtype alpha$_1$a. Alpha$_1$-blockers relax smooth muscle in BPH, producing an increase in urinary flow-rate and an improvement in obstructive symptoms.

Practical prescribing and product selection

Tamsulosin (Flomax Relief)

Tamsulosin is indicated for treatment of functional symptoms of BPH in men aged 45 to 75 years old. Men presenting with lower urinary tract symptoms, who appear to be suitable for OTC tamsulosin (see 'Hints and Tips' in Box 11.6) can be supplied an initial 14-day supply. Patients must be told that they will have to see a doctor for confirmation of the cause of their symptoms. If this takes longer than the supply of 14 days of treatment, then the pharmacist can provide a further 28 days of treatment. In addition, if symptoms have not improved within 14 days of starting treatment or are getting worse, the patient should stop taking tamsulosin and be referred to a doctor.

The dose is 400 µg daily (one capsule). Dizziness is the most frequently reported side effect (1.3% of patients). Other less common side effects reported include GI disturbances, headache and rash. As it is alpha-blocker it should not be given to patients receiving antihypertensive medicines with significant alpha$_1$-adrenoceptor antagonist activity (e.g., doxazosin, indoramin, prazosin, terazosin and verapamil).

HINTS AND TIPS BOX 11.6: TAMSULOSIN

Contraindications	Symptoms less than 3 months' duration
	Prostate surgery
	Unstable or undiagnosed diabetes
	Problems with liver, kidney or heart
	Postural hypotension
	Eye operation of cataract planned
	Recent blurred or cloudy vision that has not been investigated
Automatic referral	Men who report dysuria, haematuria or cloudy urine in the past 3 months, or who are suffering from a fever that might be related to a urinary tract infection
Symptoms-check questionnaire	This incorporates a quality-of-life score and the International Prostate Symptom Score. Low scores on both scales suggest mild symptoms and a good quality of life, and tamsulosin would not be appropriate
	http://www.myilearn.co.uk/flomax/resources/documents/Flomax_Relief_SQ.pdf

Further reading

Rees J, Bultitude M, Challacombe B. The management of lower urinary tract symptoms in men. Brit Med J 2014;348:g3861 http://dx.doi.org/10.1136/bmj.g3861.

Simpson RJ, Lee RJ, Garraway WM, et al. Consultation patterns in a community survey of men with benign prostatic hyperplasia. Br J Gen Pract 1994;44:499–502.

Websites

Prostate Help Association: www.prostatehelp.me.uk

Royal Pharmaceutical Society Guidance (members only): http://www.rpharms.com/practice--science-and-research-full-guidance/otc-tamsulosin-full-guidance.asp

Chlamydia treatment

Background and prevalence

Chlamydia trachomatis is the most common sexually transmitted bacterial infection in the UK, and the incidence is increasing, in part due to it being asymptomatic. At least 70% of women and 50% of men infected are asymptomatic. In 2010, people younger than 25 years old accounted for 65% of chlamydia diagnoses.

Practical prescribing and product selection

Azithromycin was reclassified in 2008. It is indicated for men and women 16 years of age or older who are asymptomatic and have tested positive for genital chlamydia infection. It is also indicated for treatment of their sexual partners without the need for a test. The dose is a single stat dose of 1 g (2 × 500 mg tablets). Side effects that might be experienced are GI upset, namely nausea, vomiting and abdominal discomfort.

Future deregulations

The number of POM to P deregulations in the last few years has slowed, while P to GSL switches have increased. This wider availability of medicines fits with current UK government policy that promotes self-care. It has resulted in the number of medicines sold only through pharmacies shrinking. The lack of POM to P switches over the last 5 to 10 years is partially a result of burdensome regulatory

Table 11.6
Possible future deregulated medicines from POM to P

Product license extensions	
Hydrocortisone	Available from 2 years of age in Australia and in different strengths
Products available OTC in other countries	
Salbutamol	Available in Singapore, New Zealand
NSAIDs	Mefenamic acid available in Australia/New Zealand
Trimethoprim	Available in New Zealand
Metoclopramide	Available in Australia/New Zealand
Non-sedating antihistamines	Desloratadine and fexofenadine available OTC in Australia
Medicines supplied under protocols	
Oral contraception	Successful PGD in South London reported on January 2012
Topical antibiotics for impetigo (e.g., fusidic acid, mupirocin)	Already established PGDs through community pharmacy
Anti-retrovirals for influenza	

PGD, patient group direction.

processes. Just eight switches were seen between 2010 and 2016 (five for 'me too' products, e.g., three proton pump inhibitors, and three from new therapeutic classes – orlistat, tranexamic acid and tamsulosin). Over the same time, two products were switched back to POM (domperidone and oral diclofenac).

The future for further switches therefore appears relatively poor in the short term. It is likely that future deregulation may be a combination of:

- Product license extensions
- New switches that mirror those already available in other countries
- Those that have been used in more controlled conditions (e.g., patient group direction supply)

Table 11.6 highlights some future candidates that are potential POM to P switches.

11

Self-assessment questions

The following questions are intended to supplement the text. Two levels of questions are provided: multiple choice questions and case studies. The multiple choice questions are designed to test factual recall and the case studies allow knowledge to be applied to a practice setting.

Multiple choice questions

11.1 Which symptom is not commonly seen in benign prostate hypertrophy?

a. Urgency
b. Hesitancy
c. Straining
d. Increased frequency
e. Pain on urination

11.2 Which of the listed side effects is least commonly associated with EllaOne?

a. Abdominal pain
b. Headache
c. Skin rash
d. Nausea
e. Dizziness

11.3 Which percent of people are asymptomatic for chlamydia?

a. 10%
b. 20%
c. 30%
d. 40%
e. 50%

11.4 What would be the best differentiating feature between an insect bite and scabies in a person with lesions on the wrist?

a. Intensity of itching
b. Severity of redness
c. Symptom improvement after taking antihistamines
d. Occupational history
e. Development of papules and vesicles

11.5 Which patient group should tamsulosin not be supplied to without first confirming current medication?

a. Asthmatics
b. Diabetics
c. Those with active ulcer disease

d. Hypertensives
e. Epileptics

11.6 How long after unprotected sex can levonorgestrel be given?

a. 24 hours
b. 48 hours
c. 72 hours
d. 96 hours
e. 120 hours

11.7 What medicine is most appropriate for an 8-year-old child travelling to Calais from Dover on the ferry (3-hour crossing)?

a. Promethazine 25 mg
b. Chlorphenamine 2 mg
c. Hyoscine 150 µg
d. Cinnarazine 15 mg
e. Cyclizine 50 mg

11.8 What medicine is most appropriate for an adult travelling to the Gambia from the UK by plane (6-hour flight)?

a. Promethazine 25 mg
b. Chlorphenamine 2 mg
c. Hyoscine 150 µg
d. Cinnarazine 15 mg
e. Cyclizine 50 mg

Questions 11.9 to 11.14 concern the following medicines:

A. Chloroquine
B. Proguanil
C. Hyoscine
D. NRT
E. Levonorgestrel
F. Tamsulosin
G. Ulipristal
H. Orlistat

Select, from A to H, which of the above medicines:

11.9 Should be avoided in epilepsy

11.10 Should be avoided in patients taking verapamil

11.11 Needs to be used with caution in patients with renal impairment

11.12 Needs to be used with caution in patients with glaucoma

11.13 Affects absorption of vitamin A

11.14 May worsen psoriasis

Questions 11.15 to 11.17: for each of these questions *one or more* of the responses is (are) correct. Decide which of the responses is (are) correct. Then choose:

A. If 1, 2 and 3 are correct
B. If 1 and 2 only are correct
C. If 2 and 3 only are correct
D. If 1 only is correct
E. If 3 only is correct

Directions summarised

A	B	C	D	E
a, b and c	a and b only	b and c only	a only	c only

11.15 Orlistat cannot be taken by:

    a. People under 18 years of age
    b. People with a BMI under 28
    c. Pregnant women

11.16 Lyme disease is caused by:

    a. Ticks
    b. Viral pathogens carried by ticks
    c. Bacteria carried by ticks

11.17 What symptom/s are associated with Lyme's Disease?

    a. Rash
    b. Fever
    c. GI disturbances

Questions 11.18 to 11.20: these questions consist of a statement in the left-hand column, followed by a statement in the right-hand column. You need to:

- decide whether the first statement is true or false
- decide whether the second statement is true or false

Then choose:

A. If both statements are true, and the second statement is a correct explanation of the first statement
B. If both statements are true, but the second statement is NOT a correct explanation of the first statement
C. If the first statement is true, but the second statement is false
D. If the first statement is false, but the second statement is true
E. If both statements are false

Directions summarised

	1st statement	2nd statement	
A	True	True	2nd explanation is a correct explanation of the first
B	True	True	2nd statement is not a correct explanation of the first
C	True	False	
D	False	True	
E	False	False	

	First statement	*Second statement*
11.18	Ulipristal is 100% effective, providing the patient does not vomit within 3 hours of taking	Ulipristal works by inhibiting egg plantation
11.19	NRT can cause nausea	Nicotine directly irritates the GI tract
11.20	DEET can irritate skin	High concentrations cause greater skin irritation

Case study

Mr and Mrs J and their two children, Sammy, aged 5, and Jessica, aged 12, are going on their summer holidays. They want to know what travel sickness tablets they should take.

a. What information do you need to know before recommending a suitable product? For each question state your rationale.

You need to know:

- *Who is affected by travel sickness: this may influence recommendation, especially if it affects one of the parents who might be driving.*
- *The length of the trip: this will influence which product will be the most appropriate. It is sensible to match up the length of journey with a medicine that has the same duration of action as the trip.*
- *Medication history: patients who are taking medication for glaucoma or prostate enlargement should avoid taking OTC medicines. Additionally, medicines with anticholinergic action will potentiate the side effects of OTC travel medication.*
- *Passed medication for similar journeys: it is likely that the family have had to purchase such products in the past. It is worth finding out what they were and how well tolerated they were before potentially recommending the same product.*

You find out they are going to northern France by ferry. This is a 2-hour boat journey followed by a further 2-hour drive. Mr J gets seasick and neither of the children likes boat or car journeys. Jessica also suffers from narcolepsy.

b. What would be the best drug regimen for the family? State your rationale.

It appears that the total journey time is relatively short and a hyoscine-based product would be the most suitable product for the two children and their father. Kwells Kids could be used by everyone; Mr J would have to take 2 tablets, Jessica 1 tablet and Sammy ½ a tablet. As Jessica has narcolepsy it is necessary to see if she takes any medication to help with the condition. If she does, then checks would have to be made to ensure that Jessica could still take hyoscine.

c. What practical advice would you also offer the family?

Hyoscine will cause dry mouth and potential sedation. Sucking on sweets can compensate for a dry mouth. Sedation might be a problem for Mr J because he has to drive after the ferry crossing. He should be told about the possible effects of hyoscine. He might choose not to take the medication, although no alternative is available that does not cause possible sedation.

The two children might experience less nausea if they are kept occupied by playing games.

CASE STUDY 11.2

Ms HS walks into the pharmacy on Saturday morning and asks to buy the morning after pill.

a. What questions do you need to ask?

You need to discover:

- *Her age*
- *How long ago did she have unprotected sex or contraceptive failure?*
- *The date of her last period and was it different than normal.*

You find out she is 18 and had sex last night. She normally takes Microgynon. Her period was about 3 weeks ago and was the same as previous periods.

b. What else do you need to know?

You also need to know about her pill-taking compliance.

She says that she has not taken her last 2 days of tablets (Thursday and Friday) and does not know whether she should take today's tablet. She has 3 tablets left before the end of the packet.

c. What advice are you going to give her?

There is no need for EHC as she has forgotten to take her tablets at the end of the cycle. She should be told to continue taking the rest of her tablets but when the last tablet is taken, she should not have a 7-day pill free period but go straight on to the next packet.

CASE STUDY 11.3

Mr Heaney asks the counter assistant for advice on stopping smoking. The counter assistant refers him to the pharmacist.

a. Outline what factors should be taken into account to determine whether Mr Heaney is a suitable candidate to be given a smoking–cessation product.

Before instigation of any treatment it is important that the patient does want to stop smoking. Work has shown that motivation is a major determinant for successful smoking cessation and interventions based on the transtheoretical model of change put forward by Prochaska and colleagues have proved effective. Most patients who ask directly for NRT will be at the preparation stage of the model and ready to enter the action stage.

Mr Heaney smokes 20 cigarettes a day and craves a cigarette when he gets up in the morning.

b. Outline the treatment option/s which will be most suitable for Mr Heaney.

A 24-hour patch might be the formulation of choice for Mr Heaney to combat early-morning cravings. Alternatively, he could use a 16-hour patch and then use a short-acting type of NRT first thing in the morning to get over any cravings (e.g., inhalator).

c. What general advice will you give Mr Heaney in addition to any NRT product supplied?

Set a quit date; remove temptations; avoid environments where smoking happens. Promote healthy lifestyle advice – exercise, diet, weight control, alcohol intake.

You supply him with a week's worth of NRT and make an appointment for him to see you for further supply. On his return, you use a carbon monoxide (CO) monitor to check his adherence.

d. Outline the principles behind CO monitoring.

The best cut-off breath CO level for the determination of smoking status is 5 ppm as it gives the best sensitivity and specificity. As there is a clustering of CO levels in individuals who smoked within the last 5 hours, this cut-off level may be a useful adjunct in detecting smoking status in individuals who have smoked within the last 5 hours. However, it is lower than the usual 6 to 10 ppm, as recommended by some studies. Middleton and Morice reported a cut-off level of 6 ppm in 94% of smokers and 96% of nonsmokers in a respiratory outpatient clinic. Jarvis and Crowley demonstrated that a cut-off breath CO level of greater than 8 ppm is strongly associated with self-reports on smoking, while Tonnesen and Jorenby used 10 ppm as a cut-off.

Answers

1 = e	2 = c	3 = e	4 = c	5 = d	6 = c	7 = c	8 = d	9 = A	10 = F
11 = B	12 = C	13 = H	14 = A	15 = A	16 = E	17 = B	18 = E	19 = A	20 = B

Abbreviations

μg	microgram
ACE	angiotensin-converting enzyme
ADR	adverse drug reaction
CB	chronic bronchitis
CSM	Committee for the Safety of Medicines
DEET	diethyl toluamide
DPH	diphenhydramine
EHC	emergency hormonal contraception
FDA	Food and Drug Administration (equivalent to the Medicines Control Authority in the UK)
GORD	gastro-oesophageal reflux disease
GP	general practitioner
GSL	general sales list
h	hour
IHS	International Headache Society
HMG-CoA	beta-hydroxy beta-methyl glutaryl coenzyme A
HPV	human papilloma virus
HSV	herpes simplex virus
IBS	irritable bowel syndrome
IgE	immunoglobulin E
INR	international normalised ratio
IUCD	intrauterine contraceptive device
KCS	keratoconjunctivitis sicca
L	litre
MAOI	monoamine oxidase inhibitor
MAU	minor aphthous ulcers
mEq	milliequivalent
mg	milligram
MI	myocardial infarction
mL	millilitre
mmol	millimole
NRT	nicotine replacement therapy
NSAID	non-steroidal anti-inflammatory drug
ORT	oral rehydration therapy
OTC	over-the-counter
P	pharmacy
PD	primary dysmenorrhoea
PID	pelvic inflammatory disease
PMS	premenstrual syndrome
POM	prescription-only medicine
PV	per vagina
SSRI	selective serotonin reuptake inhibitor
STD	sexually transmitted disease
TB	tuberculosis
TCA	tricyclic antidepressant
UTI	urinary tract infection
WHO	World Health Organization

Glossary of terms

Chapter 2

Agranulocytosis: Acute deficiency of neutrophil white blood cells leading to neutropenia.

Atopy: A form of hypersensitivity characterised by a familial tendency.

Auroscopical examination: Examination of the eardrum by means of an apparatus that shines light onto the eardrum.

Cervical lymphadenopathy: Enlargement of the cervical lymph nodes.

Dyspnoea: Difficulty in breathing.

Gastro-oesophageal reflux: The back flow of gastric contents into the oesophagus.

Haemoptysis: Coughing up blood.

Malaise: General feeling of being unwell.

Orthopnoea: Difficulty in breathing when lying down.

Pleurisy: Inflammation of the pleural membranes caused by the two pleural membranes adhering to one another.

Purulent: Term used to describe a material containing pus.

Rhinorrhoea: Watery nasal discharge.

Vascular engorgement: An area of tissue that has been excessively perfused with blood.

Vasodilatation: Increase in the diameter of the blood vessels.

Chapter 3

Chalazion: Also referred to as meibomian cyst.

Conjunctivitis medicamentosa: Conjunctivitis caused by repeated administration of ocular eye drops, especially sympathomimetic agents. On withdrawal of the medicine the patient suffers from rebound redness of the eyes.

Glands of Zeiss and Moll: Both are located within the eyelid. The gland of Zeiss secretes sebum and the gland of Moll secretes sweat.

Hordeola: Commonly known as styes.

Limbal area: Area where the cornea meets the sclera.

Meibomianitis: Inflammation of the meibomian gland.

Photophobia: A dislike of bright lights.

Visual acuity: The ability to read text. For example, distance visual acuity is the person's ability to read letters across the room and near visual acuity is the person's ability to read letters close up.

Chapter 4

Conductive deafness: Sound waves are hindered from reaching the inner ear (e.g., by ear wax), resulting in distortion of sounds that impairs the understanding of words.

Effusion: Escape of fluid (e.g., exudates) from the ear.

FDA: US Food and Drug Administration (equivalent to the MCA in the UK).

Laceration: A tear in the skin that causes a wound.

Oedematous: Abnormal accumulation in intercellular spaces of the body.

Tinnitus: A noise in the ears likened to ringing or buzzing.

Chapter 5

ADRs: Adverse drug reactions.

Amenorrhoea: Absence or the stoppage of menstruation.

Haematoma: A localised collection of blood, usually clotted, in an organ, space or tissue.

Myalgia: Muscular pain.

Paraesthesia: An abnormal sensation, for example, a burning or prickling sensation.

Pericranial: Area relating to around the skull.

Purpuric rash: Rash with a distinctive red/purple colouration, caused by haemorrhage of small blood vessels in the skin.

Chapter 6

Anovulatory: Term used to describe women who do not ovulate.

Bacteriuria: Bacteria in the urine.

Dyspareunia: Difficult or painful sexual intercourse.

Dysuria: Painful or difficult urination.

Haematuria: Blood in the urine.

Menarche: Onset of menstruation.

Nocturia: Excessive urination at night.

Perianal: The area around the anus.

Perineal: The area around the perineum. The perineum describes the area between the vulva and anus.

Postmenopausal women: Women who have finished menstruating. The average age for women to be postmenopausal is 51.

Prostate gland: The gland that surrounds the neck of the bladder and urethra in men.

Pyelonephritis: Inflammation of the kidney due to bacterial infection.

Suprapubic: Area above the pubic region.

Chapter 7

Annular lesions: Skin lesions that are circular.

Diverticulitis: Inflammation of a diverticulum, which is a pouch or sac. It occurs normally after herniation.

Halitosis: Bad breath.

Suprapubic: Area above the pubis area of the abdomen.

Tenesmus: Cessation of incomplete bowel evacuation.

Ureter: Tube connecting the kidney to the bladder.

Chapter 8

Atopy: Literally means 'strange disease'. The triad of atopic dermatitis, asthma and allergic rhinitis.

Comedone: A plug of oxidised sebaceous material obstructing the surface opening of a pilosebaceous follicle, commonly referred to as a blackhead.

Crust: The term given to dried exudate.

Macules: Flat stains or spots of altered skin colour.

Maculopapular: Literally a papule developed on a macule, i.e., a mixture of the two types of lesion.

Nodule: A solid elevation whose greater part lies beneath the skin surface.

Papules: Raised palpable spots.

Punctiform: Pinpoint-like lesions.

Pustule: A pus-filled lesion.

Vesicles: Small, raised, fluid-filled lesions or blisters.

Wheal: Areas of transient dermal oedema. Classically associated with urticaria and also following insect bites.

Chapter 9

Abduction: The term used to describe movement of a part away from the median plane of the body, for example, moving the leg straight out to the side.

Ankylosis: When the joint becomes stiff or fused in a particular position.

Arthropathy: Pathology in a joint.

Articular cartilage: Cartilage occurring in the joint.

Disc herniation: Abnormal protrusion of the nucleus pulposus of the disc, which may impinge on a nerve root.

Epicondylitis: Inflammation of the epicondyle, which is the protuberance above the condyle. The condyle refers to the rounded part at the end of the bone used for articulation with another bone.

Chapter 10

Erythema: Redness of the skin due to capillary vasodilation.

Intertriginous area: Skin eruption on apposed skin surfaces.

Lichenification: Thickening and hardening of the skin.

Chapter 11

Erythrocytes: Alternative name for red blood cells.

Melanocytes: Cells in the skin epidermis responsible for producing melanin.

Index

EDINBURGH
LONDON NEW YORK OXFORD
PHILADELPHIA ST LOUIS SYDNEY